Principles of Dental Treatment Planning

Principles of Dental Treatment Planning

ROBERT B. MORRIS, D.D.S., F.I.C.D.

Private Practitioner, New Berlin, Wisconsin; Adjunct Associate Clinical Professor, Department of Clinical Oral Pathology and Diagnosis, Marquette University School of Dentistry, Milwaukee, Wisconsin

Lea & Febiger · 1983 · Philadelphia

Lea & Febiger
600 Washington Square
Philadelphia, PA 19106
U.S.A.

Library of Congress Cataloging in Publication Data

Morris, Robert B.
Principles of dental treatment planning.

Bibliography: p.
Includes index.
1. Therapeutics, Dental—Planning. I. Title.
[DNLM: 1. Dentistry. 2. Planning technics.
WU 166 M877p]
RK318.M67 617′.6′06 82-15370
ISBN 0-8121-0841-8 AACR2

PRINTED IN THE UNITED STATES OF AMERICA

PRINT NUMBER 3 2 1

To my wife Dianne, my children, Allison and Amy, and my parents, Bernard and Maysel

Preface

The secret of teaching is to appear to have known all your life what you learned this afternoon.

ANONYMOUS

The practice of dentistry offers unique challenges to one who would make it his life's work. While physically and mentally demanding, it can be spiritually as well as materially rewarding. Among the rewards of dentistry is the great satisfaction derived from seeing diseased, debilitated mouths become healthy, restored mouths as a result of treatment. A thoughtfully conceived and carefully executed treatment plan is central to this transformation. The treatment plan is the marriage of the mind's conception and the hands' execution which is so critical to the practice of dentistry.

As a general practitioner and teacher of oral diagnosis and treatment planning, I have felt a need for greater emphasis on practical dental treatment planning in dental education and practice. There is a wealth of textual material dealing with examination and diagnosis, but it touches only lightly on treatment planning. Other texts on treatment planning are weighted heavily toward oral and general medicine. This emphasis on oral medicine pervades much of dental education today, and while it is laudable to train and encourage the student to be a "physician" of the oral cavity, it does not always relate well to actual clinical dental practice. Still other treatment-planning texts rely heavily on exhaustive case examples that, while interesting, may not provide the reader with the tools to plan effective dental treatment.

Since the inception of this text, two treatment-planning texts have been published. The serious student of dentistry would do well to consult Dr. Norman Wood's contributor work for its detailed discussion of oral medicine and Dr. Laurence Barsh's text for its excellent discussion of problem-oriented record systems.

The goal of this text is to examine the process of treatment planning, to break that process into its component parts, and to identify and discuss the principles and concepts on which it is based. In addressing the "nuts and bolts" of treatment planning, it is necessary to limit the scope of the text to avoid duplication of the many fine works available on examination, diagnosis, and oral medicine. Limiting the scope of a text on treatment planning is difficult, because the discussion of treatment planning necessarily touches on the entire field of general dentistry. Indeed, a truly "complete" work would be a textbook of general dentistry, its references and bibliography including the entire body of dental literature. For that reason, this text has limited references and bibliography, and its discussions of certain topics are intentionally brief. Rather than illustrate comprehensive treatment plans, I will describe some reasonable minimums in dental treatment and concentrate on the basic tools of treatment planning. These tools should be useful for the general practitioner, for he is the primary source of most dental treatment and should be the coordinator of all phases of treatment. They should also be helpful to the junior or senior dental student who has had basic courses in oral diagnosis and radiography and some clinical experience.

The text approximates the chronologic sequence of the treatment-planning process. Chapters 1 through 3 deal with treatment planning as it involves the patient. The dentist must realize that he does not work with teeth or mouths, but with human beings who have hopes, dreams, aspirations, cares and responsibilities not necessarily focusing on their oral condition. Unless his diagnosis and plan of treatment addresses the total patient, the dentist is doomed to fail. Chapters 4 through 6 deal with the dentist's role in the treatment-planning process. The routine systematic approach employed in the information-gathering phase can be carried into the diagnostic and treatment-planning process. This section discusses data gathering, arriving at a multifactorial diagnosis, establishing a rational sequence of treatment, and planning specific procedures. Chapters 7 through 9 introduce a number of general principles, concepts, and strategies in treatment planning, especially as they are applied to complex cases.

Illustrations are used throughout the text to illuminate specific concepts or strategies in treatment planning. The strategies used in such examples are not meant to represent the only possible solution to a given problem, nor are they meant to dazzle the reader with the author's ingenuity or technical brilliance (however, having that brilliance occasionally show through is a risk I must take). In some case examples, specific fees are listed for the purpose of illustrating record systems and phasing strategies; these fees are purely arbitrary, and, as rough averages at the time of writing, will be obsolete immediately.

A word about terminology is in order: throughout this text, the pronoun "he," rather than the combined pronouns "he/she," will be used. This is done for the sake of simplicity and sexual bias is neither implied nor intended.

Finally, every attempt has been made to keep the text practical, realistic, clinically oriented, and easy to read. The result, I hope, is less a scientific treatise and more a handbook of both the art and science of treatment planning.

Milwaukee, Wisconsin ROBERT B. MORRIS

Acknowledgments

This book is in no way a one-man effort. As a student, I absorbed the knowledge and experience of countless people; I only hope that, in organizing it in a unique fashion, I can pass this knowledge on to others.

It is not difficult to single out the people who had the greatest impact on this work and who deserve my heartfelt thanks and best wishes:

Dr. Ben Karr, teacher and friend, whose interest and assistance made this book possible; Dr. William Nequette, my favorite teacher, good friend, and associate, who taught me what quality dentistry could be; and Drs. William Gabler, Gerald Feldman, and James Werwie, who kindly offered help and suggestions regarding the manuscript.

Many thanks to Robert Albertin, who ably executed the illustrations, Jeff Seipel, who converted more color slides to black and white prints than either of us cares to remember, and Marian Daniels for her help with the manuscript.

A special word of thanks to my wife, Dianne Morris, who, as editor, typist, and friend-in-need, is mainly responsible for the completion of this project.

Finally, I offer a debt of gratitude to all the excellent and dedicated dentists, researchers, and clinicians who have given of themselves so that others could learn. This text is but a small down payment on that debt.

Contents

SECTION 1 Patient-Oriented Dental Treatment Planning 1

Chapter 1 The Treatment-Planning Process 3

Chapter 2 The Role of the Patient in Dental Treatment Planning 5

Chapter 3 The Preventive Approach to Treatment Planning .. 26

SECTION 2 The Routine Systematic Approach to Treatment Planning 33

Chapter 4 Data Gathering and Records 35

Chapter 5 Diagnosis 92

Chapter 6 Synthesis of the Treatment Plan 124

SECTION 3 Principles of Complex Treatment Planning 141

Chapter 7 Phasing Dental Treatment 143

Chapter 8 Management of Complex Cases 160

Chapter 9 Establishing the Prognosis 204

Index 233

SECTION 1

Patient-Oriented Dental Treatment Planning

Patient-oriented dental treatment planning is not a new concept; it is, however, a concept that is more often discussed than applied.

It is easy within the dental profession to become so engrossed with the technical and mechanical details of what we do that we lose sight of the human element. The first principle of dental treatment planning, then, is to recognize and accept that we are dealing with fellow human beings, each with their own personality, needs, hopes, fears, and "hang ups." When we deal with patients, we must deal with the sum total of these elements, not merely with teeth, oral cavities, or orofacial complexes. Many of the procedures we perform in dental practice are mechanical in nature, but the human relationship between dentist and patient demands that they be performed *with* our patients as opposed to *for*, or worse yet, *to* them. Dentist and patient must share the common goal of oral health, which requires not only elimination of lesions and prosthetic repair of damaged or lost tissue, but the *creation and maintenance of an oral environment* that will prevent further disease and allow long-term success of treatment. The creation of this environment depends greatly on the patient's involvement in every phase of dental practice. The patient becomes involved in dental treatment in a stepwise process:

1. The dentist gathers information about the patient. This information must include not only the dental and oral findings, but also the human factors that will influence the patient's dental condition and the course and outcome of his dental treatment. As the dentist discovers the patient, the patient must be given the opportunity to discover the dentist: who he is, how he works, and what kinds of services he can provide.

2. The dentist must convey his findings to the patient. The patient must be informed of his dental and oral conditions in language that he can readily understand; he must also be made aware of the infective, hereditary, or behavioral factors that contributed to these conditions.

3. Together, the dentist and patient arrive at a goal toward which they may work. The goal may be optimal oral health achieved by stringent self-control on the part of the patient and ideal comprehensive dental treatment provided by the dentist, or immediate relief of pain and minimal "holding-type" treatment, or some intermediate goal. Once the goal is commonly agreed upon, the course of treatment that will result in the desired ends is selected.

This process will be analyzed and discussed at length in the three chapters to follow.

CHAPTER 1

The Treatment-Planning Process

The foolish man fails to learn from his mistakes. The smart man does learn from them. The wise man tries to learn from the mistakes of others.

When a skilled and experienced clinical dentist studies radiographs, diagnostic models, and clinical findings to arrive at a diagnosis and create a plan of treatment, it seems very much like a magical act. The effortlessness, speed, and insight with which the skilled dentist answers questions that others might not even consider has impressed and intimidated many a young dentist; lacking the "magic," the young dentist feels inadequate to face the challenge of comprehensive treatment planning.

How does one begin to develop such skill, finesse, and wisdom? Age and experience are wonderful aids, but sensible and effective treatment planning should not have to wait for old age. Furthermore, time is not the only key to good treatment planning, for many dentists, rather than gaining experience year by year, seem to repeat the first year's mistakes again and again.

The answer lies in the knowledge that treatment planning is not a random, intuitive process practiced by the "Merlins" of our profession, but an orderly, systematic process that can be dissected into its component parts and studied. Time and experience can accelerate the process so that it appears to be a matter of deep insight, but in fact, a routine system must be operating. In this text, I will attempt to identify the components of the treatment-planning process and develop a number of concepts upon which this process is based. I will identify a number of general principles in the hope of providing the dentist with the tools for successful treatment planning (Fig. 1–1).

The importance of treatment planning as an independent process cannot be overstated. As our knowledge of every aspect of dentistry expands, we are forced to keep up with ever more specialized information—indeed, the specialist is aptly defined as the person who "knows more and more about less and less." As this special knowledge diverges, the burden becomes ever greater on the general practitioner to be the "quarterback" of the team, the person who must ensure that each specialized step in treatment is performed in logical sequence and does in fact lead to an overall goal. To speak of prosthetic treatment planning, endodontic treatment planning, or orthodontic treatment planning is interesting, but the failure to integrate all phases of dental treatment can be disastrous. I have approached this study of the treatment-planning process with an eye to avoiding such disasters.

Effective treatment planning requires the following three components: sufficient data base, accurate diagnosis, and an effective treatment plan.

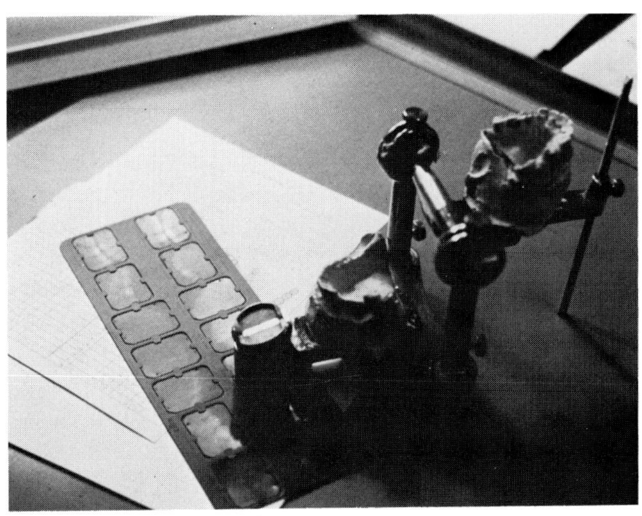

Fig. 1–1. The tools of the trade.

SUFFICIENT DATA BASE

Diagnosis and treatment require a data base that includes sufficient information about the patient's oral and systemic conditions so that the clinician can make good judgments in diagnosis. The clinician should consider all general information about a patient that might bear on their professional and/or business relationship, all significant, systemic conditions as revealed by examination and medical and dental histories that might influence the patient's oral condition and possible treatment, and, finally, all relevant oral and dental findings obtained by a complete, routine, systematic examination. These factors must be studied in sufficient depth and detail, so that their impact on the overall situation will not be ignored or underestimated.

In summary, then, the first requisite for success in dental treatment planning is the gathering of all relevant information, broad enough in scope and with sufficient detail to provide the data base necessary for an accurate diagnosis.

ACCURATE DIAGNOSIS

The second essential ingredient in successful treatment planning is an accurate diagnosis, or set of diagnoses. Many dental patients have complexes of problems that often interrelate to constitute syndromes, but just as often exist as multiple, independent pathoses. These problems need to be identified and classified by the clinician, their relationships to one another defined, and their probable etiologies established.

EFFECTIVE TREATMENT PLAN

The third criterion for success in treatment planning is that the plan address the observed and diagnosed problems effectively. Checking the results of the patient's examination to make sure that all problems have been considered in the treatment plan avoids errors of omission. The plan must deal with the causes of the problems, as well as the problems themselves, or else the disease process is likely to continue unabated and result in the failure of treatment. Finally, the plan must relate to the patient as an individual, so that the treatment will be understood and accepted, and the mutual responsibilities of patient and dentist fulfilled.

Successful dental treatment planning, then, can be capsulized as follows:

1. Gather all relevant information
2. Arrive at a diagnosis or set of diagnoses
3. Develop a treatment plan that
    a. Addresses all known problems,
    b. Deals with etiologic factors,
    c. Relates effectively to the patient

REFERENCES

1. Barsh, L.I.: Dental Treatment Planning for the Adult Patient. Philadelphia, W.B. Saunders, 1981.
2. Clark, J.W., et al.: Clinical Dentistry. Hagerstown, Harper and Row, 1979.
3. Kerr, D.A., Ash, M.M., and Millard, H.D.: Oral Diagnosis. 4th Ed. St. Louis, C.V. Mosby, 1974.
4. Mitchell, D.F., Standish, S.M., and Fast, T.B.: Oral Diagnosis: Oral Medicine. 2nd Ed. Philadelphia, Lea & Febiger, 1971.
5. Wood, N.K.: Review of Diagnosis, Oral Medicine, Radiology and Treatment Planning. St. Louis, C.V. Mosby, 1979.
6. Wood, N.K. (Ed.): Treatment Planning—A Pragmatic Approach. St. Louis, C.V. Mosby, 1978.

CHAPTER 2

The Role of the Patient in Dental Treatment Planning

The competent physician, before he attempts to give medicine to his patient, makes himself acquainted not only with the disease he wishes to cure, but also with the habits and constitution of the patient.

CICERO

Dentistry would be such fun if we just didn't have to work with patients . . . .

'MOST EVERY DENTIST, AT ONE TIME OR ANOTHER

In the distant past, dental treatment planning was directed more at mouths than at people. Of late, much discussion has centered around patient involvement in dental treatment planning. Unfortunately, much of this discussion has been lip service and has not considered the significance and ramifications of the concept.

The attitudes of dentists toward their patients have often run to extremes. At one end of the scale is the "dictator," who offers dental treatment on his terms only—"Take it or leave it." This attitude may well have been fostered by the autocratic approach in dental education and is often associated with a highly rigid, authoritarian personality. On the other end of the scale is the "mechanic," who passively performs whatever procedure the patient requests (or demands) with little attempt to establish a rational plan of treatment. Somewhere in between, we may find the glib "salesman," who is well versed in techniques of gentle persuasion and who, with elaborate multimedia presentations, may sell treatment plans a patient may not want or that he may not be able to carry out.

There are several reasons for these difficulties in patient involvement. The typical dentist, at least in days past, was often a fairly introverted type who usually practiced alone and was deeply engrossed in the intricate and technical details of clinical dentistry; he may well have had difficulty in communicating with his patients, especially when that communication involved listening. Dentists in the past had little or no formal training in applied behavioral science. Today, even with the groundwork in disciplines such as psychology, communication, and transactional analysis, dealing with people who present themselves for dental treatment is as much an art as a science. Finally, the dental-school model of diagnosis and treatment planning is often a fairly rigid set of rules about what constitutes "ideal" treatment, which in a teaching institution, can be readily applied to the patient population. Patient treatment in actual practice often involves compromises, and most schools are hesitant to teach anything less than ideal dentistry, thus the graduate dentist may adhere rigidly to the "take it or leave it" approach, or failing that, make poor compromises.

There are signs that this situation is changing. Personality stereotypes are fading as dental schools acquire more heterogeneous student populations. A greater incidence of group practice, or at the least, solo practice with multiple auxiliaries may lead to less introverted dentists. Also, dental schools are incorporating into their curricula courses that may lay the groundwork for more understanding, responsive, and communicative dentists. Without these basic qualities, patient involvement in treatment planning is impossible.

WHY INVOLVE THE PATIENT IN DENTAL TREATMENT PLANNING?

Most dental problems are a result of either caries or periodontal disease or functional problems stemming from them (missing teeth, for example). There is convincing evidence that the primary etiologic factor in caries and periodontal disease is bacterial plaque that adheres to teeth and periodontal tissues. A major contributing factor to plaque diseases is diet, particularly the action of refined carbohydrates, which aid in plaque formation and caries production. Since both plaque and diet are entirely under the control of the patient, we must accept that the bulk of dental disease is *behavioral* in nature. We cannot cope with a behavioral disease unless we can effectively deal with human behavior. This necessitates the patient's involvement in the entire process of diagnosis, treatment planning, and treatment itself.

Dental disease is seldom fatal. People can, and many do, live entire lives with dental disease without dental treatment. Many survive and prosper having lost all their natural teeth to dental disease. Although it can be argued that their lives could be fuller, happier, and more comfortable if dental disease were treated and arrested and its damage repaired, the fact remains that, for most people, dental treatment is not an absolute necessity.

Dental disease is virtually pandemic; therefore, many people accept it as a normal occurrence. Over 90% of the adult population has caries or periodontal disease.[1] In fact, periodontal disease may be as prevalent among dentists as it is among the general populace.

If we accept that the preponderance of dental disease is *behavioral, nonfatal,* and *pandemic,* it follows that, for most people, dental treatment is essentially *elective*. This is true in two senses: first of all, people can determine the state of their dental health by their plaque and dietary control or their lack of it. Secondly, treatment may be postponed or totally neglected until a problem becomes acute and painful, without substantially affecting the daily pattern of life.

The elective nature of dental treatment should not discourage or disparage the dental practitioner. The fact that dentistry is not a life-and-death matter does not demean us, nor does it detract from the great service we can perform for people or from the immense satisfaction gained from that service. What is significant is that the success or failure of this service depends on the patient's behavior, and we cannot deal with behavior without involving the patient in the diagnosis and the planning and execution of treatment.

GOAL SETTING IN TREATMENT PLANNING

To be effective in any enterprise, we must define goals toward which we will work. When we involve the patient in treatment planning, it becomes necessary to establish some common goal, or goals. Formal dental training may produce a dentist whose goal is to have 28 teeth in good occlusion and alignment; esthetics is often considered an accessory to that goal. Patients, on the other hand, may not know how many teeth they have (or would like to have), and have no conception of curves of occlusion or lateral guidance. A patient's goal may be to have a comfortable mouth and an attractive smile. We ought to consider that these goals are not mutually exclusive; however, an attractive smile may be obtained without insisting

ROBERT B. MORRIS, D.D.S.
14021 W. GREENFIELD AVENUE
NEW BERLIN, WISCONSIN 53151
TELEPHONE 782-4860

March 5, 1982

Mrs. Jane Doe
123 Pine St.
Littleton, WI

Dear Jane,

This letter is to sum up and review what we discussed at the time of your initial examination last Friday. As you had suspected, and our examination confirmed, you have a number of very serious dental problems which could lead to the loss of many or all of your teeth in time. Foremost among these is gum disease (pyorrhea) which we looked at together and discussed in some detail.

Fortunately, it does not appear to be a hopeless situation, and a wide range of treatment approaches might be considered. You indicated that you would prefer to keep as many of your own teeth as possible, provided the financial commitment is something you can handle. We will, in the next few appointments, more thoroughly assess the situation and present you with some treatment approaches and options to accomplish this goal.

Meanwhile, if you have any questions please feel free to call or ask at your next appointment.

Sincerely yours,

Robert B. Morris, D.D.S.

Fig. 2–1. Letter to patient defining goals of treatment. A verbal agreement accomplishes the same end.

on all 28 teeth. In this regard, we must be understanding of the patient's felt needs, so that the results of dental treatment will please the patient, and meet the objective standards of mechanical and biological acceptability.

Generally, it is best to establish broad goals with the patient. For example, by age 65, over one-half of the people in the United States have been fully edentulated.[1] A patient who has teeth may choose to keep rather than to lose those teeth; this can be the first common goal for dentist and patient. Later goals may concern the number of teeth to be retained as a function of the time, complexity, and expense of treatment. These goals must be decided upon mutually and may even be written down prior to final treatment planning (Fig. 2–1).

HOW THE PATIENT IS INVOLVED IN TREATMENT PLANNING

There is no set method for involving a patient in treatment planning, nor should there be, because patients and dentists are individuals with their own personalities and lifestyles. Flexibility, honesty, and especially naturalness are essential traits for the dentist who wishes to establish good communication with his patient. Certain elements of the process can be identified, however, and those essential elements are the following: dentist obtains necessary information; dentist prepares a diagnosis and presents the treatment plan to the patient; patient decides whether to accept treatment; and dentist and patient decide on timing of treatment.

Dentist obtains all necessary information. The obvious elements of the diagnostic process will be discussed at length in Chapter 4. In addition to the radiographic and clinical findings, the dentist must have an understanding of the patient's present complaint, his desires for specific treatment, and most important, his goals as discussed and agreed upon.

With this information, the dentist prepares a diagnosis and treatment plan and usually presents it to the patient on a subsequent visit. Whether this will be a formal consultation visit or a brief discussion combined with a treatment appointment depends on many factors; however, the basic elements of the discussion remain the same.

Four basic bits of information must be conveyed to the patient in terms that he can understand. First, the patient must be informed about the condition of his oral cavity, teeth, and supporting structures—that is, what problems are present that must be dealt with. If the patient has been involved in the examination and diagnostic process, this discussion becomes a review and summary and may clarify and answer any questions the patient may have. Second, the dental treatment plan should be outlined as it applies to the patient's problems. This treatment should be related to the goals established by patient and dentist and alternative treatments discussed in view of their relative effectiveness in reaching those goals. Third, the patient is presented with the cost of treatment. This should consider the patient's financial commitment and the approximate length of treatment, as well as the patient's commitment to maintain his oral health effectively before, during, and after treatment. At this point, the patient must comprehend the behavioral nature of his disease and share responsibility for its control. Fourth, the probable results of the proposed treatment are outlined. In order to form a prognosis, the dentist must make many assumptions regarding the success of the mechanical and biologic treatment and the patient's ability and willingness to control the disease state. The patient often needs some idea of what he can reasonably expect in terms of function, esthetics, and longevity.

Summarized, the dentist must present to the patient—in terms the patient can understand—the *problems* present in his mouth, the *treatment* that is available to correct them, the *cost* of treatment, in terms of time and money, and the *outlook* for the future assuming the treatment is accepted and carried out.

Based on this information, the patient must decide whether to accept the proposed treatment and the responsibilities associated with it. Contrary to some advice, this decision need not—and in some cases, should not—be made immediately. Although it may reduce the acceptance rate of treatment plans, ample time for reflection and discussion will ensure a reasoned and firm commitment to the joint effort; this can only improve the prognosis and make treatment easier for both parties. In many cases, a commitment to an entire course of treatment is neither necessary nor desirable. A patient often may opt for some preliminary procedures before deciding to proceed with an entire course of treatment (this concept is discussed at length in Chap. 6).

After a decision has been made to proceed with treatment, the patient and dentist must decide on the timing of the treatment—that is, when to begin and at what pace to proceed (this is discussed further in Chap. 7).

SPECIFIC TECHNIQUES OF PATIENT INVOLVEMENT

There are many means and methods of involving the patient in examination, diagnosis, and treatment planning, and we will not attempt to deal with all of them (some excellent articles on this topic are listed in the references). However, we will discuss those principles and techniques that seem most pertinent.

Basic Communication

When we attempt to involve the patient in dental treatment planning, we realize that effective communication is absolutely necessary. Communication, moreover, is an elusive concept that must be understood well to be applied effectively. If communication is defined as the transmission of a thought or idea from one person to another, the following processes must occur:

1. The communicator formulates a thought, idea, or series of thoughts and ideas.
2. The communicator puts these thoughts into a code to be transmitted, which may be spoken language, written words, or, in some cases, nonverbal forms.
3. The message is transmitted over some medium.
4. The receiver of the communication receives the coded message.
5. The receiver must form a thought, idea, or series of thoughts and ideas from the message he has received.

This may seem a cumbersome way of looking at something we take so much for granted, but let us look closely at some of the difficulties that can arise from a simple attempt at communication. First of all, the thought or idea conceived by the communicator may not be clear to him from the start, or the series of thoughts and ideas may not be coherent or may have contradictions. An example of this in the dental setting would be a receptionist attempting to explain a dental diagnosis or procedure to a patient without having a clear understanding of it herself. No matter how effective the communication techniques, if the thought is unclear to the communicator, it will be unclear to the receiver and the process will break down. Similarly, if the thought or idea is simply incorrect from the start, the process transmits misinformation and is self-defeating.

Encoding the Message

Assuming that the communicator is thinking clearly and wishes to communicate only those ideas he is reasonably sure of, we now come to the process of encoding the message. Again, what appears to be so simple can get us into no end of trouble. For example, if spoken language is the medium chosen, the communicator would probably avoid speaking in Greek if his intended receiver speaks only English. Yet every day, in thousands of dental offices and clinics across the land, dentists attempt to address their patients in "dentalese," the jargon of the dental profession. For a dentist to communicate effectively, he must refrain from using "dentalese" and transmit his thoughts in plain English (or whatever language he and the patient share).

Many times, this requires additional explanation and definition of terms, but if communication is worth doing, it is worth doing well. Given that a common language is established, the key to communicating well is the effective expression of the thought or idea in that language. We must, in the case of a spoken message, actually say what we mean, and accurately express the thought or idea.

When choosing words to express those ideas, another factor enters in: words have both denotative and connotative meanings. An example of this in dentistry might be the difference between the words "extract" and "pull"; both have the same denotative meanings, but their connotative meanings may differ greatly. This often happens when comparing the scientific-sounding words of Latin and Greek derivation with more common English derivatives—for example, having your employment terminated is more acceptable connotatively than being fired. Even among Latin derivatives there are connotative differences, such as the words "conception" and "impregnation," which are very close in denotative meaning, but quite different in connotation. Therefore, when a dentist/communicator encodes a message, he must be aware of the possible connotations of his words, and whenever possible, select the more neutral word.

Transmitting the Message

Transmission of the message looks fairly foolproof, but unfortunately, it is not. Anyone who has attempted to communicate verbally over an air-driven dental handpiece with a high-volume evacuator in operation and piped-in music can appreciate the problem. Without going into all the ways the transmission of the message can be garbled, suffice it to say that we cannot take for granted that a message sent is a message received.

Decoding the Message

The reception of the message depends on the receiver. He may not want to receive (hear) it or may not be able to receive it (deafness?), and communication fails again.

Having received the coded message, the receiver now must attempt to *understand* it, to form in his own mind the ideas that have been conveyed. The communication effort is imperilled by this decoding process, for connotation and denotation are involved as the receiver rapidly and quite unconsciously applies his knowledge, past experiences, and subjective feelings to the message he has received. He understands the message only in the context of that knowledge, experience, and feeling.

We now have a situation in which a thought has been encoded, transmitted, received, and understood, but we still do not have communication. The reason is obvious: the original communicator has no way of knowing whether the message has been received or understood, or whether the receiver has understood the message correctly. The last and most important element in communication, then, is the receiver's signal to the sender that the message has been received and understood; this essential element is called feedback.

Feedback

Without feedback there is no communication, for the sender must know whether or not he and the receiver share a common understanding of the ideas that were conveyed. Furthermore, feedback must be both continuous and specific to be useful.

In an act of communication, many messages are transmitted, and the understanding of each may depend on the understanding of the previous message. In such a situation, feedback must occur continually if the sender and receiver are to arrive at the same conclusion. For example, in discussing periodontal disease and its treatment with a patient, a common understanding of what a pocket is and what significance it has is essential to understanding why definitive surgery is employed and what it can accomplish. Therefore, feedback regarding pockets and their import should be obtained before proceeding with other messages.

The eliciting of a "message-received" signal is not adequate feedback. It is easy to pause in a communication and ask "Do you understand that?" and, when the patient mumbles "Yes, I guess so," charge fearlessly on in our discourse, never guessing for a moment that it is far easier for the patient to nod assent than to say, in a clear and steady voice, "I haven't understood a word you've said, Doctor." This statement is not likely to be uttered in the dental setting, because on the one hand, it demeans the patient to have to admit that he is too uneducated to understand what "the Doctor" is trying to explain to him so patiently. No one likes to admit ignorance, no one wants to look silly, no one wants to ask the "dumb question," so a nod of assent to the question, "Do you understand?" keeps the boat from rocking, but in no way assures actual understanding. On the other hand, suppose the patient does not feel ignorant because he does not understand what is being said. It is still difficult to express the fact, because the receiver may not wish to hurt or upset the sender. In response to "Do you understand?" a dentist is not likely to hear "Of course I don't understand, you pompous fool. Everything you've said has been Greek to me. When you start using plain English I'll have a chance to understand you!" On the rare occasion that a patient is candid enough to express those or similar feelings, the dentist should feel very fortunate to have the opportunity to try again, "in English this time." Patient understanding is a more precious commodity than a dentist's pride, perhaps due to the scarcity of one and the abundance of the other. Feedback, then, should consist of an acknowledgment of the message as well as an indication of whether the message was truly understood.

In its simplest and most effective form, feedback consists of the receiver repeating—in his own words—what he understands the sender to have said. This is neither as difficult nor as cumbersome as it may sound; in fact, this often accelerates communication, if the receiver demonstrates an immediate and facile grasp of the ideas being discussed. An excellent example of feedback facilitating communication might be the contrast between the following hypothetical conversations between dentist and patient.

Doctor: "Mrs. Smith, I'd like to take a few minutes to explain why your gums need some extensive treatment and what we feel should be done at this time."
Patient: "All right, Doctor."
Doctor: "Well, it's like this, Mrs. Smith: there are certain bacteria in the mouth—germs, you might say—that can act on the foods we eat and form colonies on the teeth and gums. We call these colonies "plaque." Now, if this plaque is allowed to remain on the teeth for some time and is not removed with toothbrush and dental floss at least once a day, the gums can become diseased, etc. Do you understand?"
Patient: "Yes, I guess so . . . ."

Nothing is inherently wrong with the message that the doctor is transmitting; it is accurate, clear, concise, and the language is fairly simple. The message could have been exceedingly lengthy, and, in the attempt to be complete, the good doctor could have told Mrs. Smith more than she needs or wants to know about her gums and not enough about her actual concerns.

Let's consider a second conversation:

Doctor: "Mrs. Smith, from what you've seen, heard, and read so far, and from what we have pointed out in your own mouth, can you tell me what you think your biggest problem is?"
Patient: "Well, Doctor, I can see now that my gums aren't in very good shape."

Doctor: "And what things have indicated that to you?"
Patient: "Well, your hygienist mentioned it right away, and she showed me the bleeding in between the back teeth. And, of course, you showed me the spaces between the gums—what do you call them?"
Doctor: "You mean pockets?"
Patient: "Yes, that's right. I saw in the film the hygienist showed me how the infection is in the pockets. Doctor, does this mean I might lose my teeth?"

Now we hope the doctor can reassure Mrs. Smith that her problem, while serious, is not very far advanced, and with proper care on her part and possibly some minor gum surgery, should be under control and not cause teeth to be lost.

The essential difference in the two conversations is not one of content, but of the quality of *feedback*. By posing questions to the patient that allow her to verbalize her understanding of the original message, the dentist knows immediately whether his message has hit home. The feedback is both continuous and specific; not only does it confirm that the message is received and understood, but it allows the patient to get the specific information and, perhaps, reassurance that she needs. The application of this type of communication technique will be illustrated further in this chapter (Fig. 2–2 summarizes the principles of basic communication in a hypothetical model).

This simplified model of the communication process does not include all the possible factors in the process, such as the setting in which the communication takes place, the expectations of the participants, or their subjective feelings toward one another irrespective of the message. When we carefully consider the entire process and all the factors that enter into it, we are forced to marvel that communication occurs at all! It is a sobering thought that perhaps much of the communication attempted does fail to some degree. With this in mind, we might better understand the situation in which a patient absolutely swears that the Doctor said "XYZ," while the doctor, having said no such thing, insists that he plainly told the patient "ABC." Each accuses the other of slander, malicious misinterpretation, and other crimes too numerous to mention. The problem is communication—the lack of it or failure in the attempt—and it is the type of problem that all too often results in hard feelings, unpaid fees, and litigation. Once again, the single element that tends to avoid such problems is feedback. Feedback allows us to make the appropriate correction immediately when the patient mistakes message "ABC" as "XYZ."

Effective Listening

In order to ensure feedback in our communication efforts, we must allow the receiver the opportunity to provide it; this means that we must develop the skill of effective listening. To some degree, listening has become a lost art in our modern world. In order to understand what effective listening is, we must first establish what it is not: listening is not the silence that one falls into when someone else is speaking. This silence is usually an expression of mental apathy, or at best, occupied by our thinking of what we are going to say when the other speaker stops. What effective listening requires is full and rapt attention to the message being conveyed.

To be effective listeners, we must consider the message on two levels. On a primary level, we must attempt to understand our patient's literal message.

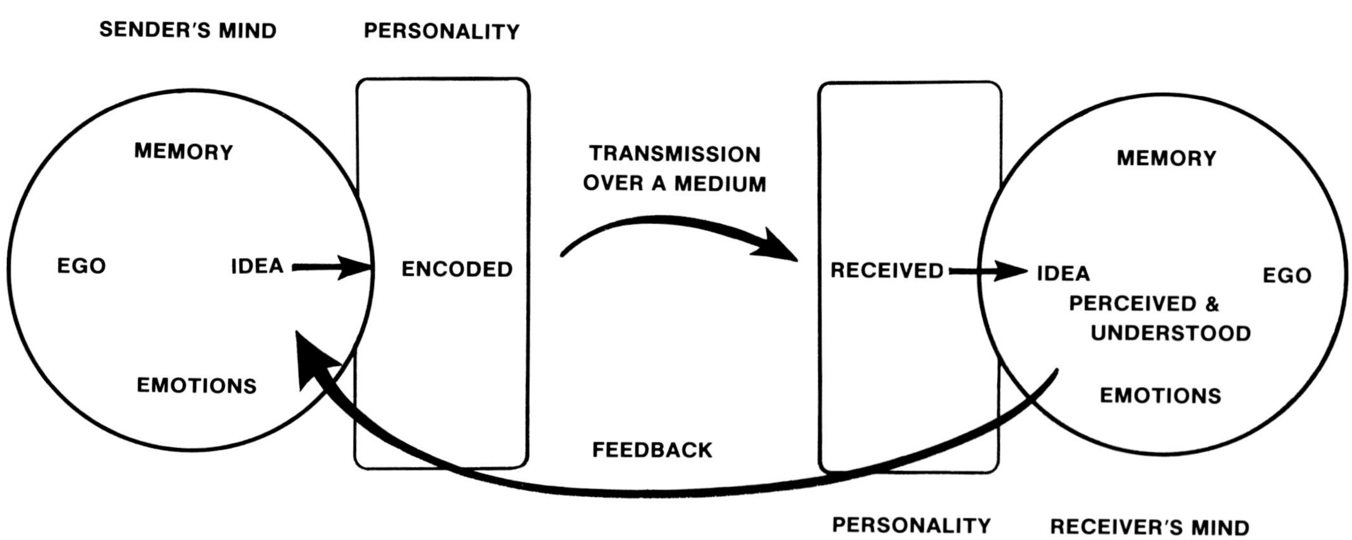

Fig. 2–2. Conceptual model of communication process.

Assuming that he may not possess effective communication skills (which we are trying to develop), he may have difficulty putting the feedback response into words. Consider also that the subject, his dental condition, may be foreign to him and not readily expressed. Finally, the setting in which the communication is occurring may be more or less threatening to the patient and adversely affect his ability to provide good feedback.

On a secondary level, we must also attempt to interpret the underlying, unspoken messages that may accompany the patient's literal message. Since our patient is not likely to be an expert communicator, the connotative message may be as important as the denotative message. For example, the patient may say one thing, but mean another:

Doctor: "I see it has been 5 years since your last dental visit. How did it get to be so long?"
Patient: "I don't like dentists."

Taken literally, this statement is absurd. The patient may really be saying "I have had bad past experiences with dentists," or "I am afraid of dentists," or, more accurately, "I am afraid that what a dentist might do to me will be painful and/or unpleasant." If we do take the statement literally, we may react emotionally or communicate about a subject that is irrelevant. Therefore, we must listen to statements such as "I don't like dentists" or "I can't afford to spend any money on my teeth" and attempt to discern their hidden messages. We can try to elicit a more accurate message by asking other questions, such as "Why do you feel that way?" or "What past experiences have you had to make you feel that way?" This encourages the patient to express a more accurate denotative message about what he thinks and feels, rather than to say one thing while meaning another.

The patient may provide feedback, but may also provide an unspoken message by the way in which he communicates. For example, a patient may be relatively noncommunicative, may not answer our questions requiring feedback, or may be very slow in responding. By refusing to answer a question, the patient may be expressing his feelings of apprehension, distrust, or confusion. It is very important that we not feel rebuffed by this lack of immediate response or uneasy when a silence follows our feedback-seeking query. If there is no response from the patient after some time (keep in mind that seconds pass very slowly when no one is speaking), the question might be repeated or restated in slightly different words. If there is still no response, we might ask whether or not the patient has understood our question. Sooner or later we are likely to get an answer, and the process can proceed from there. If the patient refuses to engage in communication, we proceed with treatment at considerable peril.

More commonly, the patient will respond to our questions, but his response will be colored by an attitude of hostility or great apprehension. Again, the dental team must understand the real message behind the expression of hostility, which may be one of great apprehension and fear. If we react emotionally to the literal messages and attitudes we perceive, we will not communicate effectively or help the patient appreciably, and develop ulcers in the bargain.

Effective listening, then, is critical to the communication process, for it enables us to interpret the feedback correctly. We must allow and encourage the patient to respond in communication and carefully consider both the literal message and the emotional components of his response.

The Setting

The setting in which the communication takes place may profoundly influence the exchange. Obviously, one would prefer quiet surroundings, free of interruption and interference. Both parties in the exchange should be physically comfortable. This involves not only a comfortable seating arrangement, but may also require that any pain or discomfort that the patient has be relieved before effective communication can occur.

The immediate relief of pain is absolutely critical to the communication process. For example, a patient having acute pain in a tooth may request (or demand) its removal. The dentist may feel strongly that the tooth can and should be retained. The rather lengthy and complicated communication required to explain to the patient why the tooth should be retained, the possible deleterious effects of its loss, the advantages of its retention, the means by which it could be treated (root canal therapy, reinforcing dowel and core, crown restoration), and the time and cost of treatment may not be possible when acute pain is present during communication. Rather than competing with this pain interference, the dentist can keep the lines of communication open by offering to relieve the pain before the patient decides whether to retain the tooth. The patient, after all, doesn't necessarily want to be rid of a tooth, he wants to be rid of the pain. If the dentist can remove the pain quickly and effectively using local anesthetic, drainage, pulpal extirpation, pulpotomy, or analgesic drugs, the question of whether and how to retain the offending tooth can be discussed on a subsequent visit in a communication setting free of pain interference.

Of equal importance in creating a good communication setting is the control of fear and apprehension. The patient often associates the dental environment with pain or other unpleasant sensations, and communication may be hampered by the patient's uneasiness. Changing or modifying the setting may help alleviate this apprehension.

Changing the Setting. A popular means of controlling fear is to carry on communication away from the dental operatory in a private office or consultation room; this removes the immediate threat of dental procedures as well as the sight of the various machines and devices with which they are performed. Such a setting should be planned and decorated with the patient's reactions in mind. The advantage of alleviating the dental threat may be lost if, in the process, we introduce other threats. For example, the dentist seated behind a massive desk with the patient's models and radiographs displayed in front of him may be threatening to a patient seated in a small chair across the desk from the dentist as if they were both in the dental operatory. It is the same feeling a dentist might get when being interviewed across a similar desk by, say, an IRS agent. We must take care, then, that when we carry communication away from the dental operatory, the setting to which we move is, in fact, less threatening.

Modifying the Setting. It may not be to the advantage of the dentist to leave the dental operatory in order to engage in communication: the dentist may feel ill-at-ease in a private-office setting, and there are any number of times when communication is necessary while the patient is in the treatment room. The setting can be modified in many ways to reduce the potential threat to the patient.

Dental instruments and handpieces can be concealed in any number of delivery systems and brought forth only when a procedure is being performed. Placing a clean napkin over instruments or instrument trays removes the visual threat to a great degree. Decoration of the operatory can do much in modifying the setting: an attractive, well-lit treatment room with plants, sculpture, and wall decorations is less threatening than a room that resembles a surgical theater with stark walls, hoses, and implements of destruction.

Dealing with Patient Fear Directly

Whether the setting is a private office or an operatory, the most effective method of controlling fear and apprehension in the communication process is to deal with it directly. The dentist should ask the patient what he is feeling, whether he is nervous or frightened, and reassure him that his is a normal and acceptable reaction. The patient should know that such feelings are common and that the dentist understands, cares, and will do everything he can to keep the patient comfortable and as free of pain as possible. This may not remove the patient's apprehension, but it allows him to deal with it, and thereby assists in creating a setting that is conducive to effective communication.

This overview of basic communication has been based on the model of verbal interaction of dentist and patient. Obviously, communication can and does occur in many other forms, and many of the principles are applicable to other communication modes. We will consider some of these in the context of various techniques of patient involvement.

Written Materials

A *preappointment letter,* which is sent to the patient prior to his first appointment (Fig. 2–3), serves

ROBERT B. MORRIS, D.D.S.
14021 W. GREENFIELD AVENUE
NEW BERLIN, WISCONSIN 53151

TELEPHONE 782-4860

Sept. 1, 1982

Dear Mrs. Smith,

This will confirm your appointment made yesterday by phone for Monday, Sept. 17th at 3:00 P.M. As you requested, we will do an examination, a cleaning, and brief consultation regarding your dental situation.

If you are coming west on I94, take the Moorland Road exit south to Greenfield Avenue. Turn left onto Greenfield and look for the small shopping center on the right (south) about 1½ miles east of Moorland Road.

To save you some time on the first appointment we have enclosed our get-acquainted questionnaire for you to complete and bring along to your appointment. We have also enclosed a copy of our welcome pamphlet which explains a little bit about our office. Please look it over and if you have any questions feel free to call or discuss them when you come.

Thank you for taking the time to complete the questionnaire, and for choosing our office. We look forward to serving you.

Sincerely yours,

Robert B. Morris, D.D.S.

Fig. 2–3. Letter to patient prior to first appointment.

to confirm an appointment and introduce the patient to the practice or clinic. Such a letter may include any or all of the following points:

1. Confirmation of the time of the first appointment and directions to the office
2. A pleasant note of welcome to the practice
3. A description of what will occur on the initial visit, including treatment fees
4. A brief description of office policy and practice philosophy
5. Forms to be filled out prior to the initial appointment, such as business information and medical history forms

An *introductory letter,* which is given to the patient upon arrival (Fig. 2–4), can be identical to the preappointment letter or somewhat more specific,

TO OUR NEW PATIENTS

Welcome to our office! It has been designed for your comfort, for we are dedicated to the proposition that dentistry can be a relatively pleasant, effective experience. We are pleased you have selected us to help solve your dental problems, because we are convinced that with your cooperation, we can show you how to personally control dental disease and maintain a healthy mouth.

Except for emergency situations requiring immediate treatment, the patient will be initially seen for a thorough examination and diagnosis. In virtually all cases, full-mouth x-rays will be taken. In some situations, diagnostic casts, a dietary analysis or other fact-finding material will be collected. This examination will not be merely limited to detecting dental decay but will include an evaluation of periodontal and other soft tissues of the mouth, occlusion of the teeth (the manner in which your teeth come together) and the effect this may have on the teeth themselves, their supporting bone, the temporomandibular joint and muscles of the face. Where indicated, we may recommend consultation with other dental specialists or your physician.

It is our desire to eliminate currently existing dental problems, but we also feel it is our responsibility to describe to you subtle changes which are apparent and which may cause serious problems in the future. This, then, is what prevention is all about. Prevention is identifying problems before they become tragedies. Prevention is learning how to control disease before it can cause irreparable loss and thereby require further treatment. Prevention can provide an attitude of success rather than the hopelessness of contimued dental repair.

At the conclusion of the diagnosis and examination, a program will be described to you that will allow you to achieve these ends. More elaborate treatment need not be entered into until you, the patient, feel confident of the continuing success of that treatment. Our hope is to help you avoid the disappointment and loss due to dental failure that often accompanies random, incomplete treatment based on inadequate analysis. In short, our ultimate goal is to teach and motivate you to achieve dental health through your own daily efforts, thereby eliminating the need for constant dental repair. We can make your mouth more comfortable, functional and attractive, but only you can make it healthy.

CER 56 – Dental Printing, P. O. Box 730, Paradise, Calif. 95969

Fig. 2–4. Introductory letter upon arrival. (By permission of Dr. Carl Rieder.)

WELCOME TO OUR OFFICE!

We thank you for choosing us for your dental care. Please take a few minutes to acquaint yourself with the understandings in this pamphlet. Please feel free to ask us about them if you have a question. We are here to serve **YOU.**

WILLIAM L. NEQUETTE AND ASSOCIATES, LTD.
PRACTICE OF DENTISTRY

14021 WEST GREENFIELD AVENUE
NEW BERLIN, WISCONSIN 53151

TELEPHONE (414) 782-4860

WILLIAM L. NEQUETTE, D.D.S.
CHARLES W. McCAULEY, D.D.S.
ROBERT B. MORRIS, D.D.S.
THOMAS S. RYPEL, D.D.S.
KENNETH J. WALISZEWSKI, D.D.S., M.S.
JAMES C. HOVE, D.D.S.

YOU CAN EXPECT FROM US . . .

A PREVENTIVE APPROACH to dental care. We now know that tooth decay and gum disease (pyorrhea) are preventable, and that good oral health need not mean ever increasing expense. We will assist you in developing your dental health practices to save you time, money and, in the end, your teeth.

A COMPLETE AND THOROUGH EXAMINATION, including all necessary dental x-rays. This is the foundation for sound and sensible dental treatment, and will be followed by an explanation of the findings and a discussion of the approximate fee.

PERSONAL AND COURTEOUS SERVICE. We feel our patients deserve the same kind of treatment we would want for ourselves and our families. If you are unhappy with the treatment you receive, please tell us.

Fig. 2–5. Preprinted welcome pamphlet.

since the patient has the opportunity to respond and ask questions (feedback) regarding the information contained in the letter.

A *preprinted pamphlet* allows specific communication about the practice but also serves as a patient-education vehicle, because its greater length allows more information to be conveyed (Fig. 2–5). It is important, however, that such mass-produced devices be carefully screened by the dental team to ensure that their information is both correct and consistent with what is being taught in the practice. Furthermore, to be relevant to the patient, the pamphlet should be referred to specifically by the dental team. Materials handed out and never mentioned again are likely to end up in wastebaskets.

Reprints or copies of brief articles of interest provide information in a very readable form. The dental team may select the source and content of these articles and update the selection periodically. Magazines will often send reprints in quantity for a nominal cost, and news clippings can be mounted or copied for perusal by the patient.

Preprinted pamphlets and reprints are valuable not only because of their informational content, but because they offer *third-party verification.* Third-party verification is an effective persuasive device to gain the confidence and acceptance of the patient. Although the patient may not fully accept what at first seems like a new idea or a different approach, having another person or source verify the information lends credibility. This occurs even if the third party is not an objective expert. For example, verification may come from a friend, neighbor, or television commercial, none of which could be considered expert sources. Objectivity is not necessarily a prerequisite, since verification can be effective from other members of the dental team (hygienist, assistant, and receptionist) who obviously are not disinterested parties.

Audio-Visual Aids

Posters are brief informational reminders or motivational messages conveyed through graphics (Fig. 2–6). The effectiveness of the devices is variable, and

WE EXPECT FROM YOU . . .

PROMPTNESS IN KEEPING APPOINTMENTS. Broken appointments deny time to other patients. We must reluctantly charge for appointments broken or cancelled with less than 24 hours notice.

RESPONSIBILITY IN PAYMENT OF ACCOUNT. We will discuss your treatment and the approximate cost before any major work is done. We feel everyone benefits when definite financial arrangements are agreed upon.

- If you maintain a zero balance by paying in full (check or cash) when treatment is rendered we are happy to extend a 5% discount on the total fee. This does not apply to treatment billed monthly, such as orthodontics, or to accounts charged through MasterCharge/VISA, which we have installed for your convenience.
- If no other arrangements are made, you will be billed by mail and payment is due in full within 10 days from receipt of statement.
- In some case, other arrangements such as installment payments, may be made with the dentist or office coordinator, but these must be agreed upon in advance of treatment.
- If you have dental insurance, you are still directly responsible for all fees, however, we ask that you read our insurance letter for details.

A SHARED RESPONSIBILITY . . .

A COMMITMENT TO YOUR ORAL HEALTH. The only person who has control over your mouth is you. We will provide the best dental treatment, the newest methods that modern dentistry has to offer, and the opportunity for you to come in for regular preventive maintenance visits. Working together, we can offer the promise of good oral health and a trouble-free mouth, but without your help we can do very little.

We hope the idea of teamwork in achieving oral health appeals to you, and we look forward to serving you in any way we can.

Fig. 2–5 ***continued.***

it is possible that a few visually striking graphics that complement the general decor of the office may be more effective than a large number of less effective messages, in which the impact may be diluted considerably. A notable exception to this might be a pediatric practice, in which posters and various visual messages that were created by children and conveyed what they have learned may be an effective form of third-party verification.

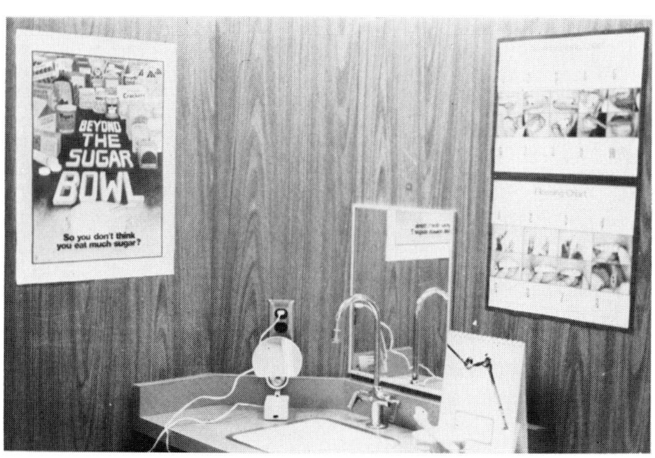

Fig. 2–6. Educational posters.

Conveying information in *displays* often may be more effective than a printed pamphlet or chart (Fig. 2–7). For example, a common device for informing patients about sucrose in the diet is a display with granulated sugar in bottles or vials that are labeled with the food name they represent. For example, a 6-ounce candy bar may contain several teaspoons of sugar and a 12-ounce sugared soft drink may contain six or more teaspoons of sugar. It is often more meaningful to the patient to visualize sugar content in granulated form than to discuss or read it in numerical terms. Other examples of patient involvement through the use of displays could include before-and-after study models in which malocclusion has been corrected, examples of recommended, versus harmful, snack foods, and cut-away models of teeth showing representations of caries and/or periodontal disease. Displays of this nature often stimulate interest and questions from the patient, and this kind of feedback is invaluable. Getting the patient involved in the problem is the first step toward the solution.

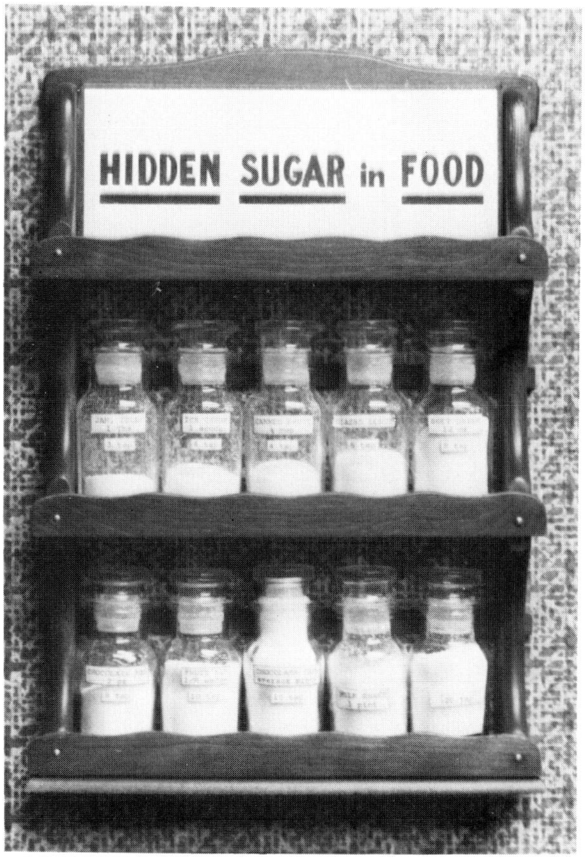

Fig. 2–7. Educational display.

Displays to be avoided are those that smack of commercialism or are obviously trying to sell some product or service. Not only is there an ethical problem with using items of this nature, but patients are likely to react to them as they would to any commercial message—with some caution and skepticism. Also to be avoided are sensational or emotional displays. For example, a jar of extracted teeth with the legend "Teeth that never knew dental floss" may be very striking, but fear is a poor long-term motivator. Also, although sections of lung tissue that show the black, tarry deposits of cigarette smoking may be used as motivation in an antismoking clinic, a person is more likely to block the image out or respond "That is something that happens to other people, not me." This reaction has been amply documented over the years, the classic examples of which are the highway-safety campaigns of the 1950's, which used lifelike recreations or actual film footage of car crashes and injured victims, much of it rather gory, especially by the standards of the times. The campaign attracted much attention, the materials were seen by many people, but the effect on highway safety was virtually nil. People may *react* to fearful stimuli, but they will *respond* to positive motivators more readily. In brief, displays of bloody extraction forceps will not result in better oral-health maintenance by the patient but may result in the patient avoiding such unpleasant reminders of his mortality.

As with any technique of patient involvement, the effectiveness of demonstration material depends on its use. The dental team should refer to the materials when counselling patients and be prepared to discuss and answer questions regarding them.

In an age of television, in which so much of life is expressed and affected by "the tube," *projection systems,* such as a television-sized sound projector, filmstrip, or videotape player, can be effective methods of patient involvement. Such devices can provide general information for numbers of people or very specific information for an individual. As with all informational materials, the films, filmstrips, or tapes should be carefully screened and selected by the dental team to ensure that their information is both accurate and consistent with what is being taught in the practice. At this time, there is a wide range of such material on the market and the quality varies tremendously. Outdated or erroneous information, poor quality production, and amateurish actors or drawings negate the effectiveness of this tool.

Since the equipment required to utilize audio-visual media is costly, it behooves the dentist and the dental team to choose it wisely. If possible, such materials should be purchased on approval or on a trial basis and screened by the dental team and their families as well as by patients, who could be asked for their reaction to the materials. It is important to evaluate the material from the standpoint of the layman, so as to avoid highly technical presentations that may look good to someone already conversant with the information, but may be technically beyond the layman.

The dentist who uses *photographs* to record treatment can often utilize them mounted or in album form to illustrate for the patient any number of concepts such as prevention (pictures before, during, and after a plaque-control program) and restoration (what a porcelain fused to gold bridge might look like). Since these materials are from the very setting in which they are used, they have immediate application and relevance.

Patient Involvement in the Examination

The most effective technique of patient involvement in treatment planning is probably the patient's active participation in his own examination. It can be accurately stated that the majority of patients have little or no idea of what is happening in their own mouths. Most people have looked at the facial surfaces of anterior teeth but have never looked carefully at their total oral cavities; they have no knowledge or understanding of what constitutes oral health or disease. For many patients, pain is the first indication of a problem and, as we know all too well, by the time most dental diseases become acutely painful, they have progressed beyond the point of simple treatment. In order to receive treatment that will be truly effective, the patient must gain an understanding of his oral condition, what constitutes health or disease, and what he must do to promote dental health and control dental disease. This understanding can be acquired in a number of ways, three of which I will describe here: patient history and interview, the use of an intra-oral mirror, and the dentist's verbalization of his findings.

Patient History and Interview

Prior to the examination, a medical history and a dental history should be obtained. The elements contained in these histories will be discussed in some detail in a later chapter; for the present, we will limit our discussion to the way in which the histories can serve to involve the patient in treatment planning.

Much of the information in a medical/dental history can be obtained by the patient completing a checklist or filling in blanks. If the questions are posed clearly and are obviously relevant to the situation, they may start the patient thinking about his oral condition. A good example of this is a dietary analysis for sugar-laden foods. Often a patient will not realize how much or how frequently he consumes sugar, but when completing a checklist he discovers the problem himself. This can also occur when a patient is asked to recall past dental problems or treatment. If a patient-completed form is concise and clear, it can be an effective means of involving the patient in diagnosis. However, if the history form is too lengthy or so involved that the patient cannot see any relevance to the questions, its effectiveness is severely reduced; indeed, it may actually cause the patient to "turn off," and be less receptive in the interview to follow.

For the patient history to be effective in involving the patient in diagnosis and treatment planning, it must be followed by an interview with the dentist or another member of the dental team in which the responses of the patient are discussed and clarified. This is quite obviously true of the medical history. For example, should the patient record a history of heart trouble, the interviewer would try to elicit specific information about the type of heart problem, when it occurred and its sequelae, and the present status of the problem. This further dialog should also clarify for the patient the reason for posing the question, which is the possible risk of heart infection (subacute bacterial endocarditis) when dental surgery is done on patients with damaged heart valves, or the possibility of drug interactions should the dentist prescribe a medication while the patient is taking another.

The dental history is even more critical to patient involvement in diagnosis and treatment planning, and the verbal review of the completed form should allow the patient to describe and expand upon past dental problems and experiences with dental treatment. This will often reveal not only what the patient has experienced in the dental setting, but how he feels about those experiences and, possibly, why he feels that way. With this tool, we hope to get a reasonable grasp of the patient's dental understanding and attitude. Is he trusting and receptive, having a history of few problems and good experiences with treatment, or is he cautious, even hostile, as a result of bad past experiences? Our entire approach to communication with patients may be based on this review of the history, and it behooves the dental team to approach the patient at his level of understanding and concern if a common ground for communication is to be established. Are there misunderstandings, erroneous information regarding dentistry and oral health that need to be corrected before effective treatment can be done? These questions may not always be addressed immediately, because direct conflict with the patient's present understanding may create a debate instead of dialog, but knowing how the patient thinks will help guide our later efforts.

A second major benefit of the patient interview is that, by openly discussing his past experiences and his feelings about them, the patient may be less likely to respond irrationally—that is, if the patient understands what factors have led to his present state, he is less likely to lash out in anger or frustration at the people who are trying to help. In the interview, the dental team can take the opportunity to make some observations on what the patient has experienced, perhaps offering some explanations as to why certain things have occurred. For example, the patient who feels (or worse, has been told) that he has "soft teeth" and, hence, cannot get away from tooth decay, may, when given a brief explanation of the causes of decay and seeing what his home care and diet have been, come to a new understanding of his oral health and be more receptive to efforts to improve it.

The patient who appears hostile to all dentists should be encouraged to discuss his "terrible experiences" with other dentists; in this way, he may conclude that perhaps one or two episodes have been primarily responsible for his attitude. By openly discussing these experiences and feelings, the patient is less likely to project them onto the dental team or to react irrationally to the dental setting. Therefore, although the litany of bad dentists, fillings that fell out, and pain that was inflicted may be time-consuming and tend to evoke defensive emotional responses from the dentist, it can be a beneficial exercise in terms of future relationships with the patient. The dentist and dental team must practice the art of "nonjudgmental listening" in order to lay the groundwork of the cooperative effort necessary for effective dental treatment.

Format of the Interview. It is certainly possible and, in some cases, necessary to obtain the entire history verbally, clarifying and expanding on the information as the history is taken. An advantage of this is that the relevance of a question can be explained immediately if the patient should question it; secondly, it presents a more personal approach to information gathering. This technique is a necessity when the patient cannot fill out a form due to language difficulty, or the inability to read, see, or write. The principal disadvantage of using the verbal interview exclusively is that it can be extremely time-consuming, whether it is obtained by the dentist or another member of the dental team. Not only does it take longer to read and answer questions verbally than to check off items on a form, but the patient must often stop and think, remembering episodes, dates, and medications, and may require some time to do so. A second disadvantage of the total verbal history is that the patient may be somewhat hesitant to disclose or discuss personal information with, for example, a dental auxiliary. A history of venereal disease or alcoholism, or various reproductive problems may be difficult for the patient to admit to and discuss with the dental team. A checklist, however, may be far less threatening, even though the same people will have access to the information, and may result in a more complete history.

The patient may fail to complete certain sections or questions of a history form; these should be investigated verbally, keeping in mind that the patient may have had some specific reason for not divulging the information. We should tactfully inquire about why the history was not fully completed so that we can anticipate, understand, and work through any difficulties the patient may have with divulging the information.

If we have a completed history form, the interview can proceed from that history. Positive answers in the history should be clarified. In order to do this, we must ask the patient questions. We should discourage yes/no responses and pose questions in such a way that the patient can expand upon the information freely. For example, if the history reveals a heart problem, we should not ask the question, "I see you indicated you have had heart problems, is that correct?" To this the patient responds, "Yes," and very little information is gained. A better question would be "I see you indicated you have had a heart problem. Could you tell me what type of problem you had and when it occurred?" Such questions require thoughtful answers and have been called, in psychologic terms, "open-ended" questions. Through such questions, the patient is unavoidably involved in the diagnosis/treatment planning process. In many cases, the entire interview can be carried out with the dentist or dental-team member asking such questions, giving the patient time to consider them before he answers. Reviewing the medical history first is advisable, because if the patient understands the relationship of general health to oral health, he is likely to respond with fewer reservations. Again, the exception here might be in the area of highly personal or potentially embarrassing information, which should be dealt with tactfully by the interviewer.

If the medical history is successfully reviewed and clarified with open-ended questions, the dental history can be elucidated similarly. In this case, however, patient involvement is even more critical and often more difficult. It is here that the biases, misconceptions, and fears of the patient tend to cloud the facts. For example, if the history indicates that it has been many years since the patient's last dental visit, we may seek to know the reasons why the patient has not sought dental care and ask the question, "I see it has been some time since you've had any dental treatment or check-ups. Why have you let it go so long?" To this the patient might reply, "I hate dentists." We have alluded to this type of exchange earlier in the chapter; it is in this type of communication situation that the dental team must maintain their patience and professionalism and ask an open-ended question such as, "What has made you feel that way toward dentists?" At this point, the principle of "Whoever talks first, loses" comes into play. We are asking the patient to confront his fears about dentists, dental treatment, and dental pain, and this is no small request. The silence that can ensue this question is deafening. The dentist who has the patience and concern to allow the patient to answer may be rewarded with a key to successful dental treatment. The dentist who pushes, threatens, or answers the question for the patient may lose that key and the patient as well.

Effective interviewing using open-ended questions

is a skill that requires much study and considerable practice. Some caution is advised when using stereotyped interview formats—"canned" questions—especially if patient resistance is encountered. It is beyond the scope of this text to go into great detail on the subject, but ample resource material is cited at the end of the chapter.

A well-designed written history can provide a good framework for the verbal interview and make the task much easier. We should also stress that, in some cases, it may take time for the patient to open himself up to the dental team. It may require some early treatment visits, which will build up the trust and confidence of the patient gradually, before deep involvement in diagnosis and treatment planning is possible. When this is the case, it is possible to plan treatment and present it in steps, or phases; this concept will be discussed more fully in later chapters.

Intraoral Mirror

The single greatest reason for the public's lack of dental understanding is that it is difficult to see into one's own oral cavity. The bathroom mirror reveals the facial surfaces of anterior teeth and, to some extent, the occlusals of posteriors to about the first molar region, seldom beyond. If the patient should attempt to visually investigate his own oral cavity, obvious disease may be ignored while normal, benign findings may be suspected or even feared unless there is a good understanding of what is seen. Thus, an ideal opportunity presents itself at the time of the dental examination, and that is to take the patient along with us on a tour of the oral cavity, allowing him to see the normal and abnormal, the health and disease. This requires only two items: a good mirror, and the dentist's desire to share knowledge and understanding with the patient in order to involve him in diagnosis and treatment planning.

The importance of the mirror should not be underestimated. Too small a mirror makes it difficult for the patient to see what the dentist is pointing out; too large a mirror may present the same problem or prevent any light from reaching the oral cavity. An ideal tool for this purpose is a magnifying mirror approximately 5 in. in diameter, with a light source attached. This type of product is available commercially and marketed under the trade name Floxite (Fig. 2–8). It can be supplied with an electrical cord or mounted on a flashlight.

For routine use in one location, the plug-in type seems most practical, because it provides good light and does not require replacement batteries. Furthermore, it can be placed on a counter or table and used for oral-hygiene practice. For situations requiring mobility, the flashlight-mounted mirror can be nearly as useful. Any good quality mirror of appropriate size, illuminated or not, can be used with good results, for even limited visualization of the oral cavity is preferable to the patient seeing only the bracket tray and dental light during the examination.

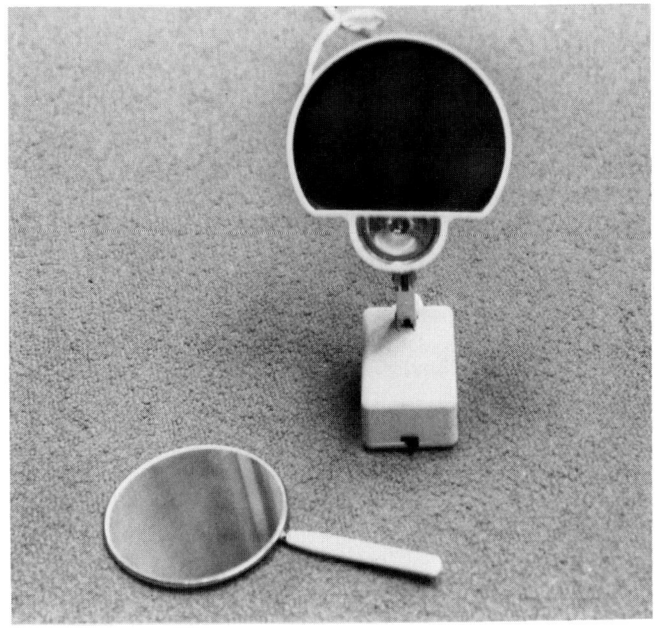

Fig. 2–8. Effective mirrors.

Verbalizing the Findings

Now that we have the patient visualizing his oral cavity, we must involve him further by verbalizing the findings of the examination. The most common failure in communication between dentist and patient occurs at this time, with the dentist speaking a language that the patient cannot comprehend—"dentalese." It seems that such an obvious concept would hardly need to be stated, yet the translation of dental jargon and terminology into lay terms poses a great problem. Prior to the first day of dental school, the dentist-to-be is gradually introduced to some fairly complex terminology through various science prerequisites. In a scientific field, it is absolutely essential that the terminology be precise and detailed, even though it then becomes polysyllabic and even more mysterious to the layman.

During his predental studies, the dentist-to-be learns to be comfortable with such Greek and Latin monstrosities, to decipher them readily, and to toss them about with style and aplomb, thus impressing friends and family. Upon entering dental school, the student is immersed in the entire body of dental jargon, and for at least 4 years, the most important communication with faculty and fellow students takes the form of "dentalese." This language is a combination of scientific and clinical terminology and dental shorthand—the "MO's," "DO's," and "RPD's," the "bi's" (bicuspids), and "skids" (discrepancy between CO and CR or IP and RP) —that is so meaningful to the dentist and dental team and so cryptic to the layman. Translating our language into plain English is a formidable task, and we must constantly be aware that we may be slipping into jargon and leaving the patient behind.

There are three basic ways of making ourselves understood by the patient. The first and best is to use terms that are correct dentally, yet in the lay vernacular as well. A lower front tooth need not be a mandibular anterior; it can remain a lower front tooth. The gums can remain gums, not gingivae, and cavities, which are well understood by both dentist and patient, need not be called carious lesions. Whenever possible in our communication with the patient, we should use terms that are commonly understood.

A second alternative is necessary when a common lay term that might be used is not correct dentally or may have connotations or shades of meaning that are inaccurate. In this situation, the dentist may use the lay term, but relate it to a more accurate word. The best example of this is the term "pyorrhea," which is recognized by many laymen, especially older individuals. These people recognize the term and readily associate it with their gums and tooth loss. In that respect, it is a good term. On the other hand, when we ask such a patient what he knows about pyorrhea, we may be told that it is something "Uncle George caught from a dirty drinking glass and 6 months later all his teeth fell out." Therefore, when using a term and attempting to transfer its meaning to a better term, we must take care that we do not transfer misunderstanding and misinformation as well. We can do so by substituting a better term, such as "gum disease," which used to be called "pyorrhea," and then briefly define and describe what gum disease is, how it occurs, and what it does.

A third alternative in selecting terms is needed when there seems to be no common lay term that comes close to the meaning to be conveyed. An example of this is the term "bacterial plaque," or just "plaque." Although the public is gradually becoming aware of the concept of plaque, and many dentists are conscientiously attempting to educate patients regarding plaque, it is still a new concept to many people. When hearing the term, however, the patient may claim to be familiar with it. Further questioning may reveal that he has confused plaque with calculus or stains, so we must not assume understanding unless we have had the patient explain his understanding in his own words. It is ineffective and unacceptable to substitute terms such as "cookie bugs" for "plaque." These terms only confuse the patient and will have to to be unlearned at some later date. Other misleading substitutes for dental terminology are "air pockets in the gums" to describe periodontal disease or "soft teeth" to explain a high rate of dental decay. Such terms are inaccurate and misleading and often do more harm than good. In such situations, it is the responsibility of the dental team to use a correct term and define it as necessary.

In summary, if we are to involve the patient in treatment planning by verbalizing our findings, we must use terms the patient can understand. Ideally, terms that are both correct and commonly understood are preferred; however, in some situations, a common term that is outdated or not quite accurate must be used with a term that is less common but more exact in meaning. If lay terminology fails, the patient may be introduced to a new term, which will have to be defined or explained.

The findings in a dental examination may be verbalized in many ways. The first and most common method is for the dentist to perform the examination in relative silence, making notations on the dental chart, and, following the examination, relate the significant findings to the patient—that is, those problems that require treatment, further evaluation or surveillance. This approach, while it is the most common, is probably the least effective in involving the patient. It does not require the patient to see and understand his oral cavity and the potential problems present therein or to take an active role in selecting an appropriate course of treatment.

A second approach is to dictate the findings out loud as the examination proceeds, pointing out both normal and pathologic conditions to the patient. This encourages patient participation, allows immediate explanation of significant findings, and should elicit questions from the patient as the examination progresses. An auxiliary member of the dental team must be present to record the findings and can also help keep the examination "on course" should the patient's questions lead to digressions. Such digressions are to be expected and should be welcomed as a sure indication of the patient's interest. In most cases, patients' questions should be answered as clearly and as quickly as possible to encourage active involvement in the examination and diagnosis.

A variation of this approach is to have the auxiliary become more involved by leading the examiner in the routine, systematic examination. The auxiliary asks questions such as "What is the appearance of the head and neck?" and "What is the condition of the lymph glands?" allowing the examiner to respond. This dialogue, which should have an almost conversational tone, may help involve the patient by its relative informality. Significant findings may be pointed out and explained both to the patient and the auxiliary; this further reduces the aura of formality and encourages patient participation. Another variation is to suggest likely or possible treatment as the exam proceeds. Thus the patient is introduced to and may begin to consider some of the possible solutions to his problems and the likely extent of treatment.

A third approach is to encourage the patient's self-discovery, which is at once the most effective and least practical method of patient involvement in examination. Ideally, the patient might be given his study casts and radiographs to peruse prior to the actual examination and be taught self-examination techniques for the soft tissue (oral cancer exam) and periodontal evaluations (plaque disclosure, bleeding points). Together, the dentist and patient might look at the oral cavity, the study casts, and radiographs, and attempt to identify significant findings. While this is not always a practical approach, it can be done, and is highly effective in terms of treatment plan acceptance. For example, if the patient has noted drifting and tipping teeth resulting from an unreplaced missing tooth, it is not difficult to explain why a fixed bridge might be necessary. Even if this technique of total self-discovery is not used, the approach can be incorporated into any examination format and still be very effective. The greatest application of the approach is in periodontal evaluation, in which the patient, with mirror in hand, is asked to visualize the gum tissues, notice differences in color, texture (firm areas versus puffy), and especially bleeding elicited by gentle probing, and describe what he sees. At the same time, the dentist can be explaining why certain areas are different in color, are puffy, or bleed easily, and what can be done about it. The importance of the patient's self-discovery in the examination cannot be stressed enough. When the patient has seen, described, and discussed pathology in the oral cavity, he has actively participated in his examination and diagnosis. Presenting a treatment plan to such patients becomes an easy task, for we can simply relate the proposed treatment to those problems seen and discussed during the examination. Often, the solutions are obvious to the patient and he may propose them himself. Following the self-discovery process, it is not uncommon for a patient to ask if he might be given instructions in home care methods that would control the plaque and thus correct the gum disease, or to ask if "a bridge or something" would prevent further tipping and eventual loss of a posterior tooth.

These three approaches to verbalizing the findings and involving the patient in the examination should not be considered mutually exclusive; they should be used whenever they are appropriate, combining and integrating any or all of the suggested techniques. The key concept here is that examination and diagnosis are not done *to*, but *with* the patient. We will succeed or fail in our dental treatment less as a result of our care, skill, and judgment, than as a result of the patient's ability and willingness to participate actively in the arrest of disease and the restoration of function.

Treatment Plan Presentation

We have already touched on this topic in relation to patient involvement in examination and diagnosis, so we need not dwell on it other than to suggest a few alternative approaches in the actual mechanics of treatment plan presentation. We must preface that with a brief discussion of dental treatment plans from the viewpoint of the patient. Basically, the patient has three main concerns regarding dental treatment: the first and foremost concern is fear; the second is necessity ("Is the proposed treatment really going to satisfy my needs?"); and the third is cost ("Is the proposed treatment affordable and worth the expense?") This final concern is the one most often expressed by patients, but while it must be addressed, it may actually be the least crucial of the three. Let us discuss the concerns in what is likely to be the true order of their importance to the patient.

Control of Fear

Fear—of pain, discomfort, the unknown—is very likely the primary reason that people do not seek dental treatment. Entering the dental office for examination often requires courage on the part of many patients. Hence, the pain potential of any proposed course of treatment is an overriding concern. The dentist who blithely proposes extraction of wisdom teeth or root canal treatment without considering the high fear potential such procedures carry, may wonder why the patient rejects the proposal. Care should be taken in this regard. The fear factor must be controlled before any treatment proposals can be considered, and the primary approach in its control is for the dentist and dental team to gain the confidence of the patient, to make him believe that they are competent and caring. The best way of doing this is for the dentist and dental team to *be* competent and caring. Many factors will serve to build the patient's confidence in the dentist and dental team. I will describe some of the most effective techniques.

Referral. A patient referred by a friend, relative, or acquaintance often has a high level of confidence in the dental staff. This is an effective form of third-party verification, and the degree of the patient's confidence depends on the nature of the referral. When a highly satisfied patient praises a dentist, extols the competence and care of the dental team, and encourages a close friend or relative to seek treatment from that team, the referred patient, while often fearful of the dental setting itself, may already possess considerable confidence in the dentist. On the other hand, when a less committed patient who seeks treatment only on an occasional basis is asked the name of his dentist, there may be very little confidence engendered in the referred patient. When considering how to approach a referred patient, it is important to determine the type of patient who referred him and the nature of the referral.

A patient referred by another dentist, a specialist, a dental school, a physician, or a pharmacist, may arrive with a high level of confidence; however, it may be directed more at the clinical competence of the dentist than at his "chairside manner"—those qualities likely to assuage the patient's fears and soothe his anxious psyche.

Courteous Treatment. There is no better means of demonstrating concern for a patient's well-being than to treat him with kindness and courtesy. Anyone who has encountered impersonal, imperious, or downright rude treatment in a health facility can appreciate the value of a warm smile, a courteous greeting, and friendly treatment by the dental team.

Professionalism. While warm and friendly treatment is important, care must be taken that professionalism is maintained. Friendly banter among the dental staff, the exchange of jokes or friendly insults in earshot of the new and fearful patient, while not unusual or improper in themselves, may lessen that patient's confidence in the dental team. A fearful patient needs to know that the dental team is concerned about him, his dental problems, and his needs, rather than last night's party or next weekend's camping trip. Anyone who has encountered immature or unprofessional behavior when seeking help for a serious problem can appreciate the need for the professional appearance and behavior of the dental team.

Skilled Hygiene Treatment. In practices utilizing the services of a dental hygienist, the patient will, in most cases, receive treatment from the hygienist prior to the presentation of a comprehensive treatment plan. If that treatment has been rendered with care, if the hygienist has been thorough but gentle and obviously concerned for the patient's comfort during the procedures, it will likely engender confidence and reduce the patient's fear when he considers the overall treatment plan. The reverse is true if the hygienist's services are painful or rendered in a rough or uncaring manner. To help in this regard, it should be the dentist's responsibility to assess the probable extent of the hygienist's treatment and the amount of sensitivity or pain likely to be encountered by the patient in its course. Sedative/analgesic premedication, topical anesthetics, or local injectible anesthetics should be used when indicated to allow the hygienist to perform effectively and thoroughly without placing the patient under stress.

Verbal Reassurance. In many cases, the simplest way to build confidence and allay fear is to address the patient's fears directly and verbally. The dentist and dental team should tell the patient that fear and apprehension are common, understandable, and acceptable. It is often effective to admit our own fears of dental treatment, "even though we know it won't hurt." With fear openly addressed, understood, accepted, and, to some extent, shared, we can then reassure the patient that most dental procedures today are painless or nearly so; we can also assure him that we will do everything we can to make him comfortable and relaxed. This reassurance is quite obvious, but often left unsaid. It can do wonders in reducing fear as a concern in treatment planning.

Environment. Reducing fear and creating patient confidence through office and equipment design is a subject that could fill a text in itself. Basically, the surroundings, office decor, and layout should be pleasant, attractive, and well-kept. Dental equipment and instruments should be concealed or made as unobtrusive as possible before, during, and after use.

These factors are by no means the only tools for building confidence and allaying fears; they merely represent the type of approaches possible in this area. It might be argued that such approaches are "practice builders," gimmicks or ploys designed to create good will and stimulate referrals. In most cases, they will serve that end; however, successful dental treatment on the scientific level depends greatly on patient involvement, which requires that we deal with fear and apprehension effectively. Any tool that accomplishes this end is as effective as any of our dental instruments. Due to better preventive methods, fluoride, and effective painless treatment, future generations of dental patients may have less fear and apprehension regarding dental treatment, and other factors may become more significant.

Satisfaction of Needs

Assuming that fear is controlled, we can then address the second major patient concern: necessity. Patients present themselves for dental treatment because they feel some need, or needs. If not addressed to the needs the patient actually feels, the most brilliant diagnosis, and the best conceived plan of treatment will fall upon deaf ears and be rejected. Two approaches should be considered here. We should attempt, whenever possible, to determine the patient's needs. The history and interview previously discussed can be instrumental in this regard. We should have a clear picture of why the patient sought dental treatment at this time, what he feels he needs or would like done, and what his expectations and goals are. Is the patient concerned about the appearance of his mouth and teeth? Is there pain or discomfort to be alleviated? Is there loss of or difficulty in function? Is there an overriding concern regarding eventual loss versus long-term retention of the teeth? Often the patient's concerns and needs may not be specifically tooth or mouth oriented, but may have to do with general physical attractiveness, comfort, or function.

We must then attempt to present a course of treatment that addresses the needs expressed by the patient. In some cases, this may be a direct application of a solution to the need. For example, if a partially edentulous patient feels a need for more teeth with which to chew food, our treatment plan should provide some prosthetic appliance to meet that need. In other cases, the plan may address the need indirectly. When the patient's concern is the appearance of his front teeth (particularly the ever-widening spaces between them), the plan may involve the same prosthetic appliance used by the first patient to provide posterior support for the flaring anterior teeth, but some explanation is needed about how this solution will address the patient's need. In yet a third situation, the patient may have a serious dental problem, such as undiagnosed periodontal disease; yet, having experienced no noticeable symptoms, he feels no need for treatment. In this situation, the second approach is essential.

The second, more effective approach is to allow the patient to discover his own dental problems, which then makes him aware of his needs, or redirects his needs toward the necessary treatment. We have already discussed this process in terms of patient involvement in the examination and diagnosis process. If the patient has participated in the discovery of oral and dental problems and understands the causes and effects of those problems, there is little question about the necessity of the treatment proposed to correct those problems.

Cost

The patient's third major concern in planning treatment is the cost. As previously noted, patients often believe this concern is uppermost in importance. If the fear of potential treatment is allayed and the patient understands and feels the need for such treatment, cost becomes much less of a concern. However, it remains a legitimate issue that must be addressed.

The question of cost, specifically dental fees, has not been addressed in most textbooks. In the rarefied atmosphere of dental academia, discussing fees seems somewhat crass. The thought of structuring a plan of treatment around a patient's ability to pay seems demeaning and unprofessional. We are, after all, highly skilled practitioners in the art and science of dentistry, and those fortunate enough to come under our care should make whatever financial sacrifice is necessary in the interest of their dental health. That being said, we should now consider the real world. In recent times, economic recessions, inflation, and general uncertainty have made cost a more significant factor in dentistry. The caring dentist must recognize and deal with this fact, like it or not.

At this time, the majority of dental treatment in the United States is rendered on a fee-for-service basis, and for the most part, the patient is solely responsible for payment of the fee. A factor that alters this relationship between the dentist and his patient is the use of prepayment plans, whereby a third party (in most cases, some type of insurance carrier) pays a portion of the fee.

Welfare or public assistance programs, Veteran's Administration dental benefits, and other similar arrangements create a different kind of relationship in which the patient, in most cases, does not pay a fee. In these instances, the responsible third party reimburses the dentist at some set level of allowable fees.

Fairly recent delivery concepts involve capitation programs or health maintenance organizations (HMO's) which involve prepayment of fees at a fixed monthly or annual rate. Each of these modes of payment creates a different relationship between dentist and patient and must be addressed.

At the present, the bulk of treatment is rendered on a fee-for-service basis, with the patient responsible to his dentist. Third-party involvement in the form of commercial insurance carriers alters somewhat, but does not change, the basic nature of this relationship. Under this system, the dentist, having presented a treatment plan and the reasons for employing it, quotes a fee for that treatment. Third-party coverage may, and in many cases should, be determined in advance, so that the patient is aware of what his financial responsibility will be prior to acceptance of the treatment plan. Then the patient must decide if he wishes to pursue the treatment. As we have stated, that decision will be based on whether or not his three major concerns have been addressed. If the patient can consider the plan without undue fear and apprehension and the need for the treatment is clear, the decision rests on the patient's perceived ability to afford the fee.

We should consider ability to pay as a continuum with extreme situations at each end. On the low end, we have the unemployed or marginally employed individual who has neither private insurance nor public assistance, who is barely able to keep body and soul together, and who simply has no money. This type of individual most often does without dental treatment, but may be forced to seek it when dental maladies become acutely painful. When such an individual says he cannot afford dental treatment, he means just that. On the other end of the continuum is the fabulously wealthy individual for whom cost is no object. At first glance, it might seem that this person would be the ideal candidate for dental treatment, but having dealt with a small number of individuals in this situation, I have learned that ability to pay is not necessarily the determining factor in accepting dental treatment. Between these two extremes, we find the majority of dental patients—indeed, the majority of the population. The United States is a country of great wealth that is widely distributed. Millions, even billions of dollars are spent yearly on consumer goods such as televisions, boats, cosmetics, cigarettes, and dog food. Credit is available to most people who simply present a small plastic card and sign their name. Therefore, for the most part, the typical patient can afford most dental treatment. The key is whether that treatment is more important to him than some other goods or services. This is determined by that individual's "hierarchy of needs."[8]

Each of us has a hierarchy of needs, a list of priorities in which greater needs take precedence over lesser ones. For most people, survival takes precedence over comfort; therefore, food, clothing, and shelter will be provided before a backyard swimming pool is installed. The dentist must consider this when presenting extensive courses of treatment to people who have mortgage payments to make and children to feed, clothe, and educate. Such patients may appreciate and desire ideal dental treatment and may in fact, be able to afford it, but if doing so might jeopardize their economic security or their ability to provide for their children, they must reject or postpone the treatment. In a later chapter, I will discuss concepts of dental treatment planning that may enable such patients to work toward ideal comprehensive dental treatment without it creating a financial crisis.

We must also consider that, for many people, dental treatment—indeed, oral health and function—is not high on their list of priorities.

The dentist must not pass judgment on patients for whom dental care is relatively unimportant, for we each have priorities that are based on upbringing, environment, education, and experience. The dental team may attempt to educate the patient and encourage him to consider dental health more seriously, but there is a limit to what can reasonably be accomplished in this regard. To introduce conflict, to argue with a patient, is counterproductive, because attitudes usually stiffen on each side, and communication is lost. Our responsibility is to offer our services; the patient is free to accept or reject them for whatever reason. We may then offer alternative courses of treatment, or decline to treat the patient if his desires (or demands) are outside the realm of ethics or good treatment. If argument and confrontation have been avoided, it should be possible for such a parting of the ways to take place amicably.

The reasons for diplomacy and restraint are obvious. First, it saves wear and tear on the gastric lining of the dentist. More importantly, we must understand that an individual's hierarchy of needs is not fixed, but ever changing; although dental care may have a low priority today, it may become terribly important in the future. If we do not confront or alienate the unmotivated patient, we leave the door open for future services to be rendered when the patient is ready. Argument and conflict may not only cause the patient to avoid our services, but may sour him on any dentist in the future.

Finally, not only do priorities change, but actual ability to afford a service may change. Certainly a large, unexpected inheritance will alter priorities, but few people experience such windfalls. More often, success in business, job promotions, retirement of past debts, and so forth will alter the patient's perception of affordability. The greatest factor of this type is the increasing availability of third party payments to defray the expense of dental care. It is not uncommon to experience a situation in which a patient was unable to afford a $200 course of treatment one year, only to return the next year and accept a

$1000 course of treatment with dental insurance paying half. In any event, the introduction of any level of third-party assistance may bring about changes in both the actual abilty to pay and the perceived ability to afford dental treatment. Thus, third-party involvement can be a boon to the patient and the dentist when addressing cost as a concern in dental treatment planning.

The primary drawback of this system is that patients will occasionally base their entire attitude towards the cost of treatment on the amount of third-party payment. Without really considering the need for treatment, patients may opt for "as much treatment as insurance will cover" in order to get their money's worth or will refuse any more treatment than will be covered in full, despite how that may affect their own oral condition. Thus, while it is helpful and often necessary to plan a course of treatment around the patient's ability to pay, and in some cases, around the availability of third-party assistance, the overall goals of treatment should be established independent of third-party payment.

Welfare or public assistance programs that do not require the patient to accept financial responsibility for the treatment have greatly benefited a vast number of people, especially children, who could not readily avail themselves of dental treatment otherwise. That being said, we must consider two major problems relating to treatment planning under such programs.

First, limitations are imposed by the third party on what type of treatment is done, to what extent it will be done, and how much of the treatment fee will be paid. Thus, we have the same problem as in fee-for-service situations with third-party involvement—namely, that treatment planning is based more on what the third party will pay than on the individual patient's oral health status and needs. Second, it seems to be the nature of human beings that our appreciation of goods and services is often inversely proportional to their cost; while a great many public assistance or V. A. patients do value and appreciate the service being rendered, many others do not. This point brings us back to the behavioral nature of most dental diseases and the unfortunate fact that, without a firm commitment on the part of the patient, long-term success of dental treatment is unlikely.

Health maintenance or capitation payment systems create yet another type of relationship between dentist and patient. Under such programs, a fixed monthly amount is paid, usually through a third party, for each person enrolled in the program. Ideally, this should cover any and all dental procedures that the patient requires. In some systems, a deductible may be required of the patient, or a surcharge levied for more extensive types of treatment, such as prosthetics involving laboratory costs. The challenge in treatment planning in such systems is that they are generally funded in the anticipation that some percentage of the people enrolled will not desire dental care and that others will not desire total comprehensive dentistry. In most systems, then, if all those enrolled sought out and demanded complete dental treatment, the capitation funds would not cover the costs of treatment and the system would collapse. With the danger of potential overutilization, the dentist may be wary of "overselling" treatment, offering more comprehensive treatment sooner than the funding will justify. To some extent, the dentist must then determine which patients receive what level of treatment at what time. This places responsibility for the cost onto the dentist, which may make for some difficult ethical choices. It should be possible, however, to provide a high level of dental care under a capitation system, and we will attempt to suggest some principles of treatment planning in such a system in Chapter 7, "Phasing Dental Treatment."

In summary, involving the patient in treatment planning requires that we address all three main concerns: fear and apprehension, satisfaction of needs, and cost. While the cost factor will vary greatly depending on the method of payment and the delivery system, the other factors may, in fact, be more significant in the patient's acceptance of the plan.

REFERENCES

1. Brown, W.E.: Oral Health, Dentistry, and the American Public. Norman, University of Oklahoma Press, 1974.
2. Cappa, E.F.: Effective patient education and communication in general practice. Dent. Clin. North Am., *14*:251–268, 1970.
3. Deneen, L.J., Heid, D.W., and Smith, A.A.: Effective interpersonal and management skills in dentistry. J. Am. Dent. Assoc., *87*:878–880, 1973.
4. Enelow, A.J., and Swisher, S.N.: Interviewing and Patient Care. New York, Oxford University Press, 1972.
5. Froelich, R.E., Bishop, F.M., and Dworkin, S.F.: Communication in the Dental Office: A Programmed Manual for the Dental Professional. St. Louis, C. V. Mosby, 1976.
6. Gold, S.L.: Establishing motivating relations in preventive dentistry. J. Am. Soc. Prev. Dent., *4*(6): 17–25, 1974.
7. Hughes, C.L. and Anderton, R.M.: Beyond manipulative dentistry. J. Am. Soc. Prev. Dent., *4*(2):40–49, 1974.
8. Maslow, A.H.: Motivation and Personality. New York, Harper and Row, 1970.
9. Morton, J.C., et al.: Dental Teamwork Strategies: Interpersonal and Organizational Approaches. St. Louis, C.V. Mosby, 1980.
10. Schulman, J.: Current concepts of patient motivation toward long-term oral hygiene: A literature review. J. Am. Soc. Prev. Dent., *4*(6):7–15, 1974.

CHAPTER **3**

The Preventive Approach to Treatment Planning

Prevention is better than cure.

ERASMUS

Preventive dentistry, in theory and practice, is presently a subject of great interest in dentistry. The accumulation of laboratory and clinical evidence identifying bacterial plaque as the chief etiologic agent in both caries and periodontal disease is primarily responsible for this interest. In confirming what many practitioners had long suspected, this evidence brings a new dimension to dental practice, for, if the primary etiologic agent can be identified, it can be controlled and the disease process itself brought to a halt. In the past, the emphasis in dental treatment has been on repairing the ravages of dental disease. Extraction of teeth, periodontal procedures that are primarily excisional, restoration of cariously involved teeth, and prosthetic replacement of lost teeth sum up the bulk of dental treatment as we know it. Failure of such treatment to deal effectively with the original etiologic factors in the disease may lead to failure of the treatment itself. Prevention is critical in the information-gathering process (examination), because etiologic factors, both primary and contributing, must be identified; it is also critical in the diagnostic phase, because etiologic factors must be related to the disease processes identified. Prevention is especially critical in treatment planning, because if dental treatment is not addressed to the etiologic factors present, the disease will continue unabated and the treatment will fail.

The first imperative in a preventive approach to treatment planning is that the dentist himself accept this concept. On the most basic level, this means that the dentist must practice effective prevention in his own mouth, control bacterial plaque and sucrose intake, be free of dental disease and have optimal restoration if necessary. Unless the dentist believes in and practices prevention, he is not likely to offer it to patients, or if he does offer it, is not likely to be credible.

Until the patient is introduced to prevention as a concept and practice, he cannot become effectively involved in the diagnosis and treatment-planning process. The importance of this involvement has been stressed previously. In order to understand the causes of dental problems and appreciate the need for preventive and corrective measures, the patient must accept and achieve at least a minimum level of understanding and effectiveness in prevention. The dentist's responsibility is to assist the patient in reaching that minimum level. This requires that the dentist carry out three basic tasks (the first two being the most critical): educate the patient in prevention, train the patient in mechanical plaque control, and motivate and reinforce the patient's preventive efforts.

EDUCATING THE PATIENT IN PREVENTION

The patient must be educated to understand the causes of dental disease.

Tooth decay and gum disease, which together account for most dental problems, are both caused by dental plaque, a sticky, whitish or colorless film that forms on the teeth and gums when the bacteria normally present in the mouth act on certain foods we eat. Plaque forms in approximately 1 day (24 hours); therefore, it must be removed daily in order to control dental disease.

Effective plaque removal requires a soft, nylon-bristle toothbrush and dental floss, both properly used so as to reach the surface of every tooth. This is a mechanical skill that must be learned, practiced, and reviewed and corrected periodically.

Diet is a major contributing factor in dental disease. Excessive or frequent use of refined carbohydrates, primarily sugars, causes more rapid plaque formation and leads to the production of acids that cause tooth decay.

These general principles represent only the basics of the patient's dental education and must be understood and accepted by the patient. How these principles are introduced to the patient is immaterial; in most cases, multiple methods may be employed. The essential element is that the patient grasp the information and understand it on his own terms. This will usually require a dialog between the dental team and the patient in which the patient is asked to express his understanding of the basic principles of dental health and disease.

TRAINING THE PATIENT IN MECHANICAL PLAQUE CONTROL

The most obvious and least understood aspect of preventive dentistry is the patient's acquisition of the basic skills of plaque control. Mechanical training can begin when the patient understands the principles of prevention and is willing to try the necessary techniques to control dental disease. The seeds of failure may be sown at this point, for if the patient does not master the basic skills of complete plaque removal, effective prevention is nearly impossible. We suspect that cursory demonstrations of brushing and flossing with little or no follow-up instruction comprise the bulk of preventive training. It is the responsibility of the dental team to demonstrate, teach, and coach the patient in the care of his own oral cavity until he can demonstrate to himself and to the dental team the ability to effectively control plaque throughout his mouth. Great flexibility is required in this task, since some patients are able to master the skills almost at once, while others may spend weeks and even months reaching their goal. The dental team must deal with each patient accordingly, offering help, encouragement, and additional plaque-removal aids when necessary. In the final analysis, a patient cannot be held responsible for maintaining oral health if he is not able to control plaque effectively.

It is immediately apparent that two classes of patients are excluded by the preceding statement. Individuals who have handicaps, limitations in physical coordination or manual dexterity, or who are retarded may be unable to fully control plaque, regardless of their motivation. These individuals must be trained to the maximum of their abilities, whereupon other methods of prevention must be applied to assist in controlling dental disease. These include, but are not limited to, the following: plaque removal by a second party (parent, sibling, etc.), multiple fluoride therapy, stringent dietary control, oral irrigation devices, and frequent preventive recall visits allowing early detection and treatment (secondary prevention).

A second group of patients excluded are those who are not interested or unwilling to spend the necessary time and effort to master plaque-control skills. Assuming these patients understand and accept the basic concepts of dental health and disease (task 1), then they are, in fact, choosing to risk dental disease. Planning treatment for such patients must be predicated upon this risk. The extent of treatment rendered to patients who elect not to control their own disease will be decided, in most cases, by the patients themselves. Such individuals may opt for emergency treatment only, or perhaps, disease control only, which includes caries removal and limited periodontal therapy. The dentist retains the right not to treat such individuals, particularly if one presents with a series of dental emergencies and refuses to pursue any kind of definitive treatment. On the other hand, a change in the patient's behavior may come with persistent counselling, encouragement, and support from the dental team. This cannot happen if the patient is refused treatment. The key question, then, is what kind of treatment, and of what length and cost, should be rendered to the nonmotivated patient. Both dentist and patient should agree to this decision, which should be made on a totally individual basis. The dentist must keep in mind, however, that although the patient may knowingly and readily accept the responsibility for success or failure of treatment, the dentist will find it just as discouraging and depressing should the treatment fail. For this reason, extensive corrective treatments such as orthodontics, periodontal surgery, and fixed prosthodontics are usually contraindicated in the nonmotivated patient.

MOTIVATION AND REINFORCEMENT

This brings us to the third basic task in prevention, which is the motivation and reinforcement of the patient's preventive efforts. We must first accept the fact that we cannot truly motivate a patient, short of threatening him with immediate punishment of one sort or another, and even then, such motivation is effective only as long as he is within reach. This might be kept in mind, as dentists have sometimes used the implied threat of pain—"Brush your teeth or we'll have to drill them again"—as a motivator, to which the patient may have been silently replying, "Not if I don't come back, you won't!"

Motivation must come from the patient himself, and the dental team can encourage it in three ways. First, the patient may be self-motivated in areas other than dental care. If the dental team can discover what factors motivate (are important to) a patient and apply them to dental health and disease prevention, they can be used to good advantage. A typical example of this might be the teenage patient who is not apparently motivated towards dental care, but who is rather strongly motivated towards the opposite sex and concerned about physical appearance and the impression he makes. Relating plaque control to an attractive smile and pleasant breath may result in much better plaque control than the threat of tooth loss by age 30 ("Who wants to live to be that old anyway?"). Other examples of applied cross motivation include relating oral health to the ability to taste and chew effectively for patients who particularly enjoy food, or challenging competitive and goal-oriented patients to improve their plaque or gingival bleeding index test scores.

Second, the dental team can instruct the motivated patient in preventive care. Often a patient will be strongly motivated to care for and keep his teeth, but may be using incorrect or inefficient methods to do so. The dentist's task here is simple and consists mainly of coaching the patient and correcting his techniques so that he can maintain his oral health effectively.

The third method of patient motivation derives from education and training in preventive methods (tasks 1 and 2) and occurs when the patient experiences a clean (plaque-free) mouth, perhaps for the first time in his life. This can be a tremendous positive motivator, especially if the patient is keenly aware that the improvement in the way his mouth looks, tastes, and feels is a result of his own efforts. This is the basis for many preventive programs that are carried out daily for some length of time. If a patient, motivated or not, can be persuaded to use effective preventive methods for 1 week, the noticeable changes that may occur (less bleeding, better taste, less odor, etc.) are in themselves powerful motivators for continuing oral-health maintenance.

Prevention should come early in the course of dental treatment. To be truly effective, however, it must continue throughout the course of treatment and follow treatment for as long as the patient has teeth he wants to keep. No matter how diligent the dental team may be in educating and training the patient in preventive methods, no matter how strongly motivated the patient may be in his commitment to good oral-health habits, a high level of oral-health care is not likely to be maintained unless these concepts and methods are continually reviewed and reinforced.

Positive reinforcement is absolutely essential to the success of dental treatment and must be regularly and periodically applied. Continued periodic reinforcement requires an effective recall system. Although we will discuss recall/maintenance treatment in a later chapter, it should be noted that recall systems should be flexible to allow intervals based on individual patient needs, and the patient should be actively involved in establishing the frequency and nature of recall visits.

Reinforcement must be a positive process. Finding fault with a patient's behavior may make the dental team feel suitably superior and may even produce a penitent patient who is chastened by the discovery of his failure, but it is not likely to help that patient practice effective prevention. It is far better to praise and reward the things that the patient is doing right (even though it may be difficult to find them), than to criticize what he is doing wrong. In preventive dentistry, as in any human behavior, people respond better to praise than to blame. We must accept people as they are without passing judgment and provide them with understanding, encouragement, and whatever help they need or desire to achieve good oral health. Good oral health can be a very positive goal. Although we often think of good oral health in terms of freedom from pain and lower dental bills, more positive benefits accrue over the long term. A clean, healthy mouth feels, tastes, looks, and smells good. Keeping one's own teeth for a lifetime has physical and emotional ramifications that make it a desirable goal.

In summary, prevention-oriented treatment planning must include three basic tasks—education, training, and motivation/reinforcement—in virtually every phase of dental treatment. The patient's ability and/or willingness to achieve and maintain good oral health will help determine whether any treatment is rendered and the type and extent of that treatment. More important, it will determine the success or failure of that treatment over the long term.

PREVENTIVE ASPECTS OF DENTAL TREATMENT

In this section, I will discuss fluoride and sealants, which are specifically preventive in nature, as well as other aspects of dental treatment that also have preventive potential.

Fluoride

No discussion of prevention-oriented treatment planning is complete without considering the role of fluorides (the reader is referred to many excellent published articles on current fluoride therapy).[13,21] Fluorides in various forms and applications have been proven effective in the control of dental caries. This effect is additive; that is, each additional application of fluoride increases the caries-preventive effects. Let us consider briefly the available forms and their applications.

The most effective form, in the epidemiologic sense, is the ingestion of the fluoride ion during the time of enamel formation, usually considered to be from birth to approximately age 12. The most common source of this fluoride is drinking water, in which fluoride may be present naturally in concentrations from trace to 25 ppm (parts per million).[17] Artificially fluoridated water supplies are supplemented to a concentration of 1 ppm. This level was determined by studies of naturally fluoridated areas and comparative DMF rates that showed a significant decrease in caries at concentrations from 1 to 1.5 ppm with no mottling. Mottling of enamel, an undesirable fluoride effect, is seen in gradually increasing severity at concentrations between 2 and 5 ppm. Fluoride found naturally in or added to drinking-water sources is effective, because it provides universal protection without requiring a behavior change in the patient and is economical.

The administration of a daily supplement can provide the benefits of ingested fluoride to people who live in areas where drinking water is not fluoridated. Patients in rural areas, suburban areas with private wells, and nonfluoridated municipalities should be identified by the dentist and fluoride supplements prescribed for children under 12. The amount of fluoride to prescribe is simple to determine. Water supplies fluoridated at a concentration of 1 ppm contain 1 mg of fluoride/L. (1 L of water weighs approximately 1,000 g, or 1,000,000 mg.) Assuming that the average intake of water is 1 L/day (about a quart), then 1 mg/day should provide roughly the same amount of systemic fluoride ion as a water system fluoridated at 1 ppm. In fact, the level will be more predictable, since water consumption may vary greatly from day to day, season to season, climate to climate. The only complicating factor the dentist must consider is that there may be some fluoride present naturally in the water, even though it is not an optimal concentration. In most locales, state or county health departments will test private water supplies for bacteriologic contamination and may, upon request, determine the fluoride concentration at the same time. This concentration may be expressed in mg/L, or parts per million, which is a comparable measurement. The dentist then prescribes the appropriate fluoride dose that will bring the daily intake into an effective (and safe) range. This can be done by supplementing children 2 years old or older with either 1 mg/day or .5 mg/day as follows: if the water supply provides from 0 to .5 ppm (mg/L, mg/day), supplement fully with 1 mg/day; if the water supply provides from .5 to .9 ppm, supplement with .5 mg/day. A water supply providing 1 ppm or more needs no supplementation. There is some controversy over exact milligram amounts, but the variation in water intake and the ample margin of safety allows us to supplement fully to ensure the maximum preventive benefits.[15] The dentist who is planning treatment should routinely determine whether his patients under the age of 12 are ingesting the optimal amount of fluoride and take steps to supplement when indicated. The supplements themselves are widely marketed and come in three forms: sodium fluoride solution, administered by drops into food or beverages, or directly into the mouth; sodium fluoride tablets, usually supplied as flavored chewables; and fluoride added to daily multivitamins. The first two forms are the most economical and can be interchanged based on patient preference and convenience. The fluoridated multivitamin is indicated when the child is taking daily vitamin supplements routinely (conveniently eliminating a second dosage), but should not be prescribed unless the vitamins are desired, due to the significantly higher cost of the vitamins.

In addition to ingested fluoride, further caries reduction can be obtained by the topical application of fluorides directly onto tooth surfaces. There are three major forms currently in use: fluoridated dentifrice, professionally applied topical fluoride, and home-use topical fluoride.

Fluoridated Dentifrice

Generally, fluoridated dentifrice employs stannous F or acidulated phosphofluoride. Those dentifrices approved by the American Dental Association (ADA) Council on Dental Therapeutics have been shown, in controlled research studies, to reduce the incidence of caries in a population group. Although the reduction is not as striking as that achieved with ingested fluoride, there is a significant benefit to be gained and nearly all patients should be encouraged to use an approved fluoridated dentifrice.

Professionally Applied Topical Fluoride

Originally, a 20% solution of stannous fluoride was applied to isolated quadrants following pumice prophylaxis. The effect was significant caries reduction and frequent vomiting post-application. Over the years, clinical research has developed lower–concentration fluorides and better flavors, which have improved the process. Incorporation of fluoride into the prophylaxis paste itself has added to total uptake. Presently, the dentist can choose from a vast selection of topical fluorides, both stannous and acidulated phosphofluorides, that are available in a wide range of forms (liquids, gels, etc.) and flavors. We must emphasize, however, that the preventive effect of topical fluoride is temporary and that to obtain maximum benefit, the fluoride should be applied at least twice a year, preferably more often.[13]

Home-use Topical Fluoride

Striking reductions in caries have been demonstrated with low-concentration topical fluorides that are used with high frequency (3 times a week or more). Other studies of home-use topical fluorides have demonstrated reductions in the decalcification associated with orthodontic bands and the actual arrest of root caries in postirradiated cancer patients. The mechanism of action is of interest as well, since neutral sodium fluoride has about the same effect with frequent use as the stannous or acidulated phosphofluorides, even though it is not taken up into the enamel matrix. In treatment planning, this therapeutic application of topical fluoride should be considered for a patient of any age who has a problem controlling caries. The following patients may warrant application of a topical fluoride:

1. Children with extreme, severe caries rates (rampant caries)
2. Children with unusually high caries rates (more than five surfaces on a regular recall visit in a span of 6 months to 1 year)
3. Handicapped or retarded patients who have difficulty removing plaque
4. Adults with unusually high caries rates
5. Adults with existing root caries on many teeth
6. Adults following periodontal surgery with exposed root surfaces
7. Postirradiated cancer patients (head and neck)
8. Patients with multiple crown margins and gumline sensitivity
9. Physically limited patients (those with arthritis or Parkinson's disease, for example) who have difficulty removing all plaque

Sealants

A more recent development in preventive therapy is the acid-etch bonded sealant system. Deep pits and fissures on occlusal, facial, and lingual surfaces can be coated with various resin materials, precluding the development of carious lesions in the susceptible sites. The noninvasive nature of such treatment, the excellent esthetic properties, and the relative ease of application are definite advantages. Good studies have proven the effectiveness of the technique and allayed fears of incipient carious lesions being trapped under the sealant and progressing undetected.[8,11,19]

A disadvantage to be considered is the likely need for reapplication of the sealant over time, at which point the cost might become significant. We must at least consider the time and money expended with this technique in comparison with the cost of the more conservative amalgam pit restorations, which have a predictable life of 10 to 20 years if they are well-placed and polished. We must further consider the possibility that teeth with high fluoride content in the enamel, well maintained and periodically treated with topical fluoride, may not develop caries even in the deepest pits and grooves, thus making sealants unnecessary. Finally, sealants are not effective interproximally, where a significant percentage of caries originates.

Early Detection of Oral Cancer

Early detection of oral cancer is a preventive service with implications far beyond caries prevention. Cytology, biopsy, and/or referral of suspicious lesions for further evaluation should always be considered and can be a life-saving service.

Orthodontic Intervention

Orthodontic intervention, especially interoceptive procedures, can help prevent future dental and periodontal problems and, in some cases, may even reduce or eliminate the need for more extensive orthodontic treatment later (Fig. 3–1).

Any dental treatment, whether it is orthodontic, restorative, surgical, or prosthetic, has preventive potential when assessed as to its ability to add to or detract from the patient's oral-health maintenance. Orthodontic appliances, especially those that are fixed, usually enhance plaque formation and complicate its removal. Orthodontic results, however, by improving arch form and function and correcting rotation and crowding, should enhance the creation and maintenance of a healthy oral environment.

Restorative Dentistry

Restorative dentistry that is well contoured, has smooth surfaces, snug margins, and easily flossed contacts, enhances oral health. Prosthetic appliances that are clean and simple in design allow for effective plaque removal. Soldered joints must allow easy passage of floss beneath them, and pontics in fixed bridges should not lap the ridge so as to create traps

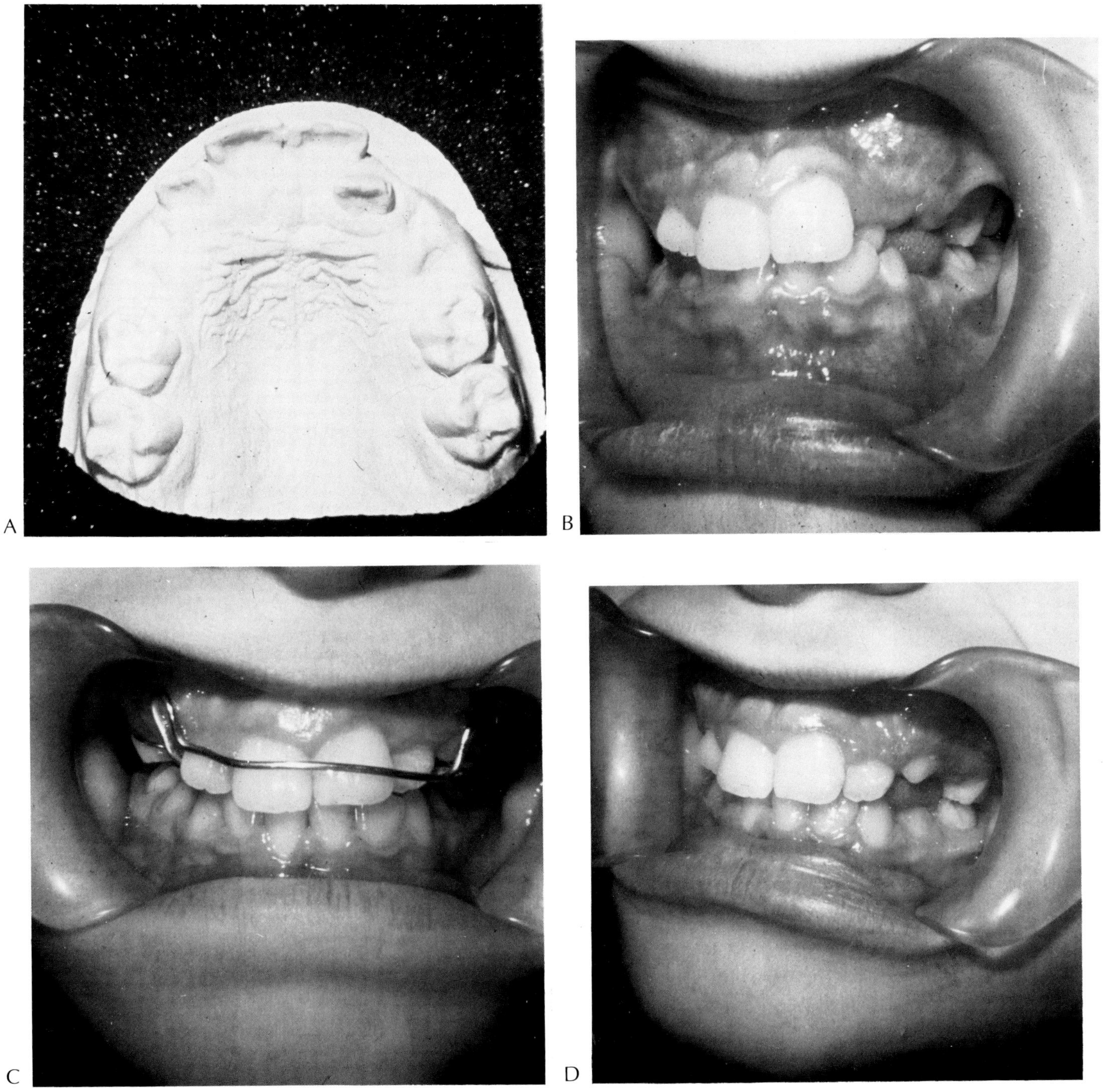

Fig. 3–1. Interoceptive orthodontics. *A*, Lingually "locked" left lateral incisor. *B*, Maxillary diagnostic cast. *C*, Simple Hawley-type removable appliance. *D*, Crossbite corrected—6 weeks treatment time.

of sepsis. Such caveats are obvious when prevention is considered in treatment planning.

Even the choice between fixed or removable prostheses should be based, at least in part, on the relative maintainability of the teeth and tissue. In most cases, a simple sanitary fixed bridge lends itself to better maintenance than a removable partial denture, in which major and minor connectors, clasps, rests, and guiding planes act as shelters for plaque formation and acrylic bases impinge on soft tissues. While it is true that the removable appliance can be taken out of the mouth to be cleaned, the metal and acrylic seldom suffer the ravages of plaque diseases. Indeed, the patient's inability or unwillingness to control plaque may preclude the placement of a prosthetic device, in that the prognosis for the remaining teeth may be better without an appliance in the mouth rather than with one that the patient cannot or will not maintain.

Removal of Third Molars

Removal of third molars is often a preventive procedure when accessibility is poor and plaque removal is impossible. Extraction of such teeth at a young age may be a simple and well-tolerated procedure; however, waiting until problems arise may expose the patient to a severe pericoronitis, the need for antibiotic therapy, and a higher risk of postoperative complications. Indeed, if third molars are retained into adulthood and cannot be effectively maintained, it is not unusual to see multiple restorations placed and *failing* before the patient decides to have the molars removed. By that time, the surgical procedure itself will be less well tolerated. Impacted or partly erupted third molars can lead to cysts, caries, or resorption on the distal aspect of second molars, and periodontal defects which can persist even after third molar extraction. Early removal may preclude or prevent many of these problems.

The dentist must consider the oral-health and preventive ramifications of any treatment decision, so that in providing a health service, he does not compromise the very environment he is trying to enhance. The preventive approach should pervade our entire practice, for in most cases, it will determine the long-term success or failure of dental treatment.

REFERENCES

1. Anderson, J.L., Hester, H.C., and Nowak, A.J.: Guidelines—adapting a simple preventive dental program for children in your office. Am. Soc. Dent. Child.: 1972.
2. Bakdash, M.B.: Patient motivation and education: A conceptual model. Clin. Prev. Dent., *1*(2):10–12, 1979.
3. Barkley, R.F.: Successful Preventive Dental Practices. Macomb, Preventive Dentistry Press, 1972.
4. Barkley, R.F., Nowak, A.J., and Curd, H.F.: Supplement number one to guidelines—adapting a simple preventive dental program for children in your office. Am. Soc. Dent. Child.: 1975.
5. Bierman, E.L.: Carbohydrates, sucrose, and human disease. Am. J. Clin. Nutr., *32*:2712–2722, 1979.
6. Biggs, J.T., Sneed, T.J., and Gougler, G.M.: Reduction of plaque through behavioral control. Clin. Prev. Dent., *1*(2):23–25, 1979.
7. Brown, W.E.: Oral Health, Dentistry, and the American Public. Norman, University of Oklahoma Press, 1974.
8. Buonocore, M.G.: Caries prevention in pits and fissures sealing with an adhesive resin polymerized by ultraviolet light: A two-year study of a single adhesive application. J.A.D.A., *82*:1090, 1971.
9. Clark, J.W.: Nutrition in dental therapy. *In* Clinical Dentistry. Vol. 1. Edited by J.W. Clark. Hagerstown, Harper and Row, 1979.
10. Corn, H., Marks, M.H., and Corn, B.M.: Educating the patient in effective plaque control. *In* Clinical Dentistry. Vol. 2. Edited by J.W. Clark. Hagerstown, Harper and Row, 1976.
11. Going, R.E., Conti, A.J., Haugh, L.D., and Grainger, D.A.: Two-year clinical evaluation of a pit and fissure sealant. J.A.D.A., *92*:578, 1976.
12. Gold, S.L.: Establishing motivating relations in preventive dentistry. J. Am. Soc. Prev. Dent., *4*(6):17–25, 1974.
13. Johansen, E.: Topical fluorides in the provention and arrest of dental caries. *In* Continuing Evaluation of the Use of Fluorides, Boulder, Westview Press, 1979.
14. Kennon, S., Tasch, E.G., Arm, R.N., and Wig, P.P.: The relationship between plaque scores and the development of caries in adult dentition. Clin. Prev. Dent., *1*(2):26–31, 1979.
15. Marthaler, T.M.: Fluoride supplements for systemic effects in caries prevention. *In* Continuing Evaluation of the Use of Fluorides, Boulder, Westview Press, 1979.
16. Nizel, A.E.: Nutrition for the caries susceptible patient. *In* Clinical Dentistry. Vol. 2. Edited by J.W. Clark. Hagerstown, Harper and Row, 1979.
17. Rich, B.C.: Optimal fluoride intake—18-year study. Report of exhibit presented at the American Medical Society's annual meeting in Atlantic City. June, 1963.
18. Rowe, N.H. (ed.): Symposium on Diet, Nutrition, and Dental Caries. Ann Arbor, University of Michigan School of Dentistry and Dental Research Institute, 1978.
19. Ryge, G.: Pit and Fissure sealants. *In* Clinical Dentistry. Vol. 2. Edited by J.W. Clark. Hagerstown, Harper and Row, 1979.
20. Schulman, J.: Current concepts of patient motivation toward long-term oral hygiene: A literature review. J. Am. Soc. Prev. Dent., 4(6): 7–15, 1974.
21. Shannon, I.L., and Trodahl, J.N.: A clinically effective chemical preventive dentistry program. Q. Natl. Dent. Assoc., *37*(1):5–15, 1978.
22. Smith, G.T.: Caries prediction tests—new approaches and problems. Northwest Dent., *57*:309–312, 1978.

SECTION 2

The Routine Systematic Approach to Treatment Planning

Most dentists are now using some form of routine systematic approach to examination and diagnosis. Proceeding in a logical, stepwise fashion, the dentist can see and evaluate all aspects of the patient's oral and systemic condition in a reasonable period of time. It is also possible to apply a routine systematic approach to the process of treatment planning. This approach entails four basic steps: data gathering, diagnosis, treatment sequence, and breakdown of procedures and fees.

DATA GATHERING

All relevant information is obtained and recorded utilizing techniques of examination that will be discussed in Chapter 4.

DIAGNOSIS

From the information obtained in examination, a diagnosis, or set of diagnoses may be made. Essentially, a diagnosis not only tells us what has happened in the patient's oral cavity, but why it is happening (Chap. 5 will deal with diagnosis more fully).

TREATMENT SEQUENCE

Dental treatment procedures that will address the conditions and causes identified in the diagnosis are listed for the patient. The order of treatment is based first on urgency—where the patient is experiencing pain, discomfort, or concern, where the disease state is posing a systemic threat, or where immediate treatment may serve to avoid more complex problems (deep caries, for example). Once the urgent problems have been addressed (often on a temporary basis), the order of treatment is based on logic and convenience, which will be discussed further in Chapter 6.

DETAILED BREAKDOWN OF PROCEDURES AND FEES

Once the sequence of treatment is established, individual procedures can be listed and fees assessed. Appointments can be outlined, and approximate treatment time determined. By adhering to this systematic approach, we ensure that our treatment plans effectively address the problems present, are thorough in scope, and rational in sequence.

CHAPTER 4

Data Gathering and Records

Trifles make perfection and perfection is no trifle.

MICHELANGELO

A routine systematic approach to examination and diagnosis is essential to ensure that all relevant information is gathered and recorded within a reasonable period of time. There is a wealth of published material describing, in great detail, every aspect of the examination procedure, and the reader is urged to consult these excellent works for an exhaustive description of the examination process. This discussion will be limited to what could be considered a reasonable minimum standard of practice at this time, in terms of what information should be included in a typical adult examination.

DATA GATHERING IN A TYPICAL ADULT EXAMINATION

The dentist needs to know whom he is treating for both business and legal reasons. Special business information should be noted. In order to effectively involve the patient in treatment planning, the dentist needs to establish a personal profile of the patient. This can be superficial, or it may be quite involved. At the least, the following information should be obtained and recorded:

Business Information

Patient's full name
Address, home and business phone numbers (when applicable)
Age
Sex
Race
Occupation
Marital Status
Party to contact in case of emergency
Third-party involvement (insurance, VA, welfare, etc.)

Personal Profile

A personal profile can be obtained with a brief subjective evaluation, or, more effectively, with an interview. Areas to be explored may include, but are not limited to, the following:

1. *Referral source.* How did the patient happen to choose you or your practice for dental care?
2. *Attitude.* How does the patient behave towards you and the dental setting? Is the patient apprehensive, hostile, and noncommunicative, or is he relaxed, friendly, and outgoing?
3. *Desires for treatment.* What is the patient interested in doing or having done to his mouth and teeth? Has the patient considered comprehensive dental treatment that might prevent so-called "emergency" situations?
4. *Family history.* Do the patient's parents have their own teeth? What dental problems seem to be common among the patient's family members?
5. *Oral habits.* Does the patient smoke? What other potentially traumatic oral habits does the patient admit to having?
6. *Socio-economic status.* What is the patient's present lifestyle and how will it influence dental treatment planning? Do not prejudge the patient's willingness and/or ability to afford good dental treatment. Socio-economic status and lifestyle may affect the dental "I.Q." of the patient, however, and consequently, the level of communication at which we must reach him.

Dental History

The patient's past experiences with dental problems and dental treatment will strongly influence our approach to dental treatment and the patient's acceptance of it. At the least, the following information should be obtained and recorded:

1. *Chief dental complaint.* What prompted the patient to seek treatment at this time?

2. *Present dental illness.* History of the present dental complaint: when did it first arise and how has it progressed up to the present?

3. *Past dental problems.* What dental conditions, diseases, pain or discomfort has the patient experienced in the past?

4. *Past dental treatment.* What types of treatment has the patient experienced in the past? How does the patient feel (subjectively) about the dental problems and treatment he has encountered?

5. *Dietary profile.* Is there an excess in the amount or frequency of sucrose (or other refined carbohydrates) consumed? Does the patient eat a balanced diet?

6. *Oral hygiene habits.* What are the patient's daily oral hygiene practices? Does the patient brush? If so, how often and with what type of toothbrush? Does the patient use dental floss? How often? What other oral hygiene aids or methods does the patient employ?

Medical History

The importance of an adequate medical history cannot be exaggerated. For the patient's health and well being and the dentist's protection, a medical history must be obtained and periodically updated. The following information should be included in the history:

1. *Patient's general health.* When was the patient's last physical examination and what were the findings? Is the patient presently under treatment for any condition? Who is the patient's attending physician? What drugs or medications *(prescription or nonprescription)* is the patient presently taking?

2. *Allergies and sensitivity.* Has the patient had a reaction to a drug, medication, or anything else (foods, pollen, bee sting, etc.)? If so, what type of reaction?

3. *Systemic diseases and conditions.* Has the patient suffered any of the following conditions? If so, when?

Cardiac condition
Hypertension
Rheumatic fever
Diabetes
Hepatitis
Reaction to local anesthetic
Bleeding problems
Nervous disorders
Kidney disease
Venereal disease
Is the patient (female) pregnant at this time?

I wish to emphasize that a medical history may be considerably more comprehensive than suggested by the preceding guidelines, and that each practitioner or clinician will have his own opinions about what is most important and what should be included in the history. These questions should serve only as minimum guidelines for the typical general practitioner. Figure 4–1 includes samples of medical histories currently in use that contain somewhat more comprehensive questions. As a rule, the history should be a printed form, either completed entirely by the patient (often more convenient) or signed by the patient, if taken orally. It is the responsibility of the dentist, however, to review the completed history and clarify all positive responses. The actual design and use of medical history and other forms will be discussed later in this chapter.

Radiographic Survey

It is beyond the scope of this text to deal in detail with radiographic interpretation and diagnosis as such, but some general observations can be made regarding the role of the radiographic survey in diagnosis and treatment planning. It goes without saying that dental radiographs are an absolutely essential tool in diagnosis and treatment planning, and the dentist who renders any but the most superficial dental treatment without them does so at his peril—and the patient's. Keeping that in mind, the number, type, and frequency of dental radiographs should be based solely on diagnostic need, rather than on any standing routine. For the new patient, there are two general types of radiographic examinations that may be performed: emergency radiographs and a comprehensive radiographic survey.

An *emergency radiograph* deals only with the area involved in an acute dental or oral condition. It may be limited to one periapical film or may include several films, or types of films, but its purpose is to provide sufficient information for an immediate diagnosis of the acute condition so that effective and appropriate emergency treatment may be rendered.

In the adult patient with an intact or nearly intact dentition, the *comprehensive radiographic survey* normally requires sufficient periapical films (usually 14 or more) to cover both dental arches, including teeth and edentulous spaces. In addition, bite-wing films of the interproximal areas should supplement the periapical views. In place of the periapical views, a panographic film supplemented with bite wings and any necessary, individual periapical films may

Medical History (By auxiliary)

Date of Birth: __________
Blood Pressure: __________

What is your general physical health? __________

Do you have any heart history? __________
Are you diabetic? __________ How well controlled? __________
Do you have any kidney or liver history? __________
Have you had any recent serious illness? __________

Do you have any history of excessive emotional stress? __________

Are you taking any medication? __________
Are you allergic to any drugs? __________

A Physician's Name __________ Last visit __________

GET ACQUAINTED QUESTIONNAIRE: CONFIDENTIAL

So that we may render the best treatment
please answer all questions fully.

NAME __________ AGE __________ DATE OF BIRTH __________

MEDICAL HISTORY

When was your last physical exam? __________ (approx.)

Are you seeing a physician at this time? yes no
If so, for what? __________

Are you taking any medication or pills of any kind? yes no
If so, what? __________

Are you allergic or do you react to anything (drugs, food, etc.) yes no
If so, what? __________

Name of your family doctor: __________

Party to notify in case of emergency: __________

address: __________

Do you now, or have you ever had (circle yes or no):

Rheumatic Fever	yes	no	High or Low Blood Pressure	yes	no
Heart Trouble	yes	no	Reaction to Local Anesthetic	yes	no
Arthritis	yes	no	Epilepsy or Seizures	yes	no
Diabetes	yes	no	Fainting Spells	yes	no
Hepatitis	yes	no	Nervous Disorders	yes	no
Venereal Disease	yes	no	Tuberculosis	yes	no
Anemia	yes	no	Malignancy or Tumor	yes	no
Bleeding Problems	yes	no	Radiation Therapy	yes	no
			(female) Are you pregnant?	yes	no

B

Fig. 4–1. Examples of health histories. *A*, An abbreviated medical history that may be too brief, as a number of significant areas are omitted. *B*, An adequate medical history, if reviewed orally with the patient.

MARQUETTE UNIVERSITY SCHOOL OF DENTISTRY

HEALTH QUESTIONNAIRE

Name____________ Date________ Reg. No.________

Height____________ Weight____________

Physician's Name________ Address__________ Phone______

Have you ever been in the hospital? Yes No
For what reason?____________

My last physical examination was: Date:
Results? ____________

Are you being treated by a physician now? Yes No

Are you taking any medications or pills of any kind, prescription or nonprescription? Yes No
What? ____________

Are you allergic to, or have you had any ill effects from any particular drug, medicine or anything else? Yes No
What?____________

Do you have a history of narcotic use or alcoholism? Yes No

Have you or any member of your family had diabetes? Yes No

HAVE YOU EVER HAD?

Asthma	Yes No	History of heart murmur	Yes No
Tuberculosis	Yes No	Rheumatic fever	Yes No
Anemia	Yes No	Venereal Disease	Yes No
Hepatitis or Jaundice	Yes No	Fainting Spells	Yes No
Blood Transfusions	Yes No	Nervous Disorders	Yes No
X-Ray Therapy to head or neck	Yes No	Arthritis	Yes No
Epilepsy or seizures	Yes No	Kidney or Liver Involvement	Yes No
High or Low Blood Pressure	Yes No	Any form of tumor or malignant growth?	Yes No
		Do you wear contact lenses	Yes No

Have you ever had heart trouble? Yes No
Do you have pain in chest on exertion? Yes No
Do you get short of breath easily? Yes No
Do your ankles swell often? Yes No
Do you require extra pillows when you sleep? Yes No
Do you fatigue easily Yes No
Do you wear a pacemaker? Yes No
Have you had heart surgery? For what:____________ Yes No

Have you had abnormal bleeding from a cut or tooth extractions? Yes No
Female: Are you pregnant at the present time? Yes No Delivery Date______
Blood Pressure: ____/ ____ on ____/____/____

C Patient's Signature____________ Student's Signature____________

Fig. 4–1 ***continued.*** C, A fairly typical dental-school medical history.

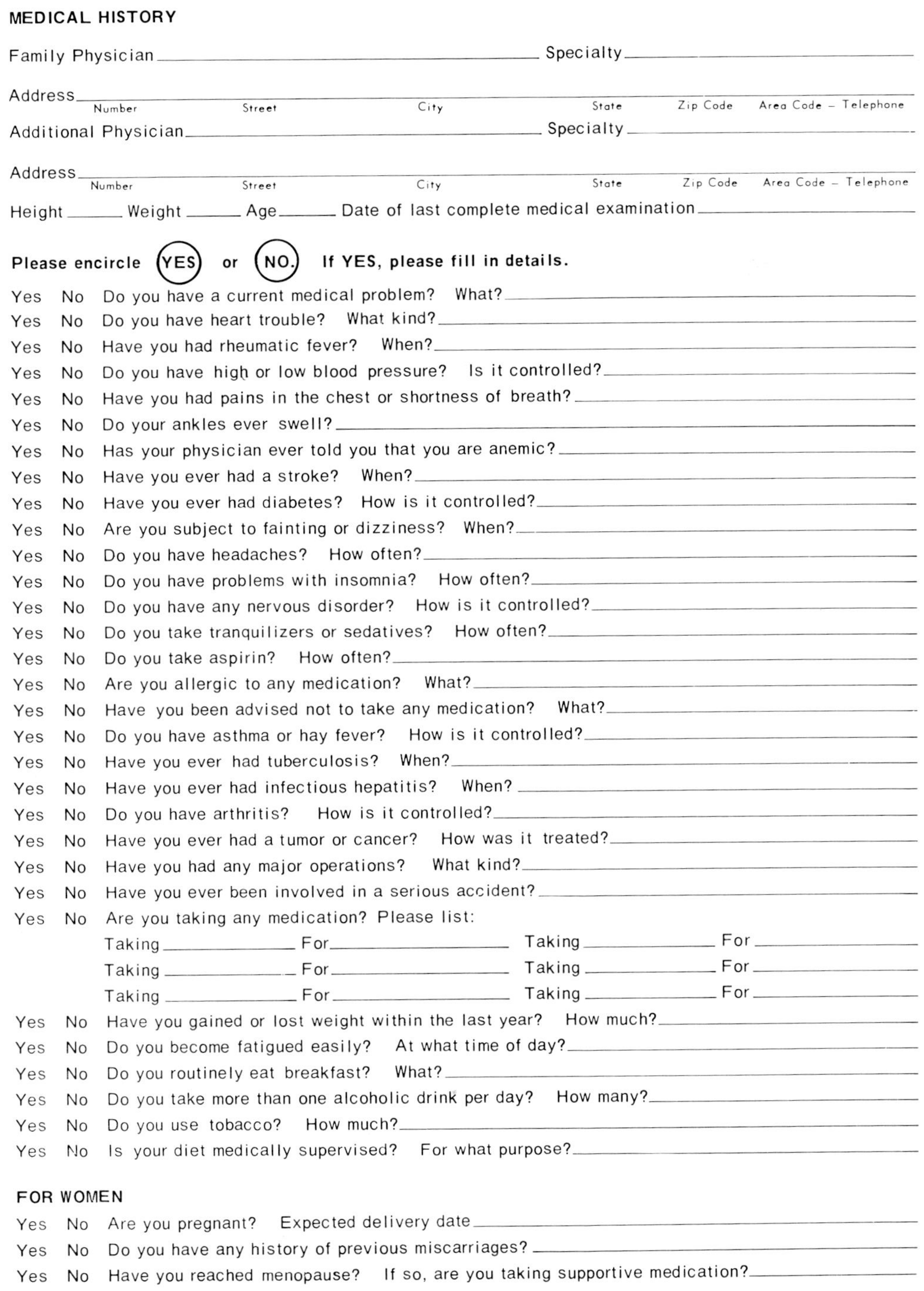

MEDICAL HISTORY

Family Physician ______ Specialty ______

Address ______
Number Street City State Zip Code Area Code – Telephone

Additional Physician ______ Specialty ______

Address ______
Number Street City State Zip Code Area Code – Telephone

Height ______ Weight ______ Age ______ Date of last complete medical examination ______

Please encircle (YES) or (NO.) If YES, please fill in details.

Yes No Do you have a current medical problem? What? ______
Yes No Do you have heart trouble? What kind? ______
Yes No Have you had rheumatic fever? When? ______
Yes No Do you have high or low blood pressure? Is it controlled? ______
Yes No Have you had pains in the chest or shortness of breath? ______
Yes No Do your ankles ever swell? ______
Yes No Has your physician ever told you that you are anemic? ______
Yes No Have you ever had a stroke? When? ______
Yes No Have you ever had diabetes? How is it controlled? ______
Yes No Are you subject to fainting or dizziness? When? ______
Yes No Do you have headaches? How often? ______
Yes No Do you have problems with insomnia? How often? ______
Yes No Do you have any nervous disorder? How is it controlled? ______
Yes No Do you take tranquilizers or sedatives? How often? ______
Yes No Do you take aspirin? How often? ______
Yes No Are you allergic to any medication? What? ______
Yes No Have you been advised not to take any medication? What? ______
Yes No Do you have asthma or hay fever? How is it controlled? ______
Yes No Have you ever had tuberculosis? When? ______
Yes No Have you ever had infectious hepatitis? When? ______
Yes No Do you have arthritis? How is it controlled? ______
Yes No Have you ever had a tumor or cancer? How was it treated? ______
Yes No Have you had any major operations? What kind? ______
Yes No Have you ever been involved in a serious accident? ______
Yes No Are you taking any medication? Please list:
Taking ______ For ______ Taking ______ For ______
Taking ______ For ______ Taking ______ For ______
Taking ______ For ______ Taking ______ For ______
Yes No Have you gained or lost weight within the last year? How much? ______
Yes No Do you become fatigued easily? At what time of day? ______
Yes No Do you routinely eat breakfast? What? ______
Yes No Do you take more than one alcoholic drink per day? How many? ______
Yes No Do you use tobacco? How much? ______
Yes No Is your diet medically supervised? For what purpose? ______

FOR WOMEN

Yes No Are you pregnant? Expected delivery date ______
Yes No Do you have any history of previous miscarriages? ______
Yes No Have you reached menopause? If so, are you taking supportive medication? ______

D

Fig. 4–1 *continued.* *D*, A rather exhaustive medical history that is more than adequate. (By permission of Dr. Carl Rieder.)

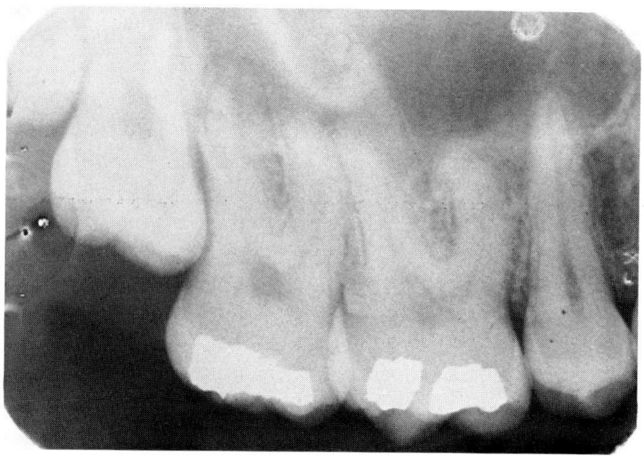

A

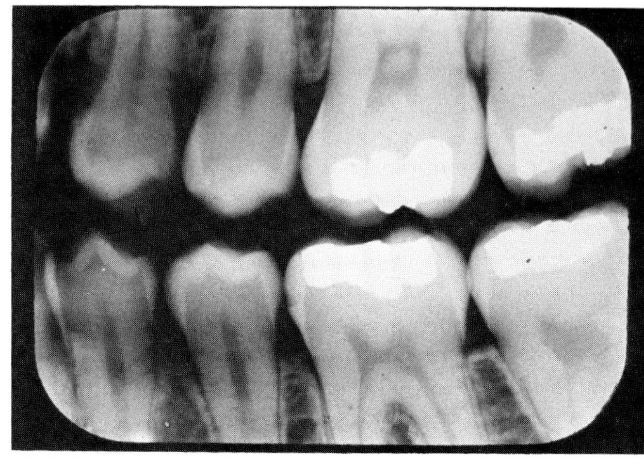

B

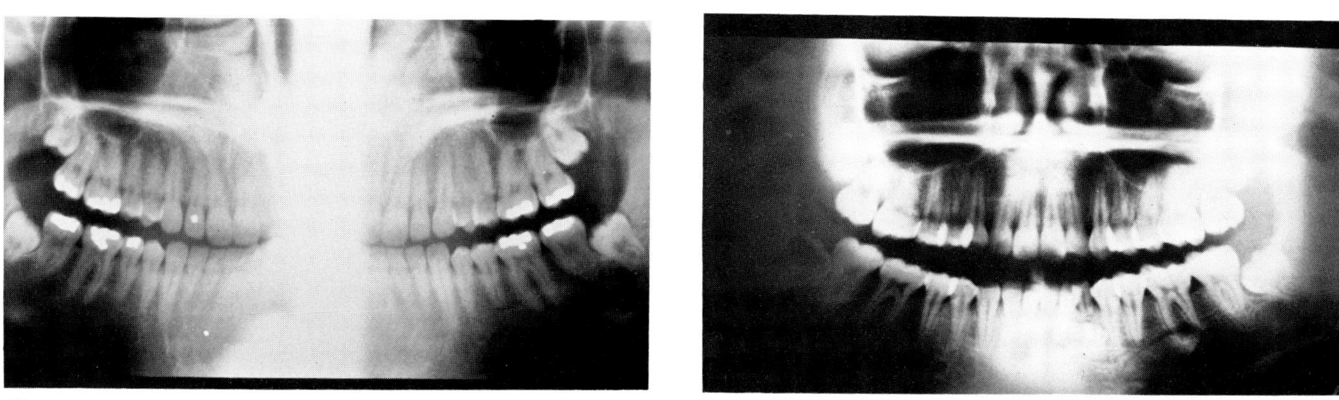

C

Fig. 4–2. Common types of dental radiographs. *A*, Standard periapical film (also available in narrow size) for constricted anterior arches. *B*, Standard bite-wing film. Note the generally good alignment through the proximal contact areas and the well-defined mesial caries on the lower first molar. A second bite-wing film, positioned more distally, would generally be indicated for effective diagnosis. *C*, Two types of panographic films.

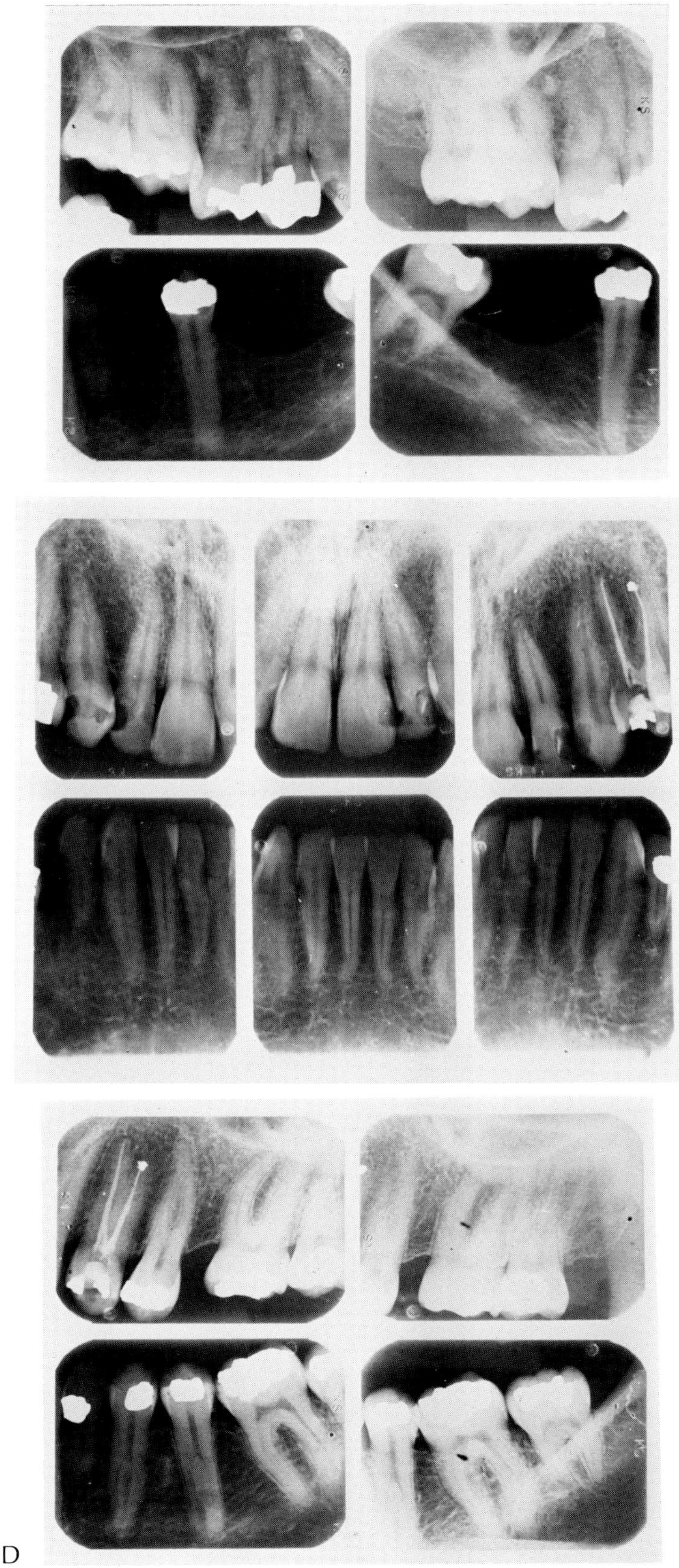

D

Fig. 4–2 *continued.* *D*, Full-mouth periapical series.

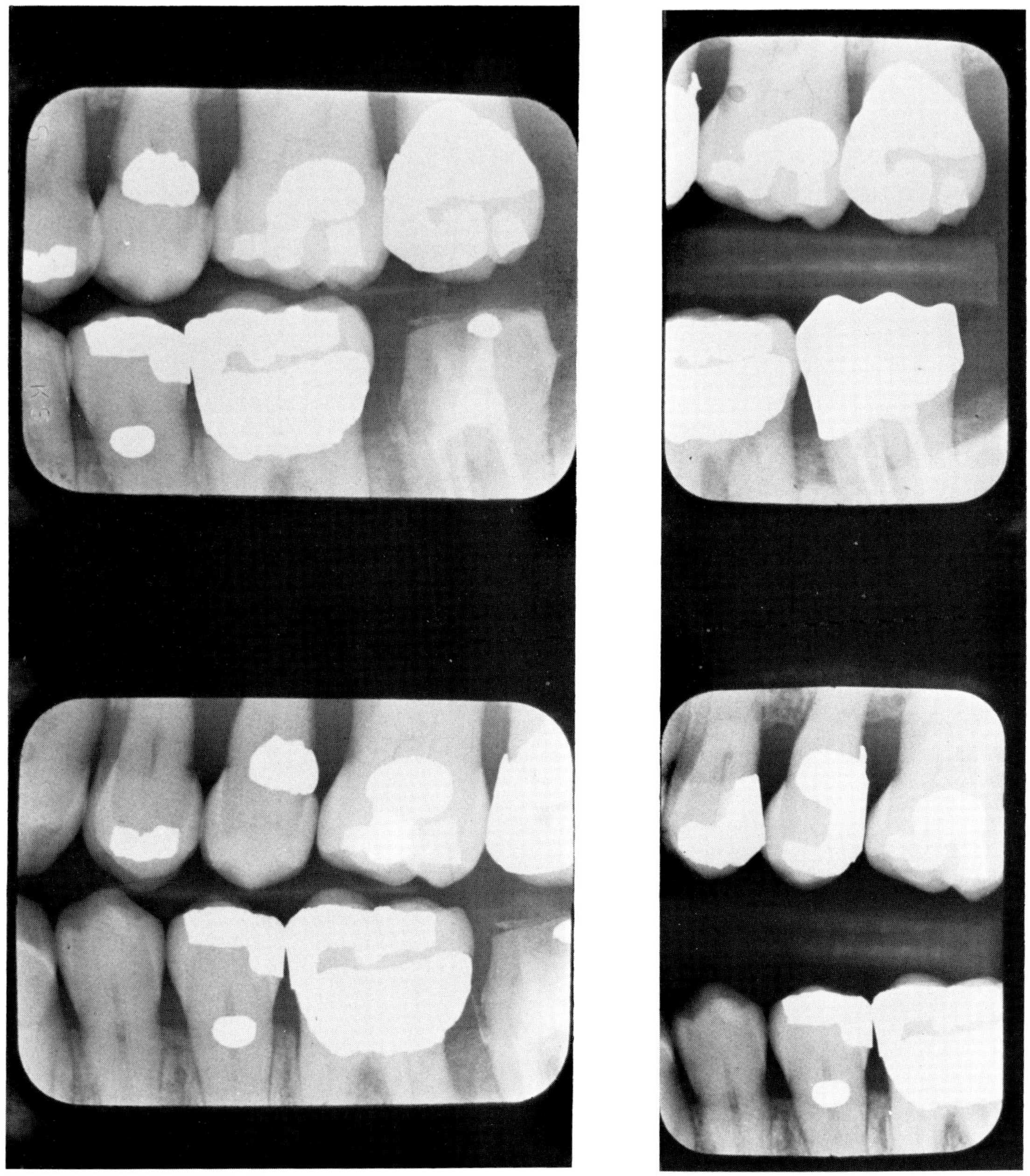

E

Fig. 4–2 *continued.* *E*, (Left) Standard bite wings on periodontally involved patient. Note difficulty of asessing bone level on maxilla. (Right) Vertical bite wings, same patient. Note the consistent depiction of the alveolar bone level.

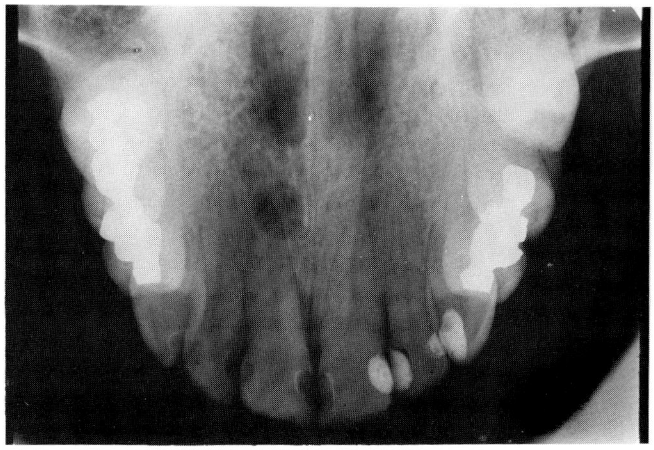

F

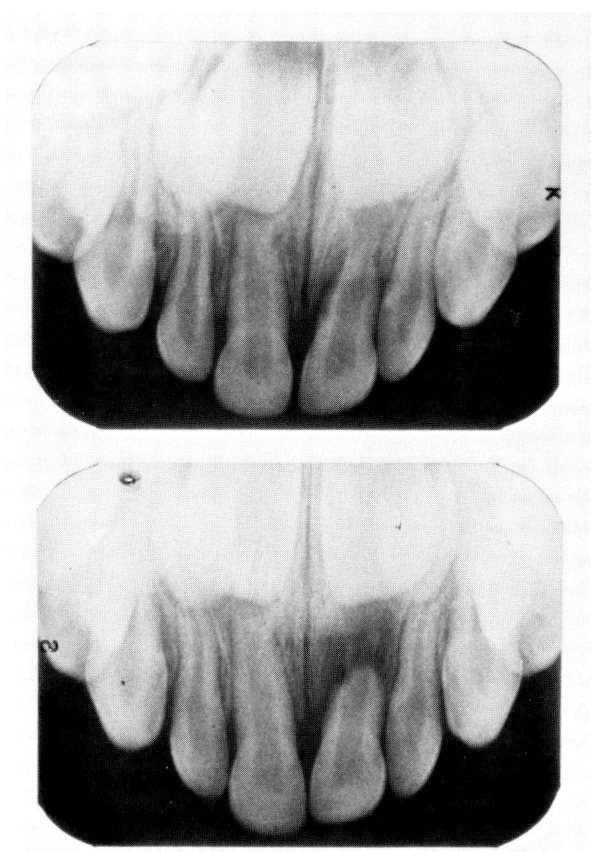

G

Fig. 4–2 *continued.* *F*, Occlusal film, maxillary anterior view. *G*, Standard periapical film used as occlusal film on young patient.

be used. Generally, the somewhat poorer resolution of the panographic film compared to that of the individual periapical views limits its usefulness, especially when periodontal or early periapical problems are being diagnosed. The panoramic film does have a greater range, however, for finding abnormalities at any distance from the apices of erupted teeth. It is often necessary, then, to supplement one type of film with another.

In the edentulous adult patient, a panographic film normally provides sufficient information if it is supplemented, when necessary, by periapical views of questioned regions. Alternatively, anterior occlusal films and posterior periapicals of edentulous ridges may be used.

On the young patient, particularly one in the mixed-dentition stage, any combination of panographic, periapical, and bite-wing films may be employed commensurate with the age, stage of development, and oral condition of the individual child—the goal being to depict both erupted and developing dentition.

Once the necessary radiographic survey is obtained, its interpretation generally requires three distinct scans:

1. *Review of the dentition*. The dental arches depicted radiographically should be scanned from tooth Nos. 1 to 32 (in the adult dentition), and all missing teeth, as well as any supernumerary teeth, should be noted. A similar scan in the young patient is in order, and the panographic film is the ideal tool for this purpose.

2. *Bone and root-end pathology*. The periapical or panographic films are again scanned in a systematic fashion for any of the following conditions:

Unerupted teeth
Supernumerary teeth
Root tips and foreign bodies
Bone lesions, radiolucent or radio-opaque
Unusual root formation
Periodontal or periapical lesions
Existing endodontic fills, satisfactory or questionable in appearance

It is helpful to accomplish this scan by tracing with the eye the periodontal space of each tooth and the surrounding bone. Normal radiographic landmarks should be noted, if not recorded. Any of the above conditions or other significant findings should be recorded either symbolically or in written form. Use of dental records in this regard will be discussed in detail later in this chapter.

3. *Findings of the clinical crown and crestal bone*. Bite-wing radiographs, which are oriented parallel to the long axis of the tooth and perpendicular to the proximal surfaces of the teeth (the contact areas), are essential for the accurate determination of the following:

Caries, both frank and incipient lesions
Overhangs on existing restorations
Improper contacts, and/or proximal contours
Periodontal findings, such as horizontal and/or angular bone loss, subgingival, interproximal calculus deposits, and furcation involvements.

Vertical bite wing radiographs are an effective tool, especially in assessing periodontal status.[27] Severe bone loss may put the crestal bone nearly out of sight on a standard bite-wing film (Fig. 4–2E).

Examples of common types of radiographs will illustrate standard practice (Fig. 4–2), but the dentist must be alert to variations and new approaches that might enhance radiographic diagnosis in the future. For example, it is possible that TMJ arthrography, in which the articular disc can be demonstrated, may be of value in diagnosis of TMJ problems.

Problems in Radiographic Diagnosis

It would seem that despite current public awareness—and, in some cases, outcry—over possible excessive use of radiation in medicine and dentistry, the average general practitioner probably takes too few radiographs for his diagnosis rather than too many. This may be attributed to his concern for the patient's safety, his attempts to keep costs down, or more often, his lack of awareness that what he doesn't know *can* hurt him and that he cannot know what he does not see. Today's medical-legal climate should encourage the dentist to obtain a thorough radiographic survey on nearly every patient. More importantly, effective diagnosis and rational treatment planning depend, in great measure, on good radiographs. That being said, one must then deal with the other side of the coin—namely, despite the extremely low radiation dosage in dental radiography and the resultant large margin of safety, any radiation exposure that is not diagnostically necessary is automatically excessive.

Suggested Guidelines for Radiographic Examination

The number and frequency of dental radiographs is a matter of the dentist's clinical judgment and should always be based on the needs of the individual patient at a given time. For example, the preteenager with multiple proximal carious lesions may require bite-wing surveys at 6-month intervals until the caries have been controlled and all lesions restored. The middle-aged adult with periodontal disease may require annual full-mouth surveys to determine the progress of bony lesions and the resulting necessity for surgical intervention; after treatment, they may be required to determine the resolution or recurrence of the disease in bone. On the other hand, a young adult, having had a comprehensive survey within 5 to 8 years (ruling out such things as impacted or supernumerary teeth and cysts) and exhibiting little dental disease, may require only occasional bite-wing views, spaced 2 to 3 years apart, and perhaps individual periapical radiographs of areas if and when any symptoms arise.

Basing the use of dental radiographs strictly on diagnostic need rather than on some arbitrary and regular interval will usually result in fewer radiographs being taken, at less cost, and with less exposure to ionizing radiation. There is some risk in this philosophy, however, because dental, oral, and even systemic disease states may arise and be detectable on radiographs some time before they appear clinically. Detected early, many of these problems can be dealt with more readily and effectively than if they are allowed to progress. Recognizing this danger, the dentist should periodically look at his patient with "new eyes." Assume for a moment that your recall patient is new to the practice and you have never seen him before. Assume that the radiographs in your file have been forwarded from a previous dentist, then judge whether additional radiographs are indicated at this time. The dentist should reappraise the patient at some set interval to reduce the risk of being lulled into a false sense of security by the seemingly ever-healthy patient. That interval would vary among dentists and patients and may be as little as 3 years or as long as 8 years, with 5 years

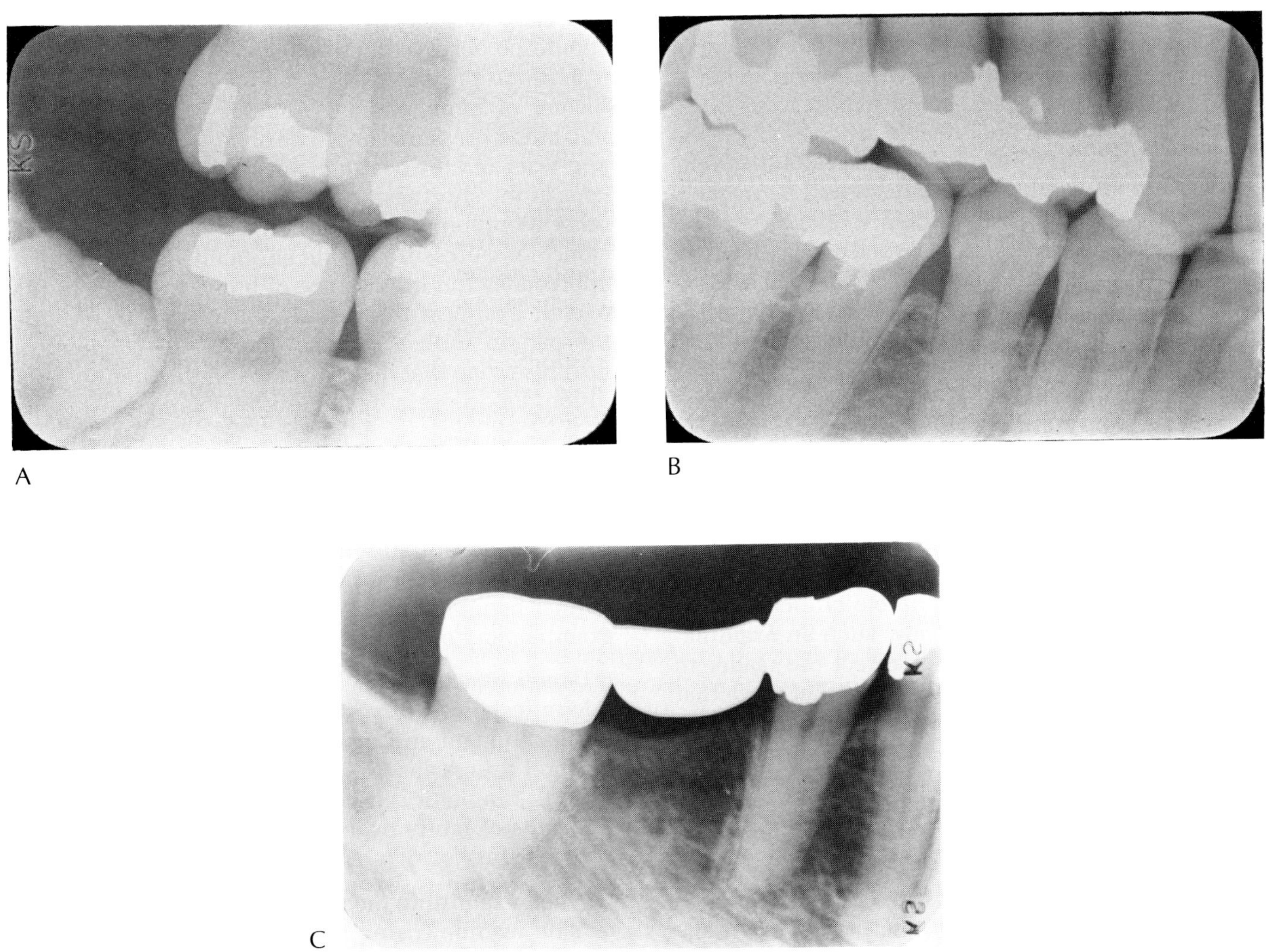

Fig. 4–3. Examples of nondiagnostic x-rays. *A*, Cone-cut bite-wing film. *B*, Overlapped and underexposed (or underdeveloped). *C*, Motion distortion.

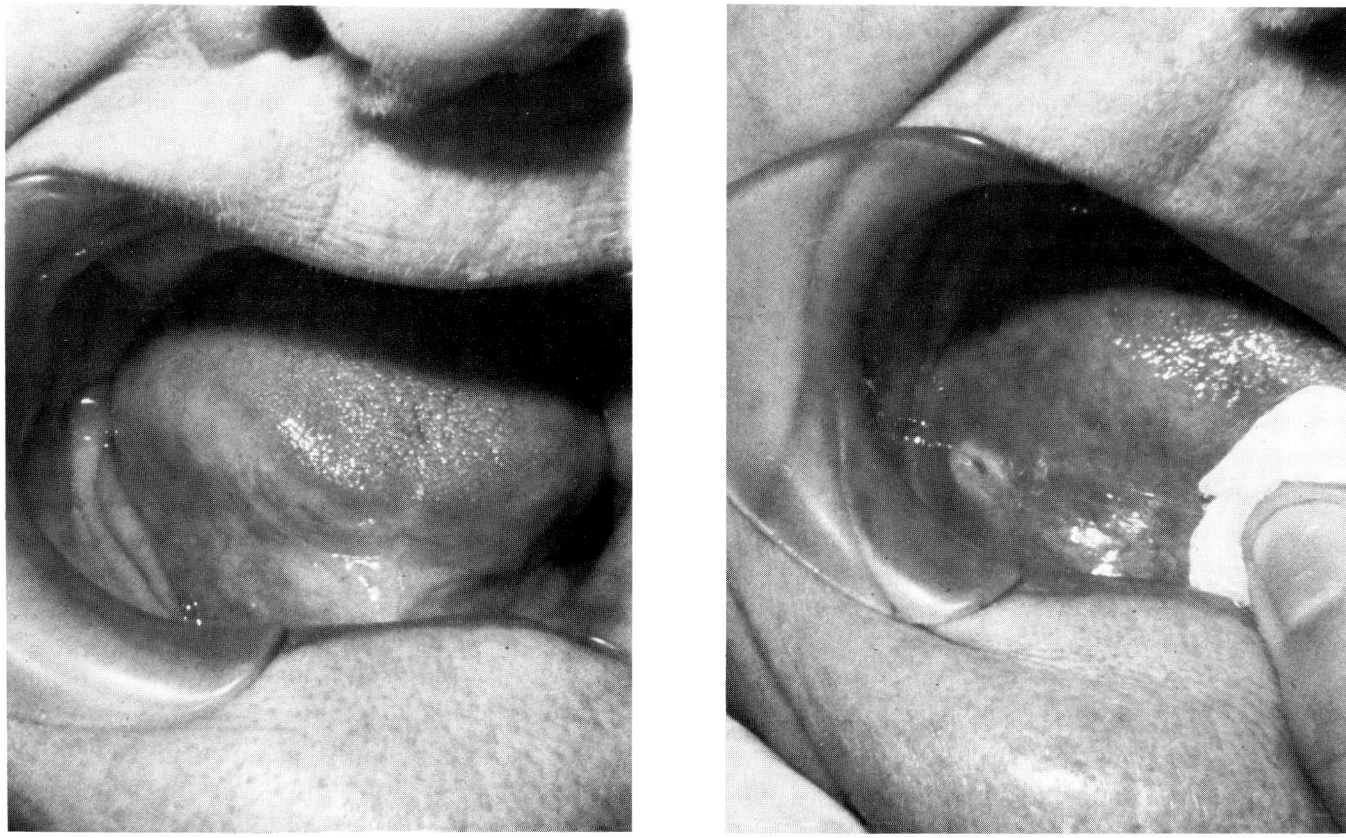

A B

Fig. 4–4. Examination of the tongue. *A*, Visualization of unretracted tongue shows nothing. *B*, Retraction (drawing tongue out and to side) reveals lesion otherwise hidden.

Oral Hygiene

This evaluation of the patient's present state of hygiene can be done at any time in the examination process, but is most relevant when related to the periodontal evaluation that completes the soft-tissue phase. There are three factors to be considered in the oral-hygiene evaluation, and all have significance to periodontal and dental health and disease:

1. *Plaque.* As the primary etiologic agent in both caries and periodontal disease, the presence of bacterial plaque on tooth surfaces is a highly significant finding (Fig. 4–5). Methods of evaluating and recording plaque deposits will be discussed later; for now, suffice it to say that both the amount and distribution of bacterial plaque should be noted. Furthermore, it is not sufficient to observe and record the presence of bacterial plaque. The patient should be involved directly in the discovery and measurement of the plaque, and the findings should be related to the patient's current oral-hygiene regimen. In other words, the patient who rarely uses a toothbrush presents an entirely different challenge than the patient who uses the brush frequently but ineffectively—not necessarily a greater challenge, but a different one.

It is often helpful to digress from the examination at this point to help the patient get a clear grasp of

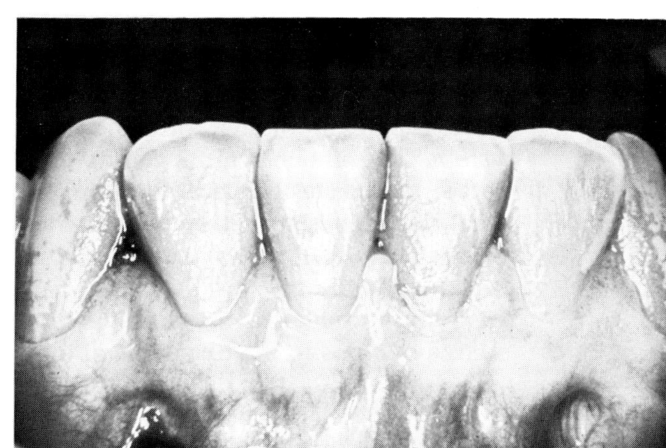

Fig. 4–5. Plaque stained with erythrocin dye.

what plaque is, how and where it forms, and its potential to induce disease in the oral cavity. With this groundwork, an understanding of periodontal problems comes more readily, and the patient is involved from the very beginning.

2. *Calculus.* Calculus was once considered a likely etiologic agent in periodontal disease due to its supposed "mechanical irritation" of the gingival sulcus. With the identification of plaque as the culprit in most dental diseases, calculus was promptly forgotten by many. Indeed, since calculus represents plaques that have calcified, in theory, totally effective plaque control should prevent the formation of calculus. In actuality, however, calculus manages to form despite the best efforts of many patients, and while it does not, in all likelihood, irritate the tissue mechanically, it certainly provides an excellent location for the formation and propagation of bacterial plaque. For this reason, a greater awareness of calculus, particularly that which forms subgingivally, is necessary. The presence, general location, and relative amount of calculus should be noted and recorded.

3. *Stain.* At once the most noticeable and least clinically significant material to be found collecting on the teeth, stains can arise from any number of sources. Aside from intrinsic staining due to fluorosis or tetracycline therapy, most stains on teeth can be traced to some dietary or habitual source, such as coffee, tea, or tobacco. Some stains, however, appear to have no readily detectable source and may be produced by certain strains of bacteria. From a didactic standpoint, unless the stain material is thick and tarry, it is of little clinical significance. To the patient, however, the unsightly stain may cause considerable concern, and if we are involved with treating human beings, we should share that concern. Indeed, since removal of certain stubborn or heavy stains requires a great deal of time and effort, we should note their presence as an aid in planning the length and frequency of prophylaxis appointments.

While plaque, calculus, and stain are, to a great degree, related to the daily home care of each patient, it is not an absolute and directly proportional relationship. As yet, we do not understand why some individuals seem to form very little plaque, or form it slowly, while others seem to show matrix formation in well under the average time, 24 hours. We have long observed rapid and heavy calculus formations in some patients and little or no calculus in others, seemingly independent of plaque levels and oral hygiene. While heavy smokers and tea drinkers, for example, most often present with stain, some do not; young children with no apparent stain-producing vices may have large amounts of dark stain.

In evaluating the oral hygiene status of each patient, we must consider all the pertinent factors in the health equation before we can intelligently relate the patient's level of oral hygiene to the oral health or disease we discover. A useful tool for assessing the patient's level of health maintenance will be described further in this chapter.

Periodontal Evaluation

When considering long-term treatment planning, the periodontium is probably the single most significant factor which we must deal with. Indeed, over the long run, dental treatment for the typical adult patient will succeed or fail, and dentition will be retained or lost more on the basis of periodontal health than on any other single factor. Because of its great significance to treatment planning, we will address the overall problem of periodontal disease as well as the periodontal evaluation that should be part of every complete dental examination.

We live and practice in a time when the dental health of the population is undergoing rapid and drastic changes. Dental caries, in years past the most significant factor in tooth loss, has been greatly curtailed, due in large measure to fluoridation of public water supplies. Indeed, it is not unusual to see patients in their late teens who ingested optimal amounts of fluoride through public water supplies or supplemental drops or tablets, had topical applications of fluoride in the course of routine dental checkups, used fluoridated dentifrices, and carried out reasonably effective plaque control with toothbrush and dental floss, with no tooth decay whatsoever.

While frequent exposure to sucrose and other fermentable carbohydrates can alter this fact greatly, efforts are now being made to create an awareness of and institute some controls over sugar consumption. With dietary control, maximum utilization of all forms of fluoride therapy, and effective plaque control, dental caries can be nearly eliminated. We are seeing this trend in both epidemiologic statistics and clinical observation.

Unfortunately, the old joke, "Your teeth are fine, but your gums have got to go" is rapidly becoming all too true. The incidence of periodontal disease among the population has not changed appreciably; it still affects 80 to 90% of the population over age 30 and is responsible for most tooth loss after the age of 30. Although slow in onset, its effects are devastating to the dentition and difficult to overcome. Osseous defects cannot be filled with silver amalgam as cavities due to caries can; it seems that a number of dentists have tried, though, judging by the gross overhangs frequently seen on radiographic examination. The failure of the dental profession thus far to deal with periodontal disease in the population (which is not to say that we have not dealt with it effectively in some individual cases) may reflect a problem of attitude rather than aptitude. We have, in fact, many modalities and approaches that have proven effective in preventing or arresting periodontal disease, but there are several possible reasons why we, as a profession in a population, have not been more effective in doing so.

First, as was mentioned early in this text, the pandemic nature of periodontal disease, the fact that nearly everyone has it, can make it appear normal. This is especially true of periodontal disease in that its incidence among the dental profession is apparently no less than that among the general populace (this information is based on screenings at dental meetings). Unless we understand and appreciate what periodontal health looks, feels, and tastes like in our own mouths we are unlikely to appreciate the significance of the disease in our patients. As outlandish as it may sound, many practitioners simply fail to recognize periodontal disease in any stage other than that of acute abscesses, which cannot be easily overlooked.

Second, there seems to be an attitude among many in the dental profession that periodontal disease, while not exactly normal, is inevitable, a logical consequence of aging, and difficult, if not impossible, to treat effectively. This attitude might better explain the lack of application of periodontal therapies that may be effective. This attitude is understandable, given the tremendous incidence of periodontal disease and the undeniable fact that periodontal therapy applied late in the course of the disease can and often does fail. The patient is often unable or unwilling to carry out the stringent plaque control regimen that might have prevented the disease had it been applied earlier in life; plaque control will be even more demanding and difficult following the bone loss and soft-tissue alterations of periodontal surgery. This fatalistic view, often held by the patient population as well, tends to greatly inhibit the diagnosis and treatment of periodontal disease even in its early stages, when success is most readily attainable.

Third, and possibly most significant, is a general feeling of inadequacy among general practitioners in dealing with periodontal lesions. This attitude is fostered by a tendency to view any periodontal involvement short of frank periodontitis as relatively insignificant: "It's only a little inflammation" or "It's only a little bleeding" or "It's only 3 millimeters." The frequent incidence of such "little" problems tends to reinforce their insignificance. By the time the disease progresses to a point of alarm, with deep pockets and bone loss, the practitioner suddenly realizes that while he may recognize the problem, its solution may be beyond his capabilities. This feeling that periodontics must entail sophisticated mucogingival surgical techniques, such as osseous recontouring and grafting, discourages many general practitioners. Most undergraduate dental school curricula do not provide students with a facile grasp of these techniques. Furthermore, there is often substantial disagreement among specialists in the field of periodontics about which modalities should be employed and a lack of good, long-term statistics on the relative success or failure of definitive periodontal procedures. Although plaque has been identified as the primary etiologic agent in the disease, the contributing factors are countless, and host resistance plays a tremendous role. The general practitioner, then, is faced with a dilemma. Unlike caries, the treatment of which is part of the basic training of every general practitioner, advanced periodontal disease may be recognized, but the treatment is beyond—or apparently beyond—his capabilities. The logical course in this situation is to refer the patient to a periodontal specialist for treatment.

Unfortunately, a logistical problem exists that renders this solution somewhat ineffective. Many communities and locales throughout this country have no available specialist in periodontics. Even when such practitioners are available, the backlog of patients would be unmanageable should all or even most of the population suffering from periodontal disease suddenly seek or be referred for treatment. There is some resistance on the part of patients to "go to a specialist" for treatment, especially if there are distances involved and the treatment is likely to involve multiple visits over a period of time.

There are three possible solutions to this dilemma. One could argue for the creation of more graduate programs in periodontics, thus producing more specialists to deal with the population. Assuming this is feasible, there still remains the distribution question, and the fact that a referral must be made and the patient agree to see another practitioner.

A more practical approach is to train the general practitioner to do more periodontal procedures. Dental schools could increase and upgrade their clinical exposure to definitive periodontal therapy, and graduate dentists could be encouraged, or even required, to participate in the many excellent continuing education programs in periodontics. The American Academy of Periodontology does, in fact, propose that the general practitioner carry out a great deal of definitive treatment in uncomplicated cases. We have seen general practitioners with interest and skills in periodontics act as periodontists to fellow dentists in communities without a limited-practice periodontist.

While these measures might be effective over a period of time in addressing the dilemma, a third approach is necessary, which would be by far the most effective. It is necessary for all dentists to reorient their conception of what constitutes periodontal disease, to stop thinking of periodontal disease in terms of deep pockets and bone loss occurring in late middle age, and recognize that gingival inflammation in childhood, adolescence, teenage years, and early adulthood is periodontitis in the making. We are all acutely aware that an early carious lesion should be treated so as not to lead to extensive loss of tooth structure and/or pulpal involvement. We should be just as stringent in addressing early periodontal lesions, perhaps more so, because there is no recovery from severe bone loss, no root canal therapy or cast restoration that can restore the periodontium to full form and function. We must recognize and deal with gum disease whenever and wherever it appears, and make our patients aware of their condition, and where it can and probably will lead. If this is done early enough in the disease, dramatic results are not uncommon. This awareness requires a thorough periodontal evaluation of each and every patient (Fig. 4–6).

The periodontal evaluation should consider the color and texture of the gingival tissues, any loss of papillae and/or stippling, and any changes in architecture. The condition and width of attached gingiva should be noted, as well as the presence of frenum attachments, especially those that encroach upon the gingival margin due to their unusual height or the

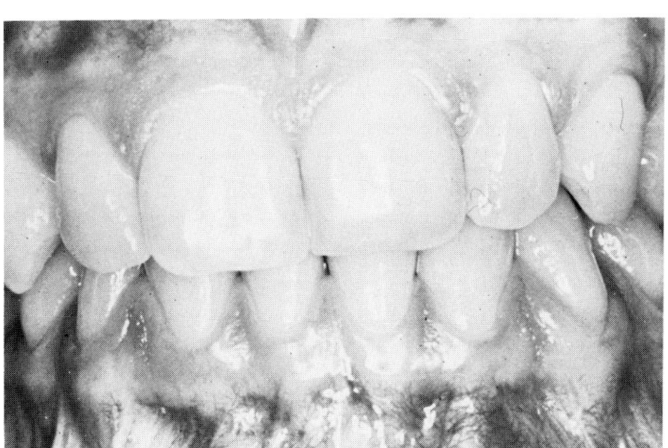

Fig. 4–6. A normal, healthy periodontium—not a common finding among adults.

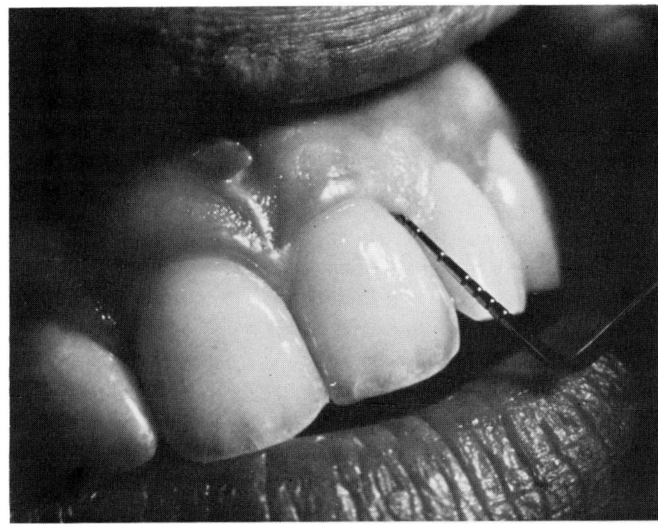

Fig. 4–7. Use of the periodontal probe (anterior view).

recession of the gingiva. Mobility is a critical factor in the periodontal evaluation, particularly as it relates to occlusal traumatism, which can play a tremendous role in the course of periodontal disease. A complete periodontal probing with a calibrated periodontal probe is an essential part of the examination when any signs of periodontal involvement have been observed. (Fig. 4–7).

These signs are many, of course, but there are three "early warning" signs that should be considered carefully. First, any evidence of inflammation, which is reflected by the color or texture of gingival tissues, is a significant sign. Second, any bleeding of gingival tissues, whether spontaneous or elicited by gentle probing or dental floss, may indicate disease. Third, any pocket nearly 3 mm deep or greater should be considered a potential periodontal lesion and investigated further.

Most periodontal disease does not come upon people in late middle age, but develops slowly over a period of time—often decades. Therefore, early signs of incipient periodontal disease are likely to be present in childhood, early adolescence, and the teenage years and must be dealt with at that time if periodontal disease is to be prevented. Aspects of treatment planning specifically related to periodontal disease will be discussed in a later chapter.

Dental Examination

Despite the generally laudable efforts to stress oral medicine in dental education, the essence of dentistry is still teeth, and the great many patients who will present themselves to us will expect attention to be focused on their teeth. In fact, much of what we do in terms of the periodontal and functional condition of the mouth is relevant to teeth—their function, appearance, and retention. The risk entailed in downplaying the tooth orientation of yesteryear is that we may fail to do the sound, basic, operative dentistry our patients expect and deserve; yet overemphasizing the teeth not only risks errors of omission but can result in a certain degree of complacency about the dental examination. We must strive for a happy medium in which we accord the dental examination its proper importance in the practice of dentistry without becoming haphazard in its execution. During the dental examination, the dentist should chart existing restorations, carious lesions, and defective restorations.

Charting Existing Restorations

The location and type of all restorations that are present in a patient's mouth should be charted; this can be done quickly by utilizing an auxiliary to record the findings. Charting existing restorations is important for three reasons.

First, it is the dentist's best means of separating what restorations he has placed from those that someone else placed previously, should misunderstandings arise over failed restorations or symptomatic teeth. Merely having a record of what restorations one placed may not be enough, so it can be very helpful on occasion to refer to a chart of existing restorations to refresh our memories and if necessary, the patient's.

Secondly, treatment planning is aided greatly by a complete chart of existing restorations. When diagnosing caries on a radiograph, for example, it is very helpful to know whether the existing restoration, which is visible on the radiograph, is small and conservative or broad and includes cusps, and has buccal or lingual extensions not discernible on radiographs. Having such information already charted enables us to decide whether an amalgam restoration is likely to suffice, or whether a casting is preferable or definitely indicated. In the case of radiolucent restorative materials, a complete charting may allow us to distinguish between a restoration and proximal caries.

Third, and most important, a complete and accurate charting of all dental restorations can be invaluable in the event of a tragedy—fire, airplane crash, or foul play. In many cases, positive identification of a badly burned or decomposed body can be made only through dental records, and incomplete or poorly kept records may deny a bereaved family the positive identification of a loved one.

Charting Carious Lesions and Defective Restorations

Both radiographic findings and clinical findings are correlated here, keeping in mind that even though good clinical judgment may dictate that a questionable area be simply watched for a period of time, the fact that it is questionable ought to be recorded.

It is essential to good treatment planning that careful observation and recording be carried out to include radiographic and clinical evidence of caries and defective restorations.

Radiographic evidence of caries:

1. Obvious dentinal caries, encroaching upon the pulp, requiring prompt treatment
2. Obvious dentinal caries, not encroaching upon the pulp, requiring treatment within a reasonable period of time
3. Incipient, or so-called "enamel" caries, not visible radiographically in the dentin (although likely involving the dentin) that may require restoration or re-evaluation on periodic recall

Clinical evidence of caries:

1. Large carious lesions, visible to the naked eye, requiring prompt treatment
2. Caries detected with dental explorer that are obvious and unmistakable—that is, they are unquestionably present in the dentin and require treatment within a reasonable period of time
3. Incipient caries, detectable only with careful probing of pits or margins, that may represent only a deep pit or less than ideal margin and thus require either restoration or re-evaluation on periodic recall

Defective restorations:

1. Marginal defects, present from original placement or arising from deterioration of restorative material or fracture of enamel, that allow frank penetration with the explorer and thus, even though they are not necessarily carious, require replacement
2. Marginal defects allowing little or no penetration of the explorer that require periodic re-evaluation
3. Improper contact interproximally, either gross, open contacts contributing to obvious periodontal inflammation or broad, rough hypercontacts preventing effective cleansing with dental floss and requiring replacement of the restoration
4. Improper contacts that, assuming the restoration to be otherwise sound, might be corrected by conservative procedures such as adding proximal contact to silver amalgam by cutting a small box into the existing restoration and adding more amalgam or reducing hypercontacts with finishing discs and/or strips.

5. Improper contacts that, while not ideal, are not deemed serious enough to correct—that is, contacts that are present without signs or symptoms of periodontal inflammation but should be observed on periodic recall.

6. Improper contour, either gross under contour, which leads to loss of function, supereruption, or periodontal damage, or gross over contour including overhangs, which leads to periodontal inflammation and requires replacement of the restoration

7. Improper contours that can be modified with conservative treatment (discing, trimming, etc.) so as to allow retention of the otherwise sound restoration

8. Improper contours that, while not ideal, are not presently creating any observable functional or periodontal problems and may be observed on periodic recall

It is obvious that findings of radiographic caries, clinical caries, and defective restorations depend on subjective clinical judgment to a great degree. What seems acceptable to one clinician may be wholly unacceptable to another. While there is no instant solution to this problem, there are some guidelines that clinical experience has proven useful.

Quality of Diagnostic Tools

It is absolutely essential in diagnosis that the tools employed be of top quality. Simply stated, blurred or overlapped radiographic films will allow only the grossest pathologies to be diagnosed. Dull, blunted, or broken explorers create the same problem in the clinical dental examination. The tremendous loss of tactile sense that occurs when a poor-quality instrument is used allows only gross caries or open margins to be detected. This is not a matter of clinical judgment. Clinical judgment can only be applied when accurate observations are made. Poor-quality diagnostic tools make accurate observation impossible (Fig. 4–8).

The solution is relatively simple: use only new or freshly sharpened explorers in the dental examination. This can be done by reserving a few such instruments and marking them, using only the marked instruments in examinations. Remove the markings at the first sign of dulling and replace the less-than-factory-sharp instrument with another. The dulled instrument can be resharpened (although its temper is often lost in the process) and used in the day-to-day practice of dentistry, in which an instrument with uniform temper and sharpness is not required.

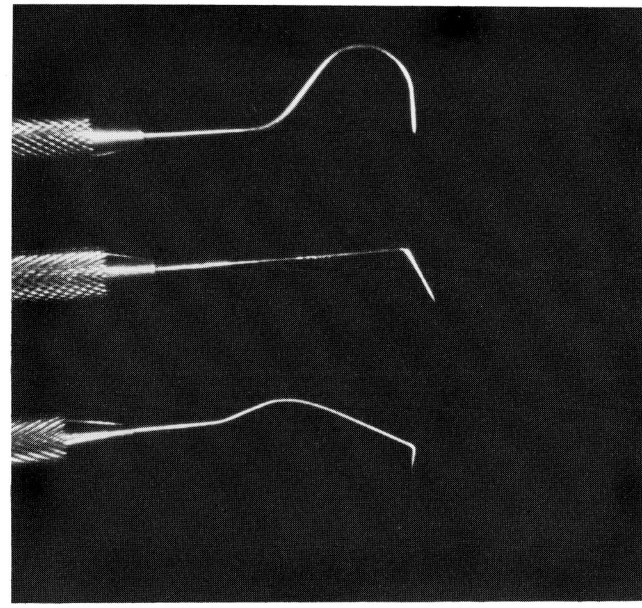

A

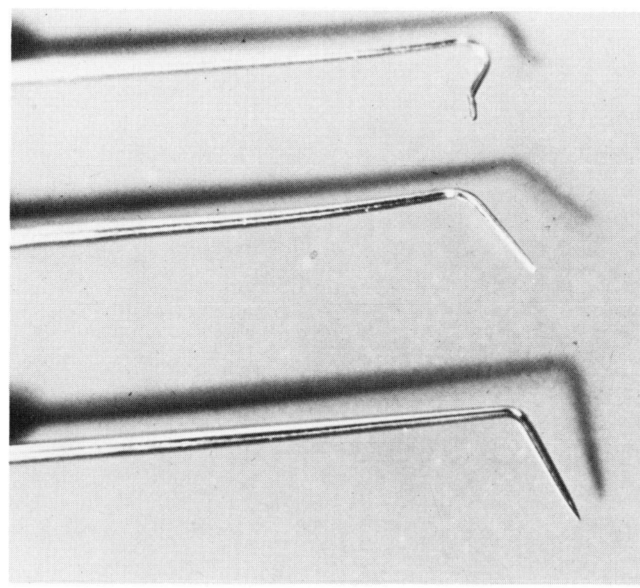

B

Fig. 4–8. *A*, Different configuration explorers are helpful in different clinical situations. *B*, Explorers do not improve with age, as the top instrument proves. Compare the center, dull explorer with the factory-sharp instrument below it.

Clinical Judgment Based on Observed Pathology

Given a set of observations derived from high-quality diagnostic tools and techniques, subjective clinical judgments can be made regarding caries and defective restorations. The decision to treat must be an individual one, based on specific findings and the individual examiner's judgment. Often that decision will be influenced by the general state of health or disease observed in a given patient. For example, a questionable carious lesion may be watched and re-evaluated in an otherwise caries-free mouth, but should probably be treated if there are numerous definite lesions.

Clinical Judgment Based on Predicted Patient Behavior

A questionable lesion might be watched if the patient has demonstrated good plaque control and reasonable dietary patterns and can be depended upon to return for re-evaluation. When heavy or generalized plaque is present, and/or a high frequency or amount of sucrose is in the diet, and/or the patient is a transient or has not returned for recall visits in the past, a questionable lesion should probably be restored.

In any event, a patient should be informed of a clinical-judgment decision to watch and re-evaluate a questionable lesion or restoration. Not only does this stress to the patient the importance of returning on recall, but it also prepares him for the possibility of further treatment. This can be very important when a patient is making great efforts to control dental disease and might be very dismayed to find those efforts apparently going for naught. If we can make the distinction between apparently new lesions and those that we had been suspicious of and were watching, we may provide a more positive reinforcement of the patient's efforts.

Charting Tooth Mobility

A brief evaluation of relative mobility should be done routinely, because occlusal traumatism may be present in what appears to be a normal, healthy mouth. A more rigorous evaluation is indicated whenever periodontal involvement is observed and mobility greater than normal is assigned some value and recorded. Particularly significant are findings of mobility on teeth that are normally very stable—canines and first molars, for example. Since a number of factors can produce mobility, the examiner should establish, insofar as possible, the likely cause. Some of the common causes include the following:

1. *Primary occlusal traumatism.* The tooth may be high in closure, due to faulty restoration of the tooth *or an opposing tooth.* The tooth may be taking excessive lateral forces in excursive movements, which is often seen with upper first premolars in a non-cuspid rise situation. The teeth may all be taking excessive occlusal forces in the patient who clenches or bruxes, and exhibit a generalized mobility. In any event, primary occlusal traumatism suggests that greater than normal forces are being applied to the tooth, which results in mobility.

2. *Secondary occlusal traumatism.* A tooth exhibiting mobility under normal function due to loss of supporting tissue is undergoing secondary occlusal traumatism and may require splinting or other reinforcement; the tooth may, in fact, function well for an indefinite period, even though slightly mobile.

3. *Periapical involvement.* Pulpal involvement can produce mobility of varying degrees of severity ranging from slight mobility and extrusion due to a transient hyperemia to gross mobility associated with severe bony defects created by large periapical lesions. Because mobility can be produced by a wide variety of conditions, it should be carefully evaluated and recorded.

Charting Pulpal Response

Pulpal testing is indicated any time a patient reports having symptoms with a tooth or teeth. This includes reaction to temperature, sweets, or function (biting, chewing), or spontaneous sensations of tenderness, pressure, or pain. In addition, pulpal testing is indicated on discolored teeth (unless the cause is obvious), teeth with large carious lesions, deep caries, as seen radiographically, and teeth with a questionable periapical radiographic appearance.

Electric Vitality Tester (Pulp Tester)

Probably the most commonly used tool for pulpal evaluation, the electric vitality tester sends electrical impulses of increasing amplitude into the tooth, and the numerical value of the first detectable sensation by the patient is recorded. It is necessary to place the electrode tip on unrestored enamel over dentin, which communicates with pulp; often test cavities are necessary to find such dentin. A number of teeth must be tested to establish a range of normal responses. Ultimately, the information obtained from the electric pulp tester is rather limited. Maximum power with no response probably indicates a nonvital tooth, provided that the impulses actually reach the pulp chamber. Immediate response at low power may indicate a hyperemic tooth, especially if other teeth in the area react at higher settings, but one would expect such a tooth to be thermal sensitive as well.

Commonly available testers include manual types, in which the power setting and time of application are selected by the operator, and digital read-out models, which impart a pulsating impulse of steadily increasing amplitude (Fig. 4–9). Although the digital read-out models do apply current to the teeth more

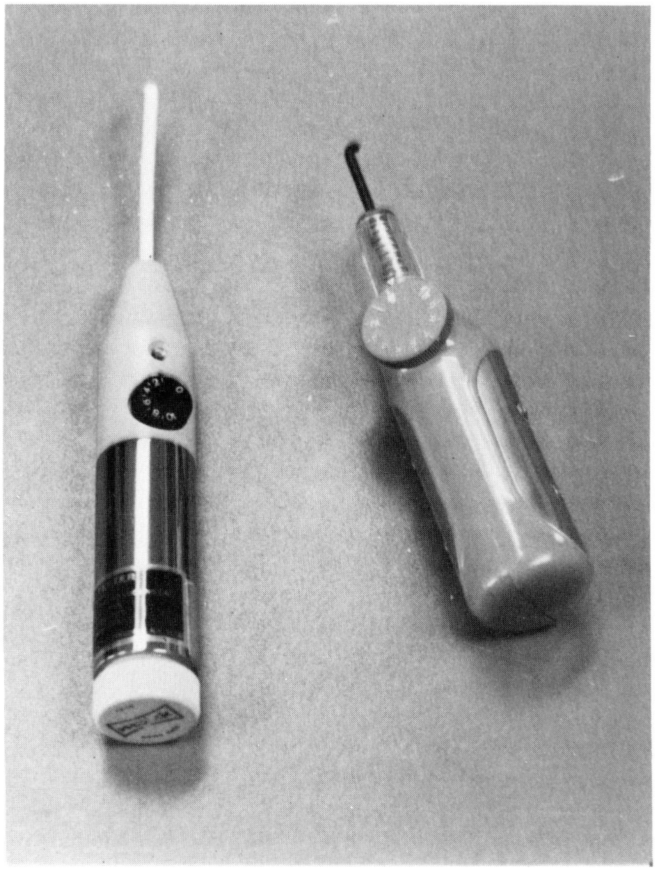

A

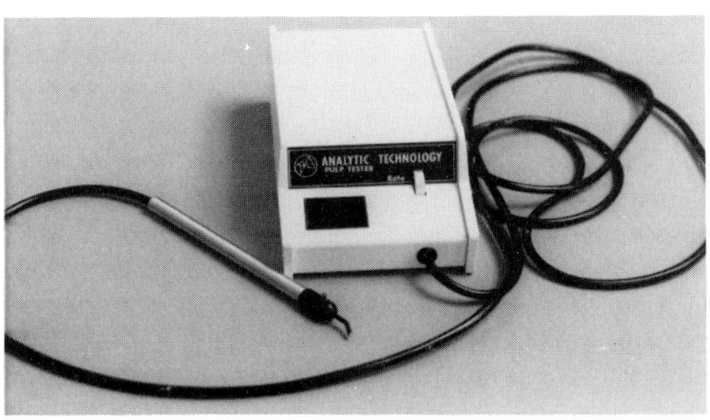

B

Fig. 4–9. *A*, Typical manually adjusted pulp testers. *B*, Digital read-out model, which automatically increases the impulse strength at the rate selected by the operator.

uniformly, variations in the teeth themselves (enamel thickness, restorations, amount of secondary dentin) make numerical differences insignificant. Other means of testing pulpal response are essential for accurate diagnosis.

Thermal Testing

The application of heat and cold to the tooth can be a very helpful technique in determining pulpal status. Heat can be applied via an instrument heated over a flame, by thermoplastic dental compound similarly heated, or by the ball tip of an electrosurgical unit at low power. Extreme caution is advised with the latter method, however, as damage can result from excessive radio current applied to a tooth. Cold applications can be delivered with ice chips, a frozen anesthetic carpule filled with water, or an ice pencil made by filling a drinking straw with water, sealing the ends with wax, and freezing it. These highly localized applications of heat and/or cold can be of great help in identifying which tooth (or teeth) is pulpally involved and in the diagnosis of the specific pulpal pathology present.

Percussion

Lightly tapping a tooth at an angle to the long axis with a mirror handle or other suitable instrument may elicit information, as may the placement of an orange wood stick or small rubber wheel on the occlusal surface of a selected tooth, which the patient will bite. In the case of a suspected fractured cusp, light tapping on individual cusps can be employed not only to identify which tooth is symptomatic, but to allow dislodgement of a fractured cusp and subsequent restoration.

Patient Symptoms

Often of more value than any clinical test is a careful reading of reported symptoms—reactions to heat, cold, mastication, and sweets, for example—which should be recorded when charting pulpal response.

Functional Evaluation

Having carefully considered and recorded findings of the dentition, teeth, and periodontal structures, one must then observe and describe how the system works, how the teeth, periodontium, temporomandibular joint, and all the muscles and muscle groups function together in the stomatognathic system. It has been stated that the practice of dentistry is the practice of occlusion, and if we broaden the scope of the term "occlusion" to cover the overall functioning of the stomatognathic system, that definition is apt. The consequence of this general principle is that a dentist who renders dental treatment without a good understanding of the function of the system is merely a mechanic who tempts failure. This discussion of the function of the stomatognathic system will not attempt to project any particular theories over any others, nor urge any specific treatment regimens, because the literature is becoming rich with such information. Rather, in this text, I will delineate a reasonable minimum approach in terms of what factors ought to be considered and what information ought to be recorded in order to make an adequate diagnosis on which to base further treatment. This approach will rely on research already in the literature and on many years of clinical experience in dealing with the system on a daily basis.

Static Occlusal Relationships

Static occlusal relationships with the teeth in normal closed contact (centric occlusion, intercuspal position, acquired centric) must be observed and recorded. The most common classification system, the Angle system, notes relationships of Class I, Class II (Divisions 1 and 2), and Class III. This classification of molar relationship should be noted on both sides, as should the vertical and horizontal overlap of the anterior teeth. In addition to the jaw-to-jaw relation, individual tooth relationships, crossbites, diastemas, rotated teeth, or transposed teeth should be noted. It is also helpful while observing the static occlusion to note the presence and severity of crowding, the esthetic appearance of the anterior teeth, and the patient's feelings about the appearance of his teeth. A diastema between central incisors may be an agonizing disfigurement to one patient, a source of pride in a familial trait to another, or a feature scarcely ever thought of by yet another. We must be careful not to impose our own value judgments of the esthetic appearance of the dentition upon a patient, for we may create problems that were not there to begin with; nor should we dismiss too quickly a patient's complaint about an esthetic situation that we find perfectly pleasing. If closing a diastema, for example, will provide a patient with greater peace of mind and a better self image, treatment may well be indicated, even though the problem seems insignificant to us.

In observing and noting the features of the static occlusion, we must remember that they may not represent the true jaw relationship, but may instead be an accommodation of sorts. We must then be careful to relate our static findings to the dynamics of the system and determine whether the bite we observe is, in fact, healthy, normal, and in harmony with the TMJ and the muscles of mastication.

Centric Relation. Centric relation (CR), also known as retruded contact position (RCP), and hinge position, should be located on each patient. This can be done using one of a variety of methods, the most common of which includes the following:

1. The point of the chin is grasped with thumb and forefinger (Fig. 4–10 A), and pressure is applied in a retrusive direction, with slight opening/closing movements. The retrusion is facilitated by having the patient draw the tongue back and up to the posterior

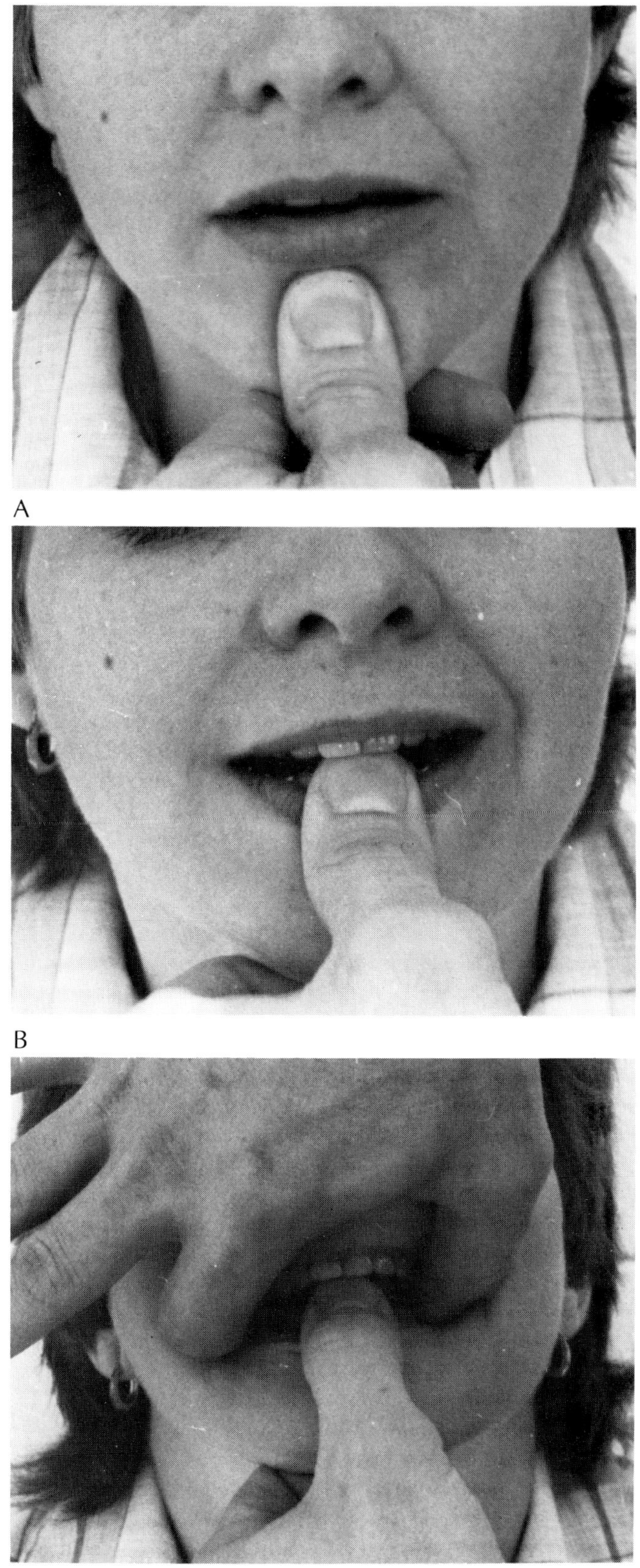

A B C

Fig. 4–10. Location of centric relation position. *A*, Thumb-to-chin method. *B*, Thumb-to-teeth, using thumbnail as "ramp." *C*, Thumb-to-teeth, using other thumb and forefinger as a "bite plane."

palate. A modification of this method employs the thumb as a ramp between upper and lower anterior teeth (Fig. 4–10 B), which allows the opening/closing motions to be carried out without cuspal contact (and proprioceptive defense reflexes) and tends to ease the mandible into retrusion by striking the thumbnail at an angle. An augmentation of this method utilizes the thumb and forefinger of the other hand (Fig. 4–10 C) as posterior bite plane; the thumb and forefinger are laid along the plane of occlusion on each side and allowed to interpose slightly while opening/closing movements are carried out. Apparently, this further reduces proprioceptive defenses preventing closure on a single point, and in most cases, is quite effective in locating the retruded position.

2. Approaching the patient from behind, the dentist can cradle the mandible in both hands (Fig. 4–11), his little fingers resting under the inferior border on each side.[10] Gentle retrusion can then be guided during opening/closing movements using tongue position to aid the process. Method 1 or 2 can be enhanced by muscle fatiguing—that is, by exercising the opposing musculature prior to retrusion. The patient is asked to protrude the mandible forcefully and repeatedly, after which retrusion may be facilitated.

Most patients can be positioned in CR, or RCP, using one of these simple methods. A pure hinge motion should be sensed in the opening/closing movements, and the position should be maintainable without undue force applied by the operator. Once the hinge motion is obtained, the patient is asked to close lightly to contact one tooth. This initial contact in the retruded or hinge position is noted, and the patient is then asked to close fully. The difference, if any, between the first contact in retruded position and full closure should be noted. This discrepancy by itself is not necessarily pathologic. We know, however, that such a discrepancy can be contributory to TMJ disorders, occlusal traumatism, and various other problems, or may be a symptom of such problems. While there is usually some such discrepancy in the "normal" individual, a difference of more than 1 mm or a discrepancy that results in a lateral shift of the mandible to gain intercuspation should be noted. Individual tolerance plays a great role in this situation. Some patients tolerate and function well with gross discrepancies between CR and centric occlusion (CO), while others experience disabling symptoms with the slightest deflection. Furthermore, this tolerance can change with time, and one may see young adults develop functional problems stemming from occlusal discrepancies present since childhood.

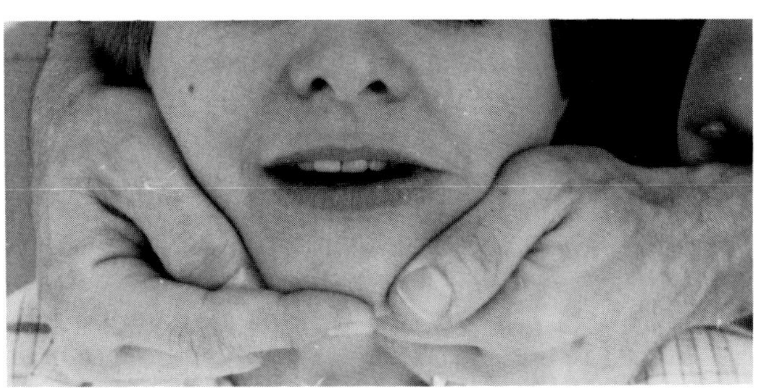

Fig. 4–11. "Cradle" method to locate centric relation.

Also significant is our dependence on the CR position as a reference and starting point in restorative dentistry. A patient may function satisfactorily in an acquired occlusion, but should multiple crowns or bridgework be required, we have no way of knowing how the patient will tolerate our attempts to harmonize the prostheses to that naturally acquired occlusion. To be safe, we must often restore an occlusion in CR, which we know from experience is a functionally acceptable position. Thus, it behooves the dentist to note whether there is a discrepancy between the acquired occlusion and retruded position, particularly if there are signs or symptoms of pathology in the stomatognathic system, or if any extensive occlusal restorations are contemplated.

A potentially significant finding is the inability to locate the retruded position due to muscle tension or pain. A variety of other, more sophisticated, methods for achieving full retrusion are available, one of the most common being a bite plane. This appliance, when cemented or clasped to the upper teeth, provides contact for the lower teeth against a smooth surface, free of intercuspation or lateral interferences. In most cases, 3 to 10 days of use will produce a relaxation of the musculature and allow retrusion. It should be noted that such muscle tension may be a sign of dysfunction in the system, and careful evaluation is indicated. It should also be noted that occlusal disharmony of long duration that has resulted in considerable accommodation by the neuromuscular system may prevent full retrusion into hinge position even with the use of bite plane and other techniques. We have observed patients whose mandibular position continued to change over months and even years as interferences were removed, until a full retrusive position was obtained. The dentist must be careful not to assume that he has located CR just because there is an apparent resistance to further retrusion, especially when retrusion is difficult to begin with.

Dynamic Occlusal Relationships

The dynamic functioning of the occlusion is of comparable importance in the diagnosis process. The patient should be asked to move the mandible into left and right lateral excursions, maintaining light tooth contact. This can be facilitated by gently stroking the patient's upper lip in the direction of movement desired, or, if all else fails, by giving the patient a mirror with which to observe his lateral movements and facilitate making those movements. Factors to be observed and recorded include, but are not limited to, the following:

1. *Working-side guidance.* On the working side, the side toward which the movement is being made, which tooth or teeth provide guidance? Especially significant will be the guidance in the first 1 to 3 mm of movement. This can be observed visually to some extent, but the use of articulating paper or thin occlusal indicating film is recommended to obtain more accurate findings.
2. *Balancing-side contacts.* On the balancing side, any contact in lateral excursion should be noted. This finding is best made using very thin plastic film placed between the teeth in static occlusion. The patient is then induced into initial lateral excursion and the film pulled out of the occlusion. If there is resistance to removal, a balancing contact is revealed. This can be repeated at increasing lateral distances. If balancing contacts are discovered, articulating paper may be employed to identify which slopes of which teeth are involved. While balancing side contacts are not in themselves pathologic, they may be quite significant in a number of occlusal disorders, particularly bruxism.
3. *Protrusive guidance.* From static occlusion, the patient is asked to move the lower jaw directly forward. Lateral deflections or deviations and the teeth that provide guidance should be noted. Finding guidance in the posterior region rather than in the anterior may be especially significant.

Patients present with a staggering range of occlusal patterns and relationships, few of which coincide with textbook definitions of the "ideal" occlusion. In the absence of pathology, whatever occlusion a patient has must be considered "normal" for that patient. The caution in this principle, however, is that pathology related to occlusion and occlusal disharmonies may be slow in onset, subtle in appearance, and may appear in any part of the stomatognathic system: teeth, periodontium, TMJ, or the neuromuscular apparatus (this concept will be developed further in Chapter 5, "Diagnosis"). While we utilize a stepwise approach to the examination of the system, we must keep in mind that it functions as an integrated whole and be prepared to withhold judgment until all the information is obtained.

Gross Interferences. Rather loosely defined, gross interferences are those tooth contacts in lateral or protrusive excursion, either working or balancing, which prevent the patient from carrying out the movement or require exaggerated muscular accommodation in order to do so. Typical examples of such interferences are tipped or supererupted teeth, malposed teeth, or teeth with extremely deep intercuspation or deep vertical overlap. Missing teeth or teeth held in open-bite relationships may, by their absence, create gross interferences in areas that might otherwise function normally. Dental restorations and prostheses that do not harmonize with the occlusion and the TMJ are all too often a source of gross interferences.

Space for Prostheses. Finally, the occlusion should be evaluated in terms of available space, in case prosthetic replacement is required. Thus, tipped, drifted, or supererupted teeth should be evaluated on the basis of potential room for prosthetic appliances.

Temporomandibular Joint. Closely related to the dynamic occlusion, the function of the temporomandibular joint will have tremendous impact on the stomatognathic system, and dysfunction can result in a host of problems in the oro-facial complex. Accordingly, the TMJ should be observed, palpated, and in some cases, auscultated in the routine examination process. More sophisticated evaluation is possible using techniques such as myomonitors, pantographic tracings, and tomographs. A reasonable, minimal approach to evaluating the TMJ would include the following:

1. *Motion or deviation* in lateral and/or protrusive movements should be observed and recorded.
2. *Subluxation,* in which the condylar head slips anterior to the meniscus and in some cases, the eminentia itself, should be palpated and recorded if it is present.
3. *Crepitus,* or other noises or clicking during normal joint function may be heard or palpated.
4. *Pain or tenderness* upon palpation is a significant finding. If such a condition is found when palpating the joint itself, or if other symptoms of dysfunction are reported, palpation should be carried out on the major muscles of mastication—the temporalis, masseter, and internal and external pterygoid muscles.
5. *Patient symptoms* that are elicited in the history and that may be associated with TMJ should be recorded. Typical symptoms might include pain or difficulty in chewing, difficulty in opening wide, fre-

quent dislocations, earache not specifically diagnosed as infection, ear noise, and headaches.

Patient symptoms are critical since many patients suffer severe dysfunction as a result of TMJ problems or myofascial pain/dysfunction syndrome. Such patients should be evaluated carefully and fully prior to drawing any conclusions about the probable etiology of the symptoms or rendering any treatment. A strong psychogenic influence is often seen in these disorders, and while mechanical manipulation of the dentition may bring relief, it can also precipitate further problems. A careful history of the problem, including the relationship of symptoms to time of day or periods of psychic stress may be helpful. Any and all past attempts at treatment should be reviewed as to the type of treatment rendered, its effects, and the patient's subjective feelings about it. While there is a wide range of opinion on treatment philosophy and regimen, the conscientious practitioner should not be dismayed. What is effective for one patient may not be effective for another; if one does not have a philosophic axe to grind, one can select and apply a wide range of possible solutions to the problems encountered (the reader is referred to an abundance of literature on problems of the TMJ). It is essential to keep an open mind in this and other areas of dentistry, because there is probably no single answer to many of the questions raised.

Different patients presenting with similar TMJ symptoms may be helped—some by bite-plane therapy, some by occlusal adjustment, some by drugs and/or exercise, some by counselling, and many by an intelligent combination of available modalities. Careful, thorough examination and evaluation of the TMJ are essential to the rational selection of potential treatment options.

Myofunctional Analysis

An area of some controversy in dentistry today is the relationship of muscle function, especially lips and tongue, to tooth position and overall function of the stomatognathic system. Again, it behooves the intelligent practitioner to withhold judgment and avoid a dogmatic approach. If one observes a large number of patients, noting their lip and tongue function, the inescapable conclusion is that there is some relationship between those muscle groups and the overall functioning of the system. Hopefully, the nature of that relationship will be clarified in time to come. While there may always be some disagreement among researchers and clinicians, the wise practitioner will take the knowledge and experience of all concerned and apply it to help his patients. In order to do this, the following myofunctional factors should be observed and recorded:

1. *Tongue habits.* Does the patient suck the tongue, or interpose it between the teeth when at rest?
2. *Swallowing pattern.* Where is the tongue placed during a swallow? Does the tip rest on the roof of the mouth palatal to the upper incisors, or elsewhere? Does the tongue extrude between teeth during the swallow? Is there an open bite, anterior or posterior, into which the tongue goes during the swallow? What is the response of the lip musculature during swallowing? Does it remain at rest, or is there "pursing" of the lips? Does the mentalis contract during the swallow?
3. *Lip habits.* Does the patient bite or suck his upper or lower lips? Does the lip interpose between teeth as a habit? What are the lip length and muscle tone? Are they greater or less than normal?
4. *Speech.* Are there any speech defects or abnormalities, such as lisping, sibilant (hissing "s") sounds, or difficulties in pronouncing various vowel or consonant sounds? Is there a pronounced nasal tone to the speech? Is there any history of speech problems, stuttering, or speech therapy?

By the routine observation and recording of these factors, the practitioner will gain a great deal of useful clinical information as well as an insight into the relationship of oral muscle function, which I hope will be exhaustively researched in the future. By looking closely at the system, we may be far better prepared to evaluate the literature that is presently available and the literature to come. If we accept one dogma or another, we are in the position of generations of physicians and anatomists who firmly believed that women had fewer ribs than men because the Greek philosopher Aristotle had said so. By observing and describing all aspects of the stomatognathic system, we can make a more rational diagnosis and a sound treatment plan.

Existing Oral Appliances

In cases in which the patient has had some oral appliance made—a prosthetic or orthodontic appliance, for example—the examiner should evaluate the appliance's present usefulness to the patient. Factors to be noted include, but are not limited to, the following:

1. *Age.* When was the appliance first placed? Had there been previous appliances placed? Has the appliance been altered, relined, or modified by a dentist or the patient?
2. *Condition and fit.* Is the appliance intact, or have portions (clasps, etc.) been broken? Is it cracked? Does it show signs of wear, discoloration, or other dete-

rioration? Does it adapt well to the teeth and/or tissue? Does it harmonize with the occlusion? Is it comfortable to the patient? Does the patient wear the appliance, and if so, how often?

3. *Condition of supporting tissue, teeth, and ridge.* What is the relationship of the oral structures to the appliance? What is the condition of those structures in terms of health and disease? To what extent is the appliance contributing to the health or disease of the oral structures?

Once these factors have been noted, a judgment should be made regarding the appliance. This judgment must weigh the usefulness of the appliance in providing function, esthetics, comfort, or therapeutic benefit against its potential for harm. Almost any appliance tends to irritate the oral tissues, stress the teeth it is connected to, create plaque-collecting areas, and, in general, damage the oral structures to a varying degree. A good clinical guideline is to minimize whenever possible the number, size, and complexity of oral appliances, particularly removable appliances (this will be discussed in some detail in Chap. 8).

Laboratory Aids

I will discuss laboratory aids in three categories: specific dental aids, systemic (medical) aids, and instructional or motivational aids.

Specific Dental Aids

Whenever possible, the dentist should certainly make use of available laboratory technology to improve the quality of the diagnosis. Such aids include, but are not limited to, the following:

1. *Biopsy or cytology* of suspicious oral lesions. Most pathology labs will provide specimen bottles with appropriate preservatives, and these should be readily available so that simple biopsies can be done without a lot of fuss and bother, so as not to unduly alarm the patient.

2. *Bacteriologic cultures* may be applied in endodontic therapy, but may be especially useful when combined with antibiotic sensitivity testing in severe or intractable oral infections.

3. *Fluoride-level determination* of nonfluoridated water supplies. Municipal, county, or state health departments will often do this determination in conjunction with tests for bacteriologic purity of well water at no charge.

4. *Surface smears* for Candida albicans, Spirochetes, or other specific, suspected nonbacterial organisms.

Systemic (Medical) Aids

Many systemic (medical) laboratory procedures, such as the following, are applicable in dental practice, both in promoting good dental care and in early diagnosis of systemic pathology:

1. *RIA (Radioimmunoassay)* testing to ascertain the presence of Hepatitis "B" surface antigen (HBsAg) in patients with positive histories of the disease. The infective nature of hepatitis places the dental team at great risk and threatens other patients, who may be infected through dental instruments.

2. *Wasserman test* for active syphilis, as a protection when the patient history is positive.

3. *Urinalysis* for the presence of sugars in the urine, a possible indication of diabetes.

4. *Glucose tolerance test,* which may indicate diabetes, is most often used when urinalysis reveals sugar in the urine.

5. *Blood tests:*

Serum acid phosphate
Alkaline phosphatase
Blood urea nitrogen
Blood uric acid
Blood albumin
Blood total protein
Blood globulins
Serum protein electrophoresis
Serum glucose
Serum calcium
Serum inorganic phosphorus
Blood cholesterol
Total serum bilirubin
Lactic dehydrogenase
Serum glutamic oxalacetic transaminase
Blood vitamin C
Automated multiple tests, such as SMA-12

This is by no means an exhaustive discussion of currently available medical laboratory tests for various systemic conditions. Other texts have covered that area well.[8,14] I would propose caution in this area, however. Because such tests are employed for the detection of systemic disorders not limited to the oral cavity, it may be advisable to involve the patient's physician early in the diagnostic process. My reasons for this are twofold: First, the interpretation of the results of such tests does constitute the practice of general medicine, and although the dentist might be both clinically competent and legally entitled to prescribe and interpret any or all such tests, referral to a physician early in the process would reflect positively on the dentist's judgment, if there are any medical or legal problems at a later date. Second, both the number and complexity of medical tests have mushroomed in recent years and will probably continue to do so. Many physicians find it difficult to keep abreast of the changes in medical technology. The dentist, who has a formidable task keeping abreast of developments in dentistry, is not likely to be able to keep up with internal and general medicine as well. Thus, if systemic problems are suspected on the basis of the oral examination, a physician might be better able to select the laboratory tests that will be the most reliable diagnostically, the quickest, or the most economical, and the most up-to-date. Therefore, unless the dentist is able to select wisely and interpret accurately the vast range of new tests and laboratory procedures, involvement of the patient's physician or referral to a specialist may be the most prudent action.

Instructional or Motivational Aids

A number of laboratory aids currently in use are not necessarily scientific in nature or application, but can be valuable as behavioral tools. The use of these aids requires that the dentist be careful not to misrepresent the results as hard scientific data or to use them as the sole basis for courses of therapy. We will discuss some such aids which we feel have application and some which may not.

The *modified Snyder test* gives an indication of the presence of acid-producing organisms in the saliva, relates fairly well to decay rates, and can be a graphic tool, because it is a visible indicator. Furthermore, as the patient improves his oral hygiene and carious lesions are restored, it provides positive visual reinforcement. It is a motivational tool that has some scientific validity.

Phase contrast microscopy is a visual tool that allows the patient to see the organisms present in the plaque. It is not particularly valuable diagnostically, since we know that plaque is comprised of microbes. Its shock value is enhanced if the microbes exhibit some motility, and many advocates of phase contrast use various techniques to stimulate or *simulate* that motility.

While not usually thought of as a laboratory aid, *disclosing stains* employing an erythrosin or fluorescing dye to stain plaques that adhere to the teeth are instructional and motivational, as well as scientifically sound, because plaque is the primary etiologic agent in caries and periodontal disease.

The use of these and similar aids is justified because they have some scientific validity and serve to instruct the patient or motivate him toward better oral health.

Many such tests have been judged on their scientific value and have been found wanting; consequently, they may be inappropriate for use in dental diagnosis and treatment planning. An example of such a test might be the lingual ascorbic acid test, which attempts to detect deficiencies in vitamin C. It is quick, easy to use, and can be a motivational tool. Unfortunately, it does not correlate well with more accurate vitamin C determinations, such as blood levels and tissue levels as measured with more sophisticated means. If such a test were used primarily to generate interest and awareness of good nutrition in the patient, it might be appropriate, although scientifically invalid. If, on the other hand, it is used to formulate a diagnosis of vitamin C deficiency, and vitamin C supplementation is instituted based solely on the test, such use is irrational and inappropriate.

A number of currently available tests and analyses supposedly measure levels of various vitamins and nutrients. Some use food-intake diaries kept by patients, some use samples of hair and/or nails, but few have proven scientific validity. Blood and tissue analyses done under stringently controlled conditions may serve as a basis for therapy. To base the prescription of supplemental vitamins on tests with poor validity is irrational and inappropriate; this is especially true if the dentist is also in the business of retail nutritional supplement sales.

Diagnostic Casts

Diagnostic casts (study models) are useful tools in diagnosis and treatment planning and have myriad applications. What follows is a discussion of diagnostic casts, how they may be related to one another (maxillomandibular) and to a temporomandibular joint analog (articulator), and some of the typical applications they might have in dental treatment planning.

Types of Diagnostic Casts and Their Bases

1. *"Immediate."* If casts are needed in a hurry, impressions can be made with quick-setting, irre-

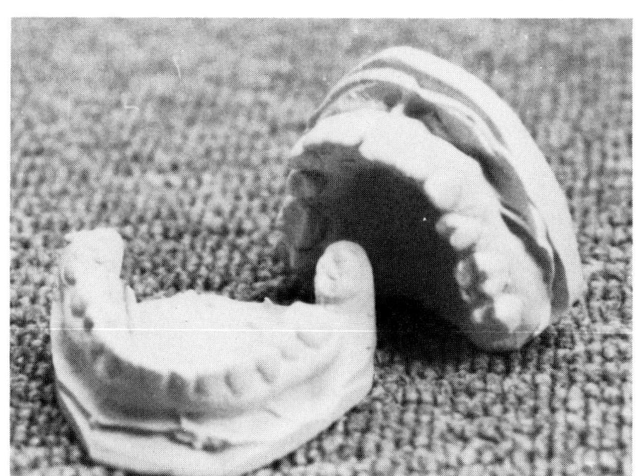

Fig. 4–12. "Immediate" study casts.

versible hydrocolloid (alginate) impression material that is poured in a quick-setting plaster or stone. Although quality may vary, useable casts can generally be produced in less than 15 minutes (Fig. 4–12).

2. *Diagnostic.* Although the same impression material may be employed, speed is usually not of the essence in producing a truly diagnostic cast. Carefully made impressions, retaken if necessary, are poured in a high-quality stone or plaster. This is the most common type of cast used in dental diagnosis and treatment planning (Fig. 4–13).

3. *High accuracy.* Casts of exceptional detail and accuracy may be required in various applications and may be produced by the use of reversible hydrocolloid or one of the rubber base (polysulfide, silicon, or polyether, for example) impression materials. Poured in an improved stone (die material), the resulting diagnostic casts are extremely faithful reproductions of the hard and soft tissues of the mouth (Fig. 4–14).

Depending upon the intended use of the diagnostic casts, the bases developed for them may take a number of forms:

1. *Arbitrary.* Simply trimmed to eliminate gross excess and permit viewing of the impressed area, arbitrary bases are probably most commonly seen on diagnostic casts. Such bases should not be so thick as to make the casts difficult to manipulate, nor so thin as to permit easy breakage. The bases should not be so broad as to prevent easy storage or mounting, nor be trimmed so closely as to lose portions of the duplicated teeth and tissues to the grinder.

2. *Orthodontically trimmed.* Bases can be much more useful if they are orthodontically trimmed. Simply stated, once the casts have been arbitrarily trimmed, they are articulated by hand or with a wax wafer, and placed together on a model trimmer. The distal aspects of maxillary and mandibular model

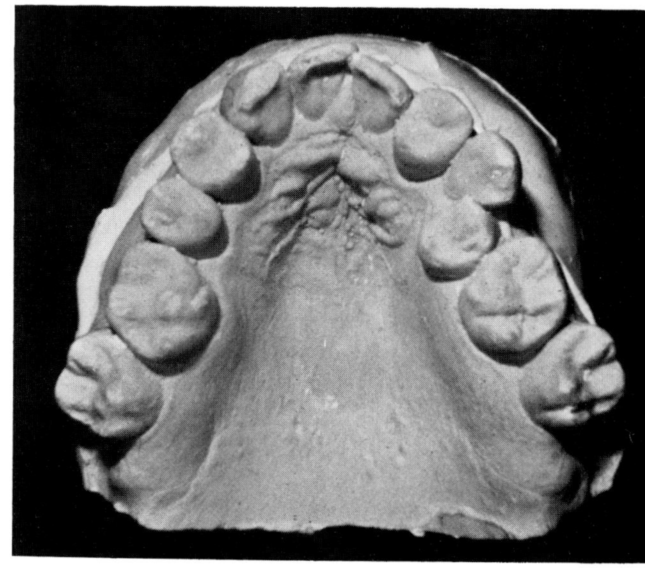

Fig. 4–14. High accuracy cast.

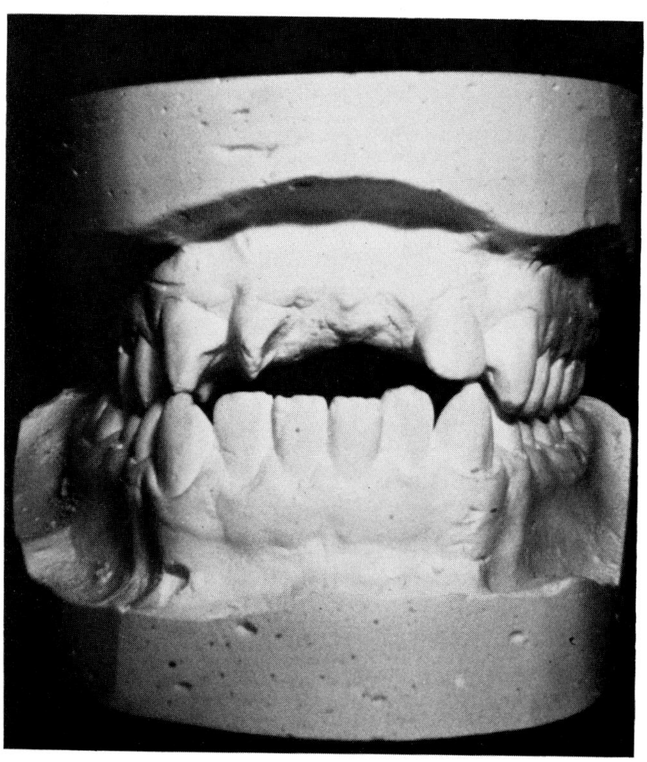

Fig. 4–13. Diagnostic casts.

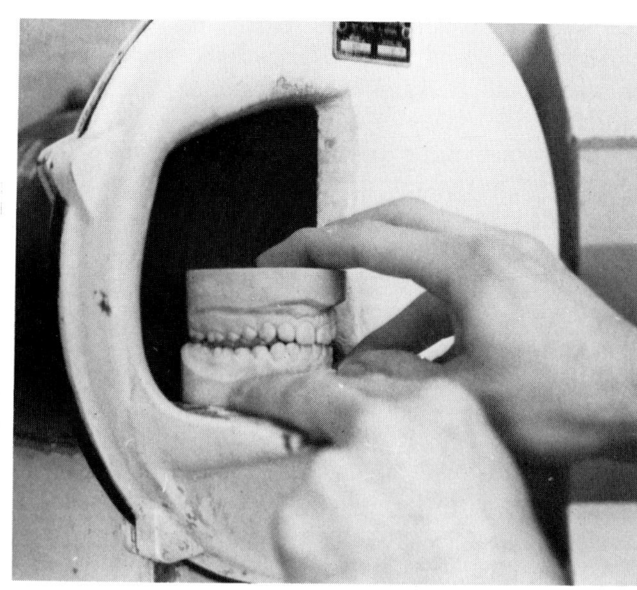

Fig. 4–15. Orthodontic trimming of diagnostic casts.

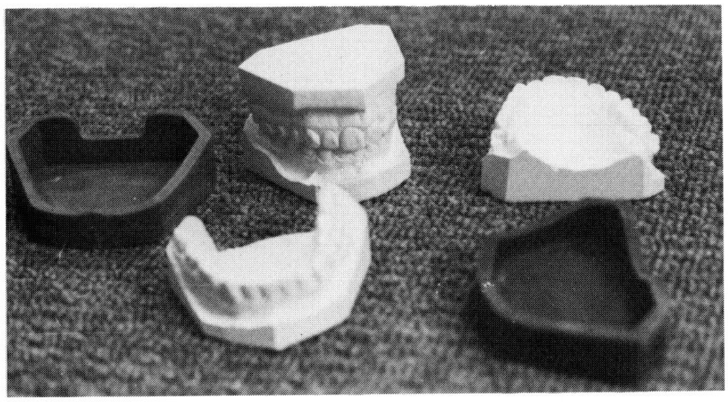

Fig. 4–16. Base formers and casts produced with them.

bases are then ground until both are flush with the trimmer wheel. The result is that the casts can be placed back down on any flat surface, brought together, and immediately rearticulated. This technique is especially useful when casts are not likely to be mounted for study or manipulation (Fig. 4–15).

3. *Base formers.* Casts intended for display or archival purposes may be made more uniform and attractive through the use of base formers. In this technique, the cast is initially poured without a base, but with retention loops or plaster lobules to secure a second pour. The anatomical portion of the cast is then placed into fresh stone or plaster in the base former, and the resulting cast looks very clean and professional (Fig. 4–16). Upper and lower bases can be oriented so that the backs are flush when the casts are articulated, just as they are in the orthodontically trimmed casts.

4. *Split casts.* Another modification of a cast base is the split cast, in which the initial base is trimmed and indexed with "V" grooves. A separating medium is applied and a second pour of some contrasting color stone is added to the base. Trimmed flush and separated, the split cast is very useful in mounting and setting various types of articulators using "check bites"—generally, wax interocclusal records of various maxillomandibular relationships (Fig. 4–17).

Relating the Diagnostic Casts

Diagnostic casts can be related to one another and/or to a temporomandibular joint analog (articulator). Often, models can simply be occluded while held in hand, provided that centric occlusion is well established. Casts can be marked or trimmed orthodontically to record this relationship. If missing teeth or

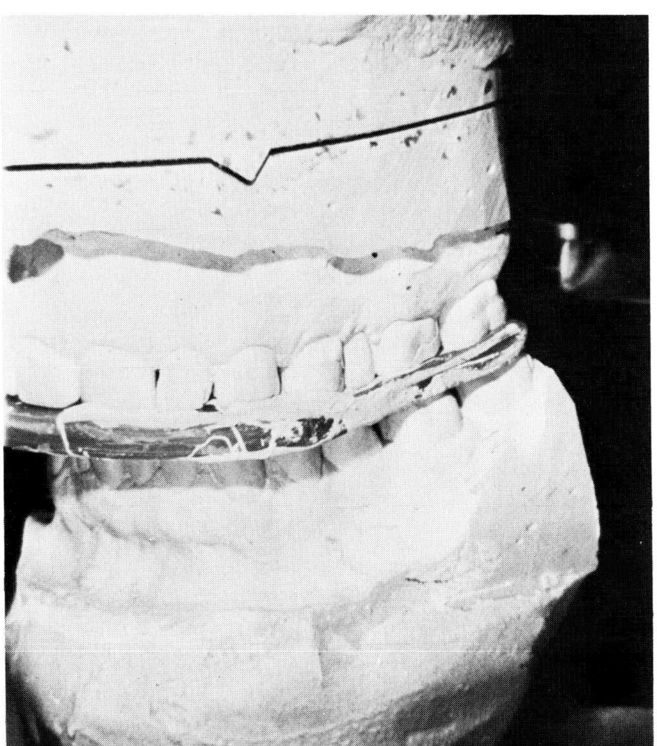

A

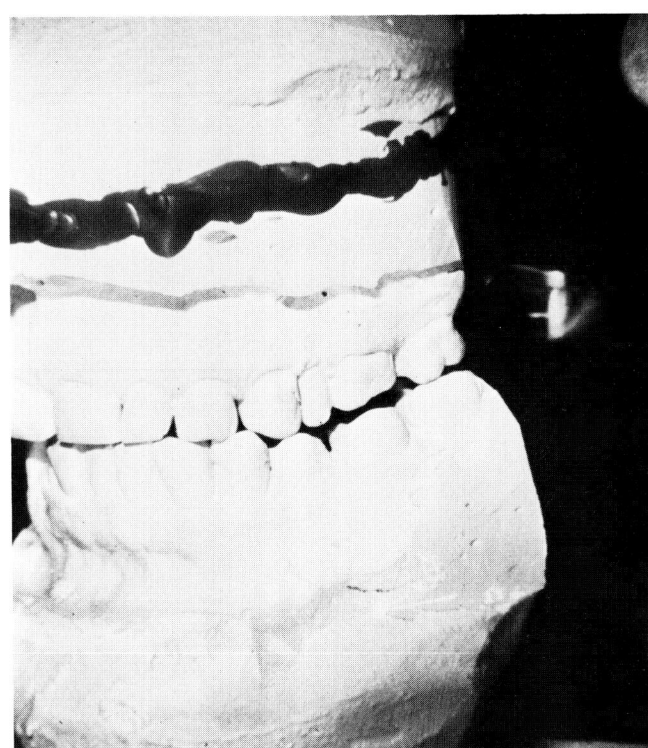

B

Fig. 4–17. *A,* Split cast placed in lateral record (check bite). Articulator would then be set so that cast and base align perfectly. *B,* Split cast reattached to base with sticky wax after articulator is set.

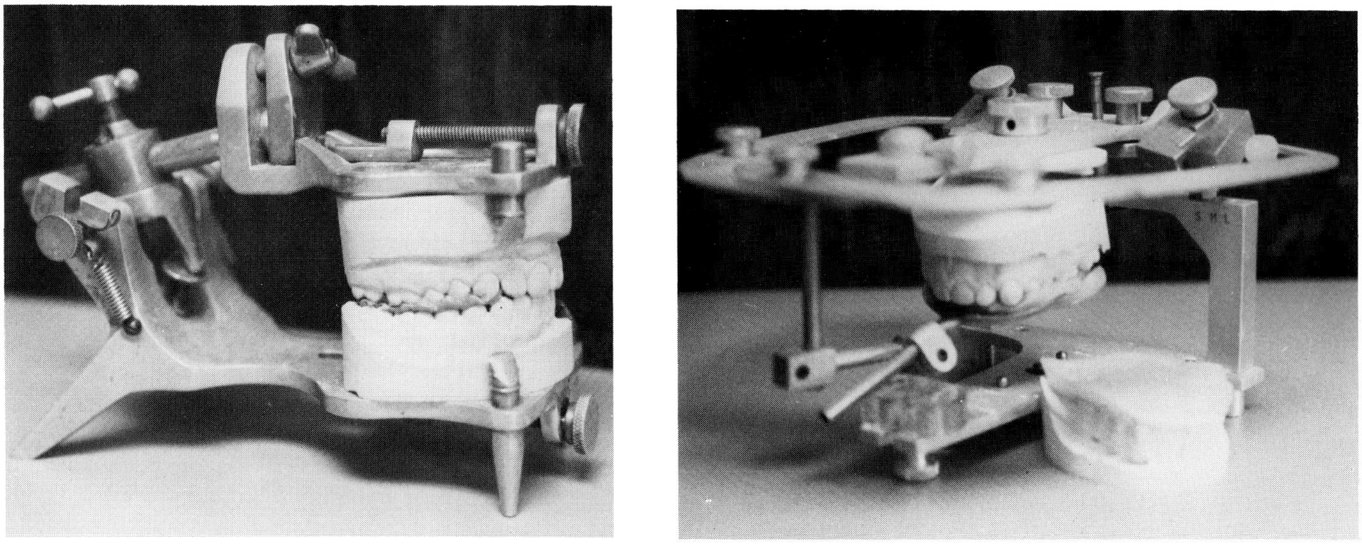

A B

Fig. 4–18. *A,* Diagnostic casts mounted on simple-hinge articulator (Galletti). *B,* Diagnostic casts being mounted on semiadjustable articulator (Whip Mix). Note that ear posts on the transfer bow relate to the articulator's axis of closure, approximating a hinge location.

abnormal occlusion make relationships difficult, a wax wafer bite taken in the mouth may be used later to approximate the casts.

The casts can be studied more easily by mounting them on an articulator, and such arbitrary mountings are often seen on simple-hinge articulators, non-plaster articulators (Galeti) (Fig. 4–18 A), or semi-adjustable articulators. It must be remembered, however, that such mountings are only a convenience and do not necessarily represent the actual relationship of dentition to temporomandibular joint and may not accurately represent even the static, maxillomandibular dental relationship. They are useful where centric relation and centric occlusion coincide well, teeth interdigitate well, and excursive movements present no potential difficulty. When the occlusion is not so simple, it becomes necessary to relate the diagnostic casts more accurately if they are to be of value in diagnosis and treatment planning.

Accurate Articulation of Diagnostic Casts

In ascending order of sophistication and accuracy, the following are some alternatives in relating the diagnostic casts to one another and to the temporomandibular-joint analog (articulator).

Centric-Relation (Retruded Position) Interocclusal Record (Wax Wafer, Wax Wafer with ZOE Wash or Aluwax) Combined with Arbitrary Hinge Location and Transfer. If one is going to use some transfer bow to relate a maxillary cast to an articulator, the interocclusal record should be in the retruded (hinge axis) position without tooth contact so as to provide some indication of CO-CR discrepancies. Methods of establishing the arbitrary axis vary and include, but are not limited to, the following:

1. Palpation of the condylar head in opening movements and approximation by that palpation.
2. Location of a point 10 to 11 mm anterior to the tragus of the ear along a line from the tragus to canthus of the eye.
3. Relating hinge position to the external auditory meatus, either directly, with ear posts, or manually, drawing tragus anteriorly and marking just anterior to the meatus (Fig. 4–18 B).

Any of these methods will give a reasonable approximation of the hinge position and, when transferred to a semiadjustable articulator, provide a closer analog to the actual situation than hand-held or totally arbitrary mountings.

Centric-Relation Records Combined with Actual Hinge-Axis Location and Transfer. This approach will duplicate the CO-CR relationship accurately. If a protrusive record is also obtained, it will allow an approximation of condylar inclination. When used with an articulator with adjustable intercondylar distance, which is capable of accepting lateral records, a very acceptable analog is created, although precise condylar movements are reduced to straight-line averages between centric and lateral positions (Fig. 4–19).

Centric-Relation Records Combined with Actual Hinge-Axis Location and Pantographic or Molded

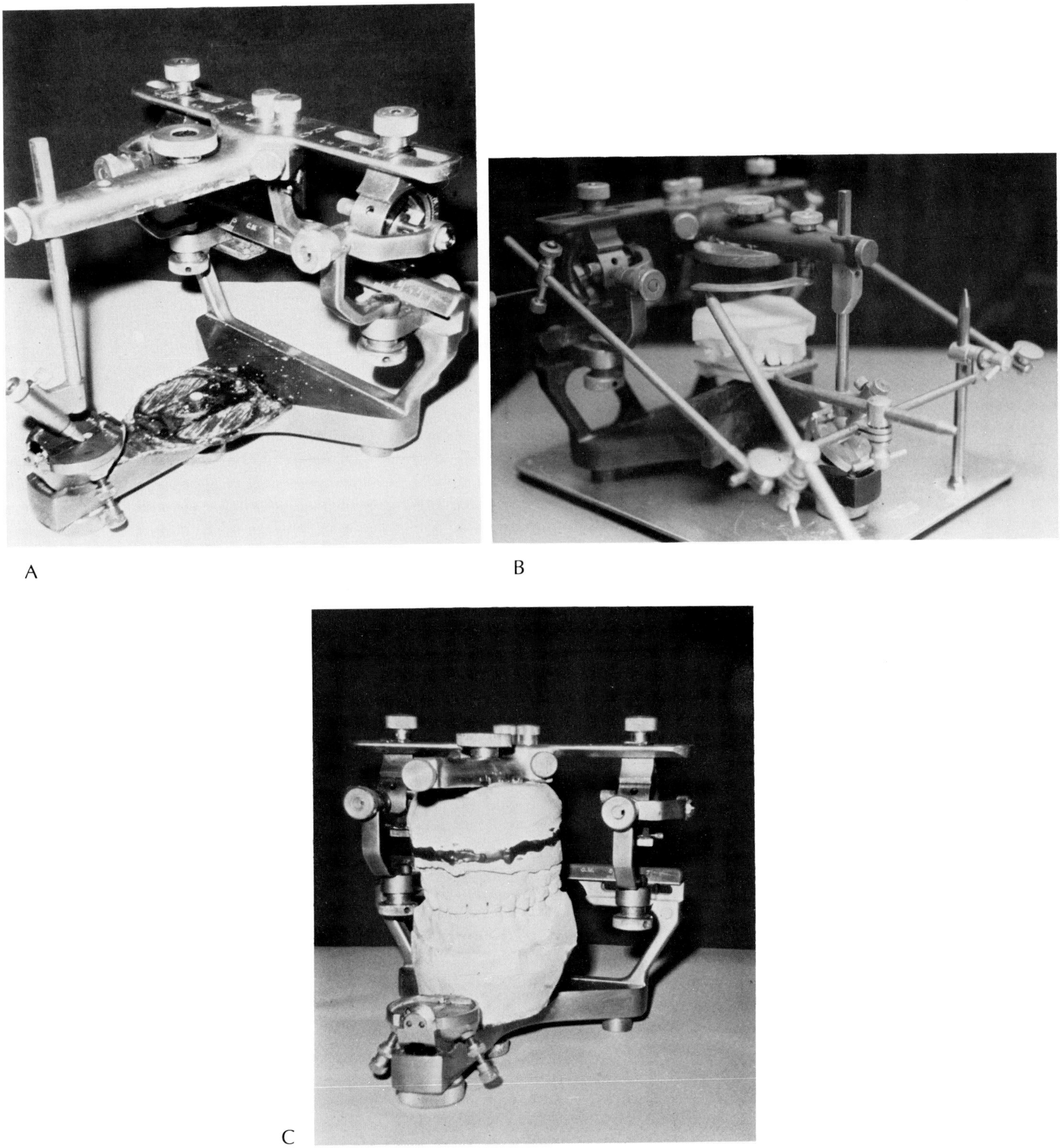

Fig. 4–19. *A*, Hanau No. 130–21 articulator. *B*, Diagnostic casts being mounted using a hinge-bow transfer of the patient's actual hinge axis. *C*, Casts mounted, using interocclusal centric relation record (not shown).

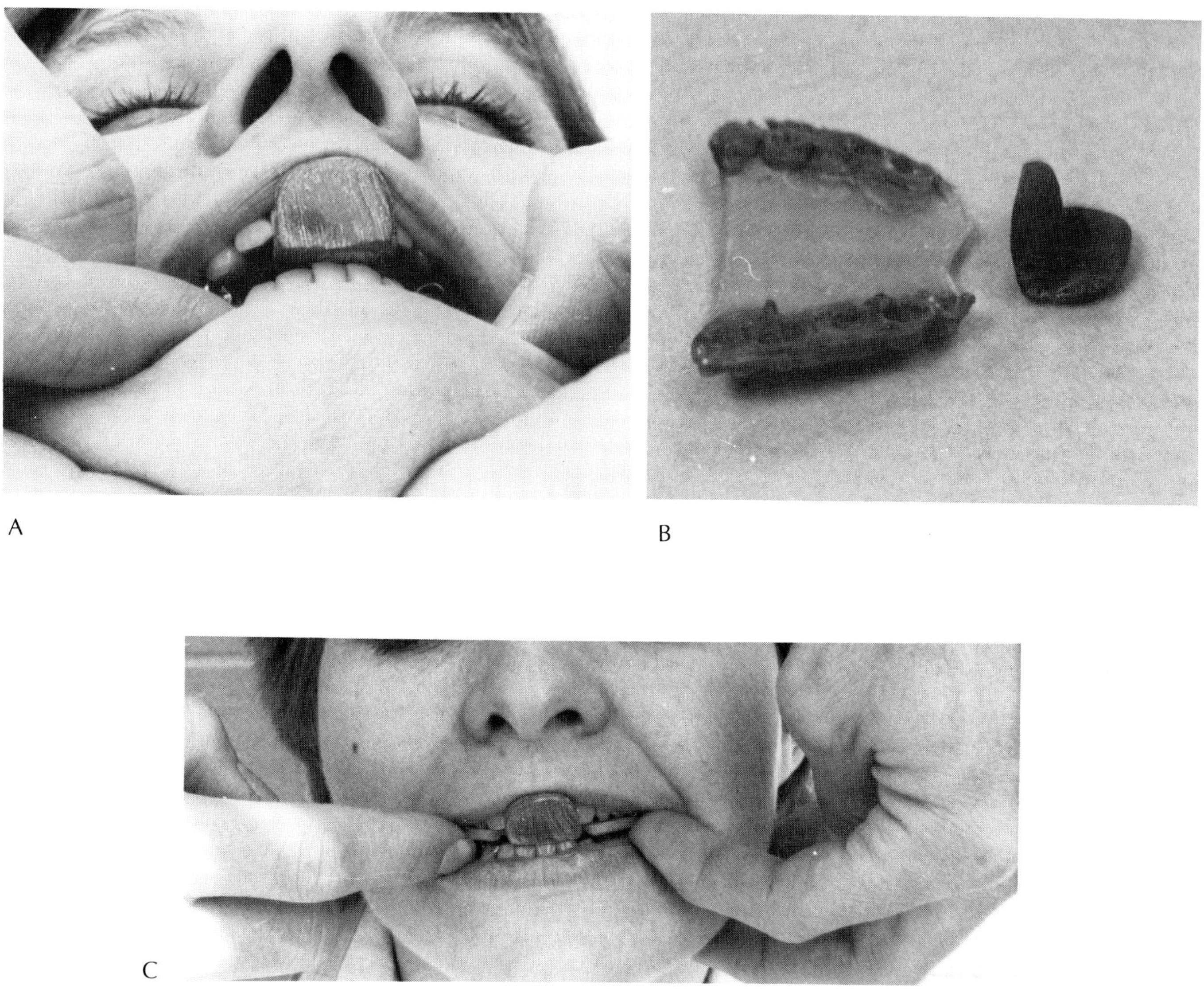

A B C

Fig. 4–20. *A*, Anterior acrylic jig seated over upper anteriors; lower anteriors contacting inclined plane. *B*, Centric relation wax record with anterior cut away for jig. *C*, Wax record being tried in mouth with jig in place.

Analog Records Transferred to a Fully Adjustable Articulator. This is certainly the most sophisticated approach in relating diagnostic casts; it is also fairly specialized, time consuming, and in most cases, impractical for typical diagnosis and treatment planning. Nonetheless, it has application in some situations, and the dentist should at least be familiar with the method and the information it can provide.

Anterior Acrylic Jig. An aid to both the location and recording of centric relation position is the acrylic anterior "jig," fabricated with cold cure acrylic over the upper central incisors. After hardening, the jig is smoothed and contoured so that it provides an inclined ramp for the lower anteriors to contact in the retruded position, keeping the posterior teeth slightly apart (Fig. 4–20 A). This helps in seating the mandible in its retruded position and can be used in combination with the actual centric wax recording by cutting away the anterior section of the bite wafer (Fig. 4–20 B).

In recording centric relation position, the patient closes into light contact with the jig, the recording material in the posterior being dead soft and thereby reducing or eliminating any reflex proprioceptive positioning of the mandible into habitual centric (Fig. 4–20 C).

The anterior jig is quick and simple to fabricate, easy to use, and greatly enhances the accuracy of the centric relation recording.

Diagnostic Wax-Ups

More specifically an aid in treatment planning, the diagnostic wax-up is an application of the diagnostic cast. A diagnostic wax-up is any alteration made on a diagnostic cast in wax to represent possible future restorations or tooth positions. It is useful in planning posterior occlusion, anterior guidance, and particularly esthetics. The example shown in Figure 4–21 illustrates solutions to challenging esthetic and functional restorative problems with the use of a diagnostic wax-up. This technique will also be discussed in subsequent chapters as an adjunct to treatment planning.

Photographs

In many cases, photographs can be useful in diagnosis and treatment planning. When constructing anterior restorations, crowns, bridges, or partial dentures, or in full denture prosthesis, old photographs obtained from the patient may be a valuable aid for the dentist attempting to mimic the natural dentition prior to its demise. However, one must be careful of the grandmother who presents her wedding photograph and holds the expectation that the proposed prosthesis will restore her youthful smile. On the other hand, catching some aspect of the patient's natural dentition is a touch of care and artistry that is often greatly appreciated by the patient and that enhances the acceptance of a dental prosthesis. Just as significant may be a patient's desire to change some characteristic of his natural dentition or of previous prosthetic efforts that has been a source of dissatisfaction. Photographs may inform us about what to avoid as well as what to strive for.

Photographs taken by the dentist—whether they are color slides or Polaroid prints—may be useful, particularly when some major change is anticipated in the patient's occlusion or appearance. Even diagnosis may be facilitated by studying a photograph, because the eye of the camera is without bias and may allow us to see things we might otherwise overlook. Such photographs may be full-face portraits, profile views, views taken from just under the chin, views of solemn expressions or smiles. Intraoral photographs are commonly employed and can be used to record many factors.

MODIFICATIONS OF THE ROUTINE SYSTEMATIC APPROACH

In outlining data gathering in a routine systematic approach we concentrated on the typical adult dental examination. It is obvious that modifications to this approach are in order when dealing with children, fully edentulous patients, or others who have special situations, problems, or difficulties. The specialist may, in fact, gloss over or omit many of the factors not germane to his area of expertise. The general practitioner, however, must consider all the factors and gather all the relevant data available for every patient. The general practitioner cannot afford to concentrate so intently upon some areas of interest and expertise that other problems go unrecognized and undiagnosed.

Since it is not within the scope of this text to outline every possible consideration in every conceivable case, the reader is referred to many excellent works dealing with subjects such as growth and development, pediatric dentistry, occlusion, and full prosthetics to embellish the general approach outlined here.

RECORDS

In this review of the routine systematic approach to data gathering, I have presented the reasonable minimum information the dentist should obtain. The individual dentist must exercise judgment about which of the factors might be omitted in certain cases and when additional data is required. Merely ob-

A B C D

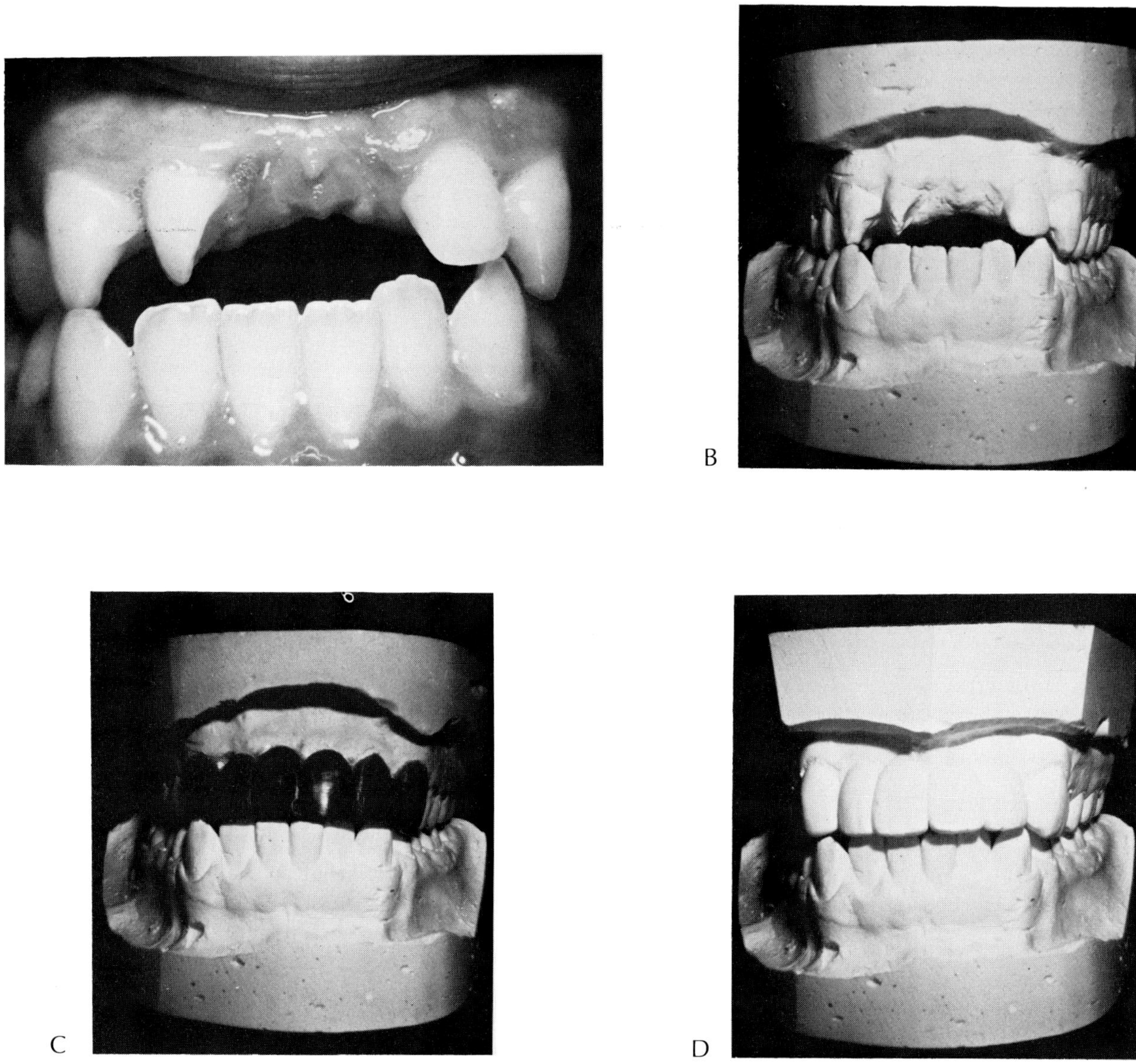

Fig. 4–21. Using diagnostic wax-ups to solve esthetic and functional restorative problems. *A*, This 18-year-old man traumatically avulsed his central incisors some years previously. Pontic space is insufficient for normal-size central incisors, the right lateral incisor is rotated, and the right canine is in end-to-end contact with the lower. *B*, Diagnostic casts are articulated and teeth prepared as for crowns. *C*, A diagnostic wax-up is developed that is both functionally and esthetically acceptable. *D*, The diagnostic wax-up is duplicated and a plaster model is made, which is the precursor of the clinical prosthesis.

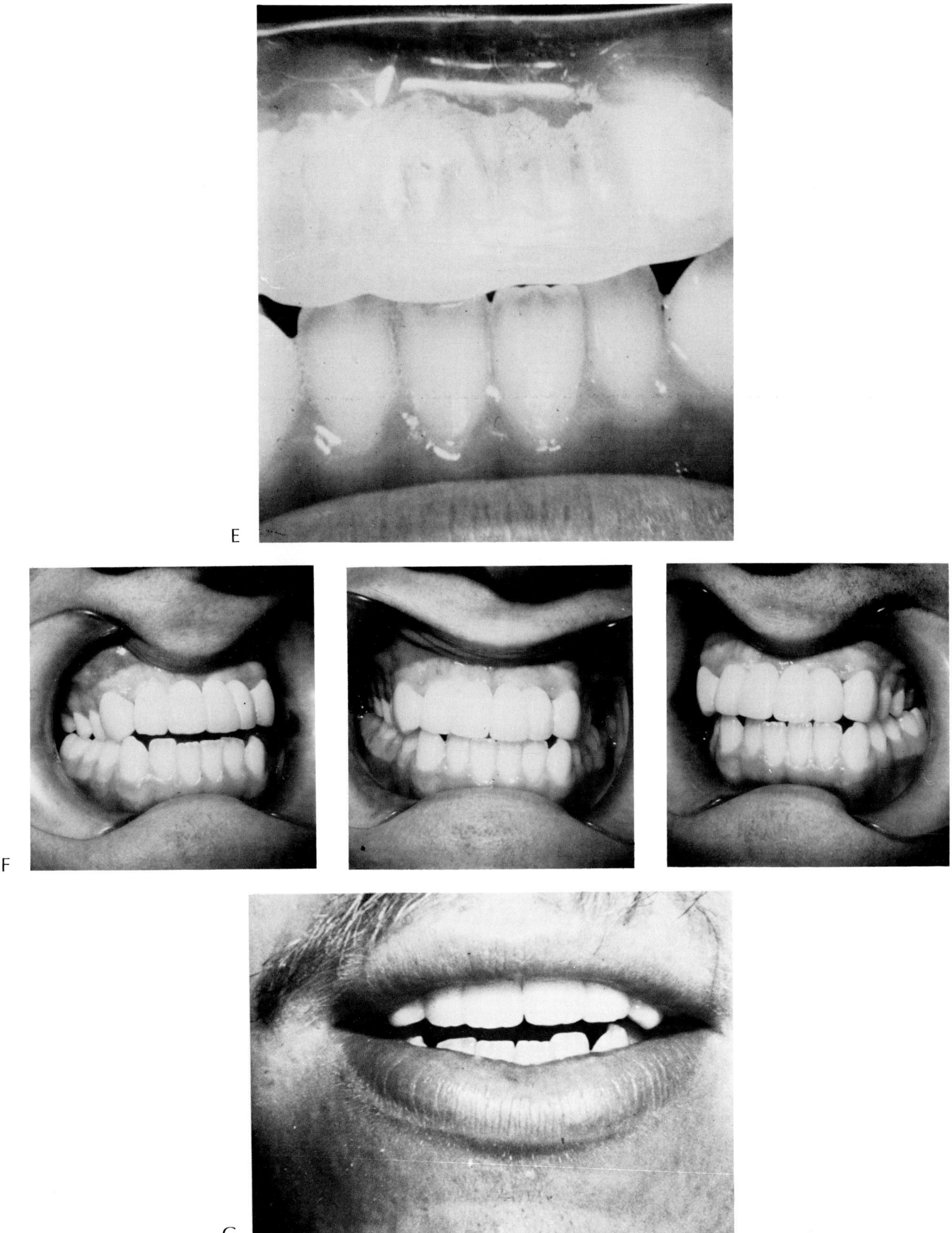

Fig. 4–21 *continued.* *E,* A thin, celluloid shim is fabricated and serves both as a guide for adequate reduction in the preparation and as a former for the temporary bridge. *F,* The clinical prosthesis, a porcelain-fused-to-gold fixed bridge. (Left) The canine has been built into the working-side group function. (Center) Anterior group function in protrusive. (Right) The steep canine overbite has been modified, and anterior group function established in lateral. *G,* Despite the initial problems, a very acceptable esthetic result has been achieved with the use of a diagnostic wax-up.

serving the various factors is useless without an accurate and complete written record. The written record is the primary tool in diagnosis and treatment planning and is essential in treatment itself. Dental records take many forms and include any or all written material (or graphic depictions) pertaining to the patient, as well as radiographs, photographs, diagnostic models, and the like.

This section will describe how records are tools in diagnosis and treatment planning, their importance from a legal standpoint, and the criteria that they should fulfill. On this basis, one can delineate guidelines for an adult dental record that contains only essential information and list its components. The selection of commerically available forms and charts, the development of custom-made record materials, and some of the legal aspects of dental records and record keeping will also be discussed.

The written dental record is the primary tool in diagnosis and treatment planning. It enables the dentist who has gathered all the pertinent information to review that information at his leisure, so that all factors observed are once again recalled. Certainly, all frank pathologic findings must be reviewed so that they may be considered in making the diagnosis and addressed in the treatment plan. Seemingly isolated pathologies often may be related and that relationship may be discovered when reviewing the record. Many findings in our examination procedure may not be pathologic or seem important until they are integrated with all the other findings, at which time patterns may emerge to reveal problems not otherwise discoverable. It is essential to review the findings of the complete, routine systematic examination and all other findings before making a diagnosis, and the written record allows us to do this. Once the diagnosis or diagnoses have been made, a plan of treatment can be formulated that also becomes a part of the dental record. Once again, the initial findings must be reviewed to ensure that the final treatment plan addresses the problems seen in the examination or discovered upon integration of the findings. The complete dental record, now including diagnosis and treatment plan, becomes the primary tool in rendering treatment, because few of us would trust to memory the types and sequences of treatment planned for a large number of patients.

Finally, all treatment rendered to a patient should be recorded, as well as any complications, changes in treatment plan, or further diagnostic discoveries. This continuing chronicle of a patient's treatment also becomes part of the permanent dental record. While it is obvious that, in most cases, treatment could not be carried out effectively without a record of what had been done, the need for detailed treatment records must be emphasized. Because further treatment may be done in an area or on a tooth months and even years later, memory alone cannot recall the conditions that existed and the treatment decisions that were made in the past. For example, our approach to treatment of a symptomatic tooth might be significantly altered if the record indicated a direct pulp cap had been attempted some years previously. Such records may be useful to other practitioners to whom the patient is referred or in the event that the patient moves.

The dental record is also a legal document. The dentist/patient relationship is in most cases a legal contract, whether written or not, and the dental record is of prime importance should any questions arise as to the nature of that contract. While we often think of the legal aspects of records primarily in terms of a defense against malpractice litigation, they are also of legal significance in other types of situations, such as the collection of unpaid fees, income tax records (for both dentist and patient), and the positive identification of deceased persons.

Criteria for All Dental Records

Given the importance of the dental record as both a tool in diagnosis, treatment planning, and treatment itself, and as a legal document, a set of criteria that all dental records should fulfill can be established.

1. *Accurate.* The need for accuracy in dental records should be fairly self-evident. For example, if the wrong tooth is marked for extraction, the results can be disastrous. Such details as the spelling of a patient's name or having a correct, current address can prevent gross errors or at least embarrassment. Inaccuracies or omissions in records tend to cast doubt on the entire record and on the integrity of the treatment.

2. *Legible.* To be of any use, the dental record must be readable, not only to the dentist, but to anyone who might need the information in the record—an auxiliary, another dentist, or even an attorney. To that end, record entries should be made neatly in ink (unless visual charting entails colored pencil, etc.) and the record protected against smudges, water spots, and the like.

3. *Complete and comprehensive.* The question of how much information should be recorded and of what detail is of prime importance. We have seen extremes in dental records, from the minimal efforts (a 5 × 7 card with a pictorial tooth chart and no room for diagnostic findings) to the maximal efforts, which are usually found in dental schools (dental

charts running to 20 or more pages that, if filled out in complete detail, would provide any reader with more information about the patient than he would really want or be able to use effectively). While it is obvious that too little recorded information is a serious defect, record systems that are extremely detailed and cumbersome may, by their very nature, discourage effective use.

Essential Components of a Record System

The record system adopted must strike a happy medium. It should allow clear and concise recording of all essential information and of a greater depth of material when necessary. In short, it should be geared to the practitioner, his routine systematic approach to data gathering, and the type of practice he is in. Any record system has certain essential components, however, and is not complete unless it includes the following:

1. *Business information* should include patient's name, address, and phone number; party responsible for the account, and so on. It is obvious that the dentist must know who he is treating and record that information.
2. *Patient history,* both medical and dental
3. *Record of soft-tissue examination* (Oral-Cancer Exam)
4. *Record of periodontal examination* should include provision for charting of pocket depths
5. *Dental chart,* pictorial or numerical, including provision for charting existing conditions, restorations, missing teeth, both clinical and radiographic pathologic findings, and restorations placed or treatment rendered
6. *Record of functional evaluation,* including occlusion, TMJ, and myofunctional findings
7. *A written treatment plan,* including approximate fees, date presented to patient, patient's acceptance or rejection, modifications, or changes made during the actual course of treatment
8. *Dental radiographs* with patient's name and the date the radiograph was taken
9. *Treatment record,* including any and all treatment rendered, procedures performed, fees charged, or conversations with patient regarding same, dated and initialed by the responsible party—dentist, hygienist, chairside assistant, etc.
10. *Other material* obtained at the discretion of the dentist should include anything he feels is pertinent to his practice or to a particular patient.

The depth of detail required is a matter of the individual dentist's judgment and must be considered very carefully if the record is to be truly comprehensive (Fig. 4–22).

It is obvious that there is no limit to the depth of detail possible in such a treatment record. The time of day, the barometric pressure, the astrological sign of the patient—all could be entered into the record. The three examples in Figure 4–22, which describe a simple, operative dentistry procedure, range from a paucity to a wealth of information. It should be apparent that the first entry is inadequate: the date fails to verify the year, and no mention is made of a base material or anesthetic. The record does not provide sufficient detail to be an effective tool. The third entry should prove completely adequate. It gives a diagnosis of the problem being treated, detailed descriptions of the procedure that was performed and of a minor complication, and a reminder of the treatment planned for the next appointment. The second entry, while considerably briefer, may also be adequate if certain conditions are met. Specifically, it can be assumed that the occlusal restoration implies a prior diagnosis of occlusal caries. "Base" may be sufficient information if the same base material is used in all or nearly all of that dentist's operative procedures. Likewise, "Anes" may be sufficient if the same local anesthetic agent is used exclusively; if two agents are used, one without vasoconstrictor, entries such as "Anes" or "Anes w/o vaso" could be made. The complication is probably described adequately in the second entry, provided that the dentist routinely informs patients of such complications and offers consistent advice on how the patient should deal with them. Should problems of a medical-legal nature arise, however, it might also be necessary to obtain testimony from a third party (chairside assistant or other auxiliary) that such information and instruction were indeed routine practices. An office manual outlining procedures, materials to be used, and routine instructions to be given to the patient might also be instrumental in supporting a sketchy dental record. The legal aspects of record keeping will be discussed in more detail later in this chapter.

At the time the record is being made, economy of time and space may appear to be of prime importance; indeed, a brief and concise record has much to recommend it. Should later developments of a dental (pain or sensitivity in the restored tooth) or legal nature (parotid tumor thought to be precipitated by the bur nick incident) require thorough recall of the procedure, it is better to have a more detailed record. Years or even months after a routine procedure is performed, memory alone will not serve. A complete and comprehensive dental record is an essential tool not only in diagnosis and treatment planning, but in the practice of dentistry in general.

Many commercially available record systems are

used in dentistry, and the typical practitioner will usually select a system of various components that he feels is workable in his practice. Certain criteria may be applied in the selection process, and these would include the following:

1. Does the record system or the various components selected provide for all the essential components of the complete dental record? For example, if there is no specific place on the chart to record periodontal pockets, recording the depths will be cumbersome.

2. Do the component areas provide sufficient depth of information? A medical history that simply asks, "Are you in good health?" is not going to provide adequate information unless it is accompanied by a fairly exhaustive oral history, which must then be written up from scratch.

3. Is the system logical in its layout and sequence? Whatever sequence is chosen by the dentist, the chart system should be adaptable to it, so that information can be easily recorded in the order in which it is obtained. This also facilitates the recovery of the information from the record at a later time. There should be a minimum of page turning and folding.

4. Is the system appropriate to the practice? A pedodontist does not need questionnaires about past full denture experiences, nor is the prosthodontist likely to require much in the way of thumbsucking history.

5. Is there a significant amount of irrelevant material in the chart? If large portions of a chart system seem unnecessary, then time will be wasted in gathering and recording trivial information or sections of the chart will be ignored, left blank, and give the distinct impression of an incomplete job.

Inasmuch as records are essential tools, it is important to select the correct tool for the task at hand. Good record systems can be assembled from commercial sources which fulfill the criteria outlined above, but the selection of the component parts is difficult, requiring careful screening of all available materials, and compromises are unavoidable. Like any tool, the more appropriate the tool to the task, the easier and more efficiently the task is performed.

For that reason, many dentists find it advantageous to design their own systems or at least some of the components of the system. There are several approaches to the creation of custom record systems, and none of them are exceedingly difficult. The simplest custom dental record is a typewritten and/or

9-21	⌊6 O/A	$ 15
9-21-75	#3 O/A, BASE, ANES. BUR NICKED RT. BUCCAL	
	MUCOSA — PT. INFORMED AND ADVISED. RBM	$ 15
9-21-75	#3 OCCLUSAL CARIES, CaOH BASE, AMALGAM	
	RESTORATION. GAVE XYLOCAINE c̄ 1:100,000	
	EPINEPHRINE VIA INFILTRATION. BUR NICKED	
	RT. BUCCAL MUCOSA WHEN PT. MOVED	
	SUDDENLY. INFORMED PT. OF SAME AND	
	RECOMMENDED SALINE RINSES IF	
	UNCOMFORTABLE. RB MORRIS DDS	$ 15
	NEXT APPT: ANTERIOR OPERATIVE	

Fig. 4–22. Three chart entries, each describing the same procedure.

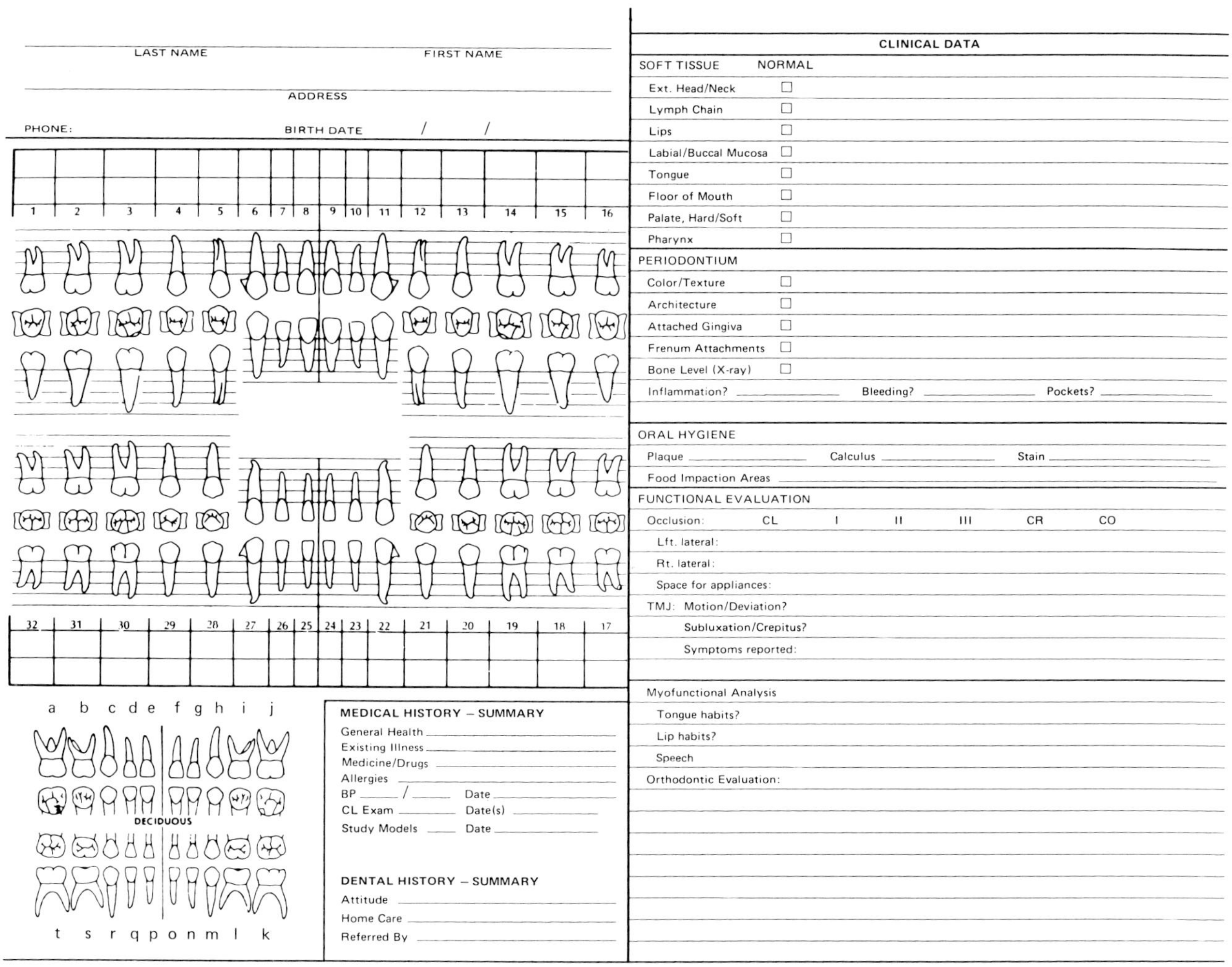

LAST NAME FIRST NAME

ADDRESS

PHONE: BIRTH DATE / /

1 2 3 4 5 6 7 8 9 10 11 12 13 14 15 16

32 31 30 29 28 27 26 25 24 23 22 21 20 19 18 17

a b c d e f g h i j

DECIDUOUS

t s r q p o n m l k

MEDICAL HISTORY – SUMMARY

General Health ______

Existing Illness ______

Medicine/Drugs ______

Allergies ______

BP ____ / ____ Date ______

CL Exam ______ Date(s) ______

Study Models ____ Date ______

DENTAL HISTORY – SUMMARY

Attitude ______

Home Care ______

Referred By ______

CLINICAL DATA

SOFT TISSUE NORMAL

Ext. Head/Neck ☐

Lymph Chain ☐

Lips ☐

Labial/Buccal Mucosa ☐

Tongue ☐

Floor of Mouth ☐

Palate, Hard/Soft ☐

Pharynx ☐

PERIODONTIUM

Color/Texture ☐

Architecture ☐

Attached Gingiva ☐

Frenum Attachments ☐

Bone Level (X-ray) ☐

Inflammation? ______ Bleeding? ______ Pockets? ______

ORAL HYGIENE

Plaque ______ Calculus ______ Stain ______

Food Impaction Areas ______

FUNCTIONAL EVALUATION

Occlusion: CL I II III CR CO

Lft. lateral:

Rt. lateral:

Space for appliances:

TMJ: Motion/Deviation?

Subluxation/Crepitus?

Symptoms reported:

Myofunctional Analysis

Tongue habits?

Lip habits?

Speech

Orthodontic Evaluation:

A

Fig. 4–23. Custom chart system. *A,* Clinical examination record and chart.

	SERVICES NECESSARY		FEES		
	1				
	2				
	3				
	4				
	5				
	6				
	7				
	8				
	9				
	10				
	11				
	12				
	13				
	14				
	15				
	16				
	17				
	18				
	19				
	20				
	21				
	22				
	23				
	24				
	25				
	26				
	27				
	28				
	29				
	30				
	31				
	32				

B

Fig. 4–23 *continued.* *B*, Treatment planning form and note space.

NAME

DATE 19 ___	SERVICES RENDERED	Fee	Balance	DATE 19 ___	SERVICES RENDERED	Fee	Balance

C

Fig. 4–23 *continued.* *C*, Procedure record.

PATIENT REGISTRATION

UPDATED
Date/Intial

For Office Use Only

DATE ______________________

PATIENT'S NAME ______________________ BIRTH DATE ______________________

NAME OF SPOUSE ______________________

IF A CHILD, PARENT'S NAME ______________________

STREET ADDRESS ______________________ PHONE ______________________

CITY ______________________ STATE ______________________ ZIP ______________________

PATIENT EMPLOYED BY ______________________ PHONE ______________________

BUSINESS ADDRESS ______________________

PRESENT POSITION ______________________ HOW LONG HELD ______________________

SPOUSE EMPLOYED BY ______________________ PHONE ______________________

BUSINESS ADDRESS ______________________

PRESENT POSITION ______________________ HOW LONG HELD ______________________

PURPOSE OF THIS APPOINTMENT ______________________ PHONE # ______________________

IN CASE OF EMERGENCY, WHO SHOULD BE NOTIFIED ______________________

WHO WILL PAY THIS ACCOUNT ______________________

PATIENT'S SOCIAL SECURITY NUMBER ______________________

SPOUSE'S SOCIAL SECURITY NUMBER ______________________

DO YOU HAVE INSURANCE THAT MAY COVER ANY PART OF OUR PROFESSIONAL SERVICES ______________________

WHOM MAY WE THANK FOR REFERRING YOU ______________________

____
(Signature of party responsible for payment)

D

Reverse side for Emergency Treatment Only

Fig. 4–23 *continued.* *D*, Registration form.

GET ACQUAINTED QUESTIONNAIRE: CONFIDENTIAL

So that we may render the best treatment please answer all questions fully.

NAME ______________ AGE ______________ DATE OF BIRTH ______________

MEDICAL HISTORY

When was your last physical exam? ______________ (approx.)

Are you seeing a physician at this time? yes no

If so, for what? ______________

Are you taking any medication or pills of any kind? yes no

If so, what? ______________

Are you allergic or do you react to anything (drugs, food, etc.) yes no

If so, what? ______________

Name of your family doctor: ______________

Party to notify in case of emergency: ______________

address: ______________

Do you now, or have you ever had (circle yes or no):

Rheumatic Fever	yes	no	High or Low Blood Pressure	yes	no
Heart Trouble	yes	no	Reaction to Local Anesthetic	yes	no
Arthritis	yes	no	Epilepsy or Seizures	yes	no
Diabetes	yes	no	Fainting Spells	yes	no
Hepatitis	yes	no	Nervous Disorders	yes	no
Venereal Disease	yes	no	Tuberculosis	yes	no
Anemia	yes	no	Malignancy or Tumor	yes	no
Bleeding Problems	yes	no	Radiation Therapy	yes	no
			(female) Are you pregnant?	yes	no

DENTAL HISTORY

Do you now, or have you had (check if yes):

Toothaches	______	Clenching or grinding the teeth, day or night	______
Bad Breath	______	Pains in or near the ear	______
Pain in Chewing	______	Other sore or painful areas in the mouth	______
Canker Sores	______		
Bleeding Gums	______		

When was your last dental visit? ______________

Did you have x-rays taken at that time? yes no

Have you had regular dental check-ups? yes no

Do you now, or have you had (check if yes):

Any missing teeth	______	Bridge(s) or Partial Denture(s)	______
Gum surgery	______	Root Canal work	______
Orthodontic treatment (braces)	______		

Have you ever been instructed on how to brush your teeth? yes no

If so, when and by whom? ______________

How often do you brush? ______________ when, usually? ______________

Type of brush: hard / soft Kind of toothpaste? ______________

Do you use dental floss? yes no occasionally

DIETARY HISTORY

Do you eat or drink between meals? ______________ during the day yes no; in the evening yes no

Does your diet include:	chewing gum	yes	no
	candy bars	yes	no
	lifesavers	yes	no
	soft drinks (soda, fruit juice)	yes	no
	cookies, cake, sweet rolls	yes	no
If you drink coffee or tea, do you use sugar?		yes	no
Do you use breath mints or cough drops fairly often?		yes	no
Do you smoke?		yes	no

E DATE ______________ SIGNATURE ______________

Fig. 4–23 *continued.* E, Medical, dental, and dietary histories.

hand-ruled master that, if taken to an instant-offset printer, can be duplicated, enlarged, or reduced quickly and cheaply.

A more professional look can be obtained by taking the rough mock-up material to a printer or a composing service, where it can be made into a camera-ready master copy, using various sizes of fine prints to create a very striking appearance. This can be used as the instant-offset master copy, which can be duplicated easily. The advantage of this approach is that the printing cost is low and desired modifications or changes can be incorporated easily onto the master.

A second approach to custom record systems is to work with a commercial supplier who will assist in the composition of a chart system and print it to your specifications. Often these companies will provide kits to assist in the design of such a system. While the cost of this approach is greater, material can be printed on oversized paper, or on heavy card stock, which the instant-offset printer cannot do.

The third approach is to custom design a system and work through a local printer. The costs of producing such record systems can be reduced if the systems are produced in quantity. It may be possible for a number of dentists to agree on a design and thereby bring the cost into line with commercially available systems. It should also be noted that cost per unit is seldom a significant expense, especially when one considers the efficiency gained by a custom-designed system. The sample charts shown in Figure 4–23 are examples of custom-design record systems for a general practice.

Additional Tools

While the system I have described fulfills the essential criteria, many additional tools can be employed in a record system as the need arises. Certainly dentists in specialty practices must tailor their systems to their areas, and it is not within the scope of this text to outline every possible type of record system for each specialty. However, several additional components will be described that the general practitioner or the specialist may find useful.

Patient Interview Record

It can be very useful to make fairly detailed notes during the initial patient interview, in addition to those normally included in the sample chart system. A narrative record of what the dentist and patient talked about (dental and nondental conversation) can be an effective tool in treating the patient. Such a record, usually done by an auxiliary using blank paper, can be used to refresh the dentist's memory about the human being whose radiographs and dental findings he might be reviewing some time later. It allows the dentist to put a "face" on the record, should days be hectic and memory fail. It also reminds the dentist of the patient's "pet peeves," which might have been elicited, or of personal items, such as an upcoming marriage or the impending birth of a grandchild. To the extent that such notes are "practice builders," a contrivance to impress the patient with our memories, they are not likely to be used routinely once the practice is established. On the other hand, if the notes represent a sincere effort to relate to the patient on human terms, if the record is made in order to more effectively plan and carry out treatment on people we care about, the patient-interview record can be an effective tool in the dental-records system (Fig. 4–24)

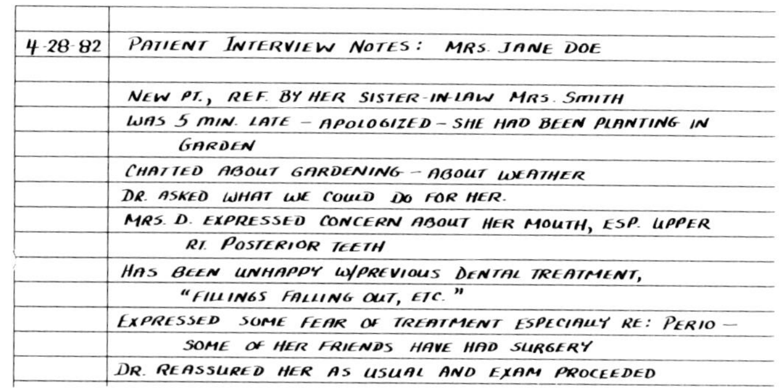

4-28-82	PATIENT INTERVIEW NOTES: MRS. JANE DOE
	NEW PT., REF. BY HER SISTER-IN-LAW MRS. SMITH
	WAS 5 MIN. LATE – APOLOGIZED – SHE HAD BEEN PLANTING IN GARDEN
	CHATTED ABOUT GARDENING – ABOUT WEATHER
	DR. ASKED WHAT WE COULD DO FOR HER.
	MRS. D. EXPRESSED CONCERN ABOUT HER MOUTH, ESP. UPPER RT. POSTERIOR TEETH
	HAS BEEN UNHAPPY W/PREVIOUS DENTAL TREATMENT, "FILLINGS FALLING OUT, ETC."
	EXPRESSED SOME FEAR OF TREATMENT ESPECIALLY RE: PERIO – SOME OF HER FRIENDS HAVE HAD SURGERY
	DR. REASSURED HER AS USUAL AND EXAM PROCEEDED

Fig. 4–24. Patient interview notes.

Special Examination Record

Another useful tool in a custom record system is the special examination form, which is used when greater depth and detail are required in a given area. An example might be a separate form for a comprehensive TMJ evaluation that is used only when needed. Such a form might list or diagram the associated muscles to be palpated and whether tenderness was found. It might include a history of patient symptoms and related findings (headaches, ear, nose, etc.) and a check list of treatment approaches to be employed (a kind of TMJ treatment plan). Many types of specialized examination records can be employed when the situation demands exhaustive information in one area but involves only a small percentage of patients in a practice (Fig. 4–25).

Oral Health Progress Record (OHPR)

An extremely useful tool in assessing the general oral-health level of the patient and following its progress over a period of time, an oral health progress record can take many forms; the example discussed

OCCLUSAL/TEMPOROMANDIBULAR JOINT EXAMINATION

PATIENT QUESTIONNAIRE

NAME ________________ SOCIAL SECURITY NO. ☐☐☐ ☐☐ ☐☐☐☐ AGE ☐☐

PLEASE CHECK ONLY ONE BOX IN EACH OF THE FOLLOWING:

13. SEX
- ☐ Male (1)
- ☐ Female (2)

14. RACE
- ☐ Caucasian (1)
- ☐ Negroid (2)
- ☐ Oriental (3)

15. MARITAL STATUS
- ☐ Single (1)
- ☐ Married (2)
- ☐ Separated (3)
- ☐ Divorced (4)
- ☐ Widowed (5)

16. EDUCATION
- ☐ Elementary (1)
- ☐ High School (2)
- ☐ Junior College (3)
- ☐ 4 Years College (4)
- ☐ Graduate School (5)

17. OCCUPATION
- ☐ Housewife (1)
- ☐ Professional (2)
- ☐ Managerial (3)
- ☐ Supervisorial (4)
- ☐ Clerical (5)
- ☐ Craftsman (6)
- ☐ Laborer (7)
- ☐ Student (8)
- ☐ Retired (9)

PLEASE ANSWER YES OR NO TO THE FOLLOWING QUESTIONS:

Yes No

18. ☐ ☐ Have you ever had orthodontic treatment?
19. ☐ ☐ Have you ever had periodontal disease (pyorrhea)?
20. ☐ ☐ Have you ever been treated for a "bad bite"?
21. ☐ ☐ Do you have extensive dental crowns and bridges?
22. ☐ ☐ Do you wear a removable partial denture?
23. ☐ ☐ Do you have missing back teeth and no replacement?
24. ☐ ☐ Have you ever been treated for problems of your jaw joint, or for facial muscle spasms?
25. ☐ ☐ Do you ever awaken with awareness of your teeth or jaws?
26. ☐ ☐ Are you aware of clenching your teeth during the day?
27. ☐ ☐ Have you ever been told that you grind your teeth during sleep?
28. ☐ ☐ Do your teeth hurt from biting?
29. ☐ ☐ Do you have any pain or soreness around your eyes, ears or other parts of your face?
30. ☐ ☐ Do you have "tension" headaches?
31. ☐ ☐ Do you ever have migraine headaches?
32. ☐ ☐ Do you frequently have neckaches or stiff neck muscles?
33. ☐ ☐ Do your jaw muscles become tired frequently?
34. ☐ ☐ Do you have difficulty in opening your mouth widely?
35. ☐ ☐ Do you have difficulty in swallowing?
36. ☐ ☐ Have you ever had arthritis?
37. ☐ ☐ Have you ever had gout?
38. ☐ ☐ Have you ever received a severe blow to the side of the head or jaw?
39. ☐ ☐ Have you ever had pain in your jaw joint?
40. ☐ ☐ Have you ever had problems with your ears, such as ringing or change of hearing?
41. ☐ ☐ Do you ever hear grating sounds from your jaw joint?
42. ☐ ☐ Do you ever hear clicking or popping sounds from your jaw joint?
43. ☐ ☐ Do you feel your bite is closed?
44. ☐ ☐ Are you presently in any pain from your jaw joint or muscles?
45. ☐ ☐ Does pain or discomfort from your jaw joint interfere with your work or other activities?
46. ☐ ☐ Are there times when you notice that this problem or pain is less or gone completely?
47. ☐ ☐ Are you afraid your problem is serious?
48. ☐ ☐ Do you feel you need treatment for this problem?
49. ☐ ☐ Do you have a problem with insomnia?
50. ☐ ☐ Do you take aspirin frequently?
51. ☐ ☐ Are you taking any tranquilizers, hypnotics, muscle relaxants or anti-depressants?
52. ☐ ☐ Do you take more than one alcoholic drink per day?
53. ☐ ☐ Do you smoke cigarettes or cigars?
54. ☐ ☐ Do you smoke a pipe?
55. ☐ ☐ Do you bite your nails, tongue or lips?
56. ☐ ☐ Do you have young children in your care?
57. ☐ ☐ Do you usually eat breakfast?

A CER 117

Fig. 4–25. Special examination records. *A,* Occlusal/temporomandibular joint patient questionnaire.

OCCLUSAL EXAMINATION

PATIENT:______________________ DATE:______________

1. **FIRST CONTACT IN CENTRIC RELATION:** R ______ | ______ L
2. **MANDIBULAR DISPLACEMENT:**
   - ☐ Anterior ________mm. ☐ To Right ________mm.
   - ☐ Vertical ________mm. ☐ To Left ________mm.
3. **LATERAL GUIDANCE FROM CENTRIC OCCLUSION:** R ______ | ______ L
4. **BALANCING INTERFERENCES:** R ______ | ______ L
   - ☐ None ☐ Early ☐ Light
   - ☐ Late ☐ Heavy
5. **PROTRUSIVE GUIDANCE:** R ______ | ______ L
   - ☐ Key-In-Lock Facets ☐ Deflection to Right
   - ☐ Posterior Interference ☐ Deflection to Left
6. **INHIBITED MOVEMENTS:**

	Slight	Moderate	Marked
☐ None			
☐ Right Lateral	☐	☐	☐
☐ Left Lateral	☐	☐	☐
☐ Protrusive	☐	☐	☐

7. **TOOTH MOBILITY:** R ______ | ______ L
   - ☐ None ☐ I ☐ II ☐ III
8. **OPEN CONTACTS:** R ______ | ______ L
   - ☐ None ☐ Developmental ☐ Migration
9. **ABNORMAL WEAR:** R ______ | ______ L
   - ☐ None ☐ Moderate ☐ Severe
10. **CUSP FRACTURE:** R ______ | ______ L
    - ☐ None ☐ Working ☐ Balancing
11. **WIDENED PERIODONTAL SPACE:** R ______ | ______ L
    - ☐ None ☐ Hour-Glass
    - ☐ Uniform ☐ Occlusal Flaring
12. **ALVEOLAR BONE LOSS:** R ______ | ______ L
    - ☐ Lamina Dura ☐ Mild
    - ☐ Vertical ☐ Moderate
    - ☐ Horizontal ☐ Severe
13. **LOCAL RESPONSE:** R ______ | ______ L
    - ☐ None ☐ Osteosclerosis
    - ☐ Hypercementosis ☐ Root Resorption
14. **PERIODONTAL EXAMINATION:** (Pocket Depth) R ______ | ______ L
    - ☐ 4 mm.+ ☐ 5 mm.+ ☐ 6 mm.+
15. **PHONETICS:**
    - "F" Position: ☐ Favorable ☐ Labial ☐ Elongated
    - ☐ Lingual ☐ Lip Strain
    - "S" Position: ☐ Favorable ☐ Class II ☐ Tongue Position
    - ☐ Class III ☐ Air Escape
16. **ESTHETICS:**
    - **Smile Line:** ☐ Complimentary ☐ Flat ☐ Reversed ☐ Distorted
    - **Spine Inclination:** ☐ Lingual ☐ Vertical ☐ Labial ☐ Rotated
    - **Dento-Facial Relation:**
      - ☐ Harmonious ☐ Prominent ☐ Strong ☐ Size
      - ☐ Discrepancy ☐ Normal ☐ Soft ☐ Position
      - ☐ Retruded ☐ Delicate ☐ Restorative Need
    - Anterior Overjet: ________mm.
    - Anterior Overbite: ________mm.

17. **MIDLINE DEVIATION:**
    - Maxillary: ☐ None ☐ Right ___mm. ☐ Left ___mm.
    - Mandibular: ☐ None ☐ Right ___mm. ☐ Left ___mm.
18. **MANDIBULAR DEFLECTION ON OPENING:**
    - ☐ None ☐ To Right ☐ To Left
    - R 15 10 5 0 5 10 L mm.
19. **MANDIBULAR MOVEMENT:** **MAXIMUM OPENING:** ________mm.
    - ☐ Normal ☐ Right Lateral ☐ Acute ☐ Hypermobility
    - ☐ Restricted ☐ Left Lateral ☐ Recurrent ☐ Chronic Subluxation
    - ☐ Painful ☐ Protrusive ☐ Chronic ☐ Spontaneous Dislocation
20. **TEMPOROMANDIBULAR PAIN HISTORY:**
    - ☐ Negative ☐ Upon Awakening ☐ Acute ☐ Slipping
    - ☐ Right TMJ ☐ During Eating ☐ Recurrent ☐ Interference
    - ☐ Left TMJ ☐ When Yawning ☐ Chronic ☐ Rubbing
21. **TEMPOROMANDIBULAR JOINT NOISE:**
    - ☐ Negative ☐ Crepitus ☐ Immediate ☐ Patient Unaware
    - ☐ Right TMJ ☐ Clicking ☐ Normal Range ☐ Recurrent
    - ☐ Left TMJ ☐ Popping ☐ Wide Range ☐ Chronic
22. **TEMPOROMANDIBULAR PALPATION:**
    - ☐ Negative ☐ Popping ☐ Externally ☐ Opening
    - ☐ Right TMJ ☐ Sore ☐ From Auditory Canal ☐ Closing
    - ☐ Left TMJ ☐ Painful ☐ Without Movement ☐ Eccentric
23. **MUSCULAR PALPATION:**
    - ☐ Negative
    - ☐ Masseter R L
    - ☐ Temporalis R L
    - ☐ Lateral Pterygoid R L
    - ☐ Medial Pterygoid R L
    - ☐ Digastric R L
    - ☐ Sternocleidomastoid R L
    - ☐ Hyoid Area R L
    - ☐ Occipital Area R L
    - ☐ Shoulder Area R L

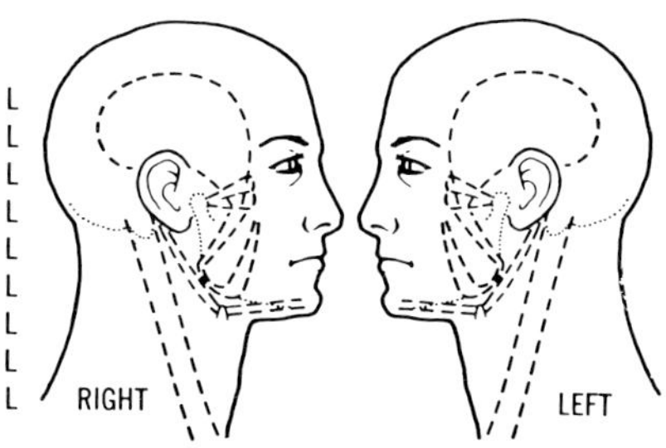

24. **MUSCULAR PAIN:**
    - ☐ Negative ☐ Facial Pain ☐ History ☐ Acute
    - ☐ Right Side ☐ Neck Aches ☐ Extrinsic ☐ Recurrent
    - ☐ Left Side ☐ Shoulder Pain ☐ Intrinsic ☐ Chronic
25. **CLENCHING TEETH:**
    - ☐ Negative ☐ During Day ☐ Anterior Bracing ☐ Acute
    - ☐ Suspected ☐ At Night ☐ Morning Awareness ☐ Recurrent
    - ☐ Patient Aware ☐ Under Stress ☐ Resultant Sore Mouth ☐ Chronic
26. **BRUXISM:**
    - ☐ Negative ☐ Retrusive ☐ Mild ☐ Acute
    - ☐ Suspected ☐ Protrusive ☐ Moderate ☐ Recurrent
    - ☐ Patient Aware ☐ Lateral ☐ Severe ☐ Chronic
27. **CHRONIC HEADACHES:**
    - ☐ Negative ☐ Minutes ________Times Per Month
    - ☐ Mild ☐ Hours Medication: ________
    - ☐ Moderate ☐ All Day Amount: ________Per Month
    - ☐ Migraine ☐ Days (_____)
28. **EMOTIONAL STRESS LEVEL:**
    - ☐ Negative ☐ Probable ☐ Medication ________
    - ☐ Questionable ☐ Pronounced OHIQ Presemex________
29. **POSSIBLE TREATMENT:**
    - ☐ None ☐ TMJ X-Ray ☐ Drug Therapy
    - ☐ Limited Restorative Work ☐ Inject TMJ ☐ Orthodontic Treatment
    - ☐ Occlusal Reconstruction ☐ Local Anesthetic ☐ Periodontal Treatment
    - ☐ Limited Occlusal Adjustment ☐ Occlusal Splint ☐ Endodontic Treatment
    - ☐ Occlusal Equilibration ☐ Muscle Exercises ☐ Surgical Consultation
    - ☐ ☐ ☐ ☐ ☐ ☐ Heat ☐ Medical Consultation

B

CER. 115 DENTAL PRINTING • BOX 730, PARADISE, CALIFORNIA 95969

Fig. 4–25 *continued.* *B*, Occlusal/temporomandibular joint examination record.

3 DAY FOOD INVENTORY

Before starting to fill out this form, please read and then follow the instructions given on the reverse, carefully.

Name__________ Date__________ Phone__________

1st Day	PROT.	Ca++	A.A.	GOOD	BAD	2nd Day	PROT.	Ca++	A.A.	GOOD	BAD	3rd Day	PROT.	Ca++	A.A.	GOOD	BAD
Breakfast						Breakfast						Breakfast					
Midmorning Snack						Midmorning Snack						Midmorning Snack					
Noon						Noon						Noon					
Between Meals Snack						Between Meals Snack						Between Meals Snack					
Evening						Evening						Evening					
Bedtime Snack						Bedtime Snack						Bedtime Snack					

CER: 152– DENTAL PRINTING, P.O. BOX 730, PARADISE, CALIF. 95969 FROM: DR. A. CHARI

C

Fig. 4–25 *continued.* C, 3-day food inventory. (All by permission of Dr. Carl Rieder.)

The foods you eat have much to do with your general and oral health. To help in evaluation of your diet, please record in detail the food and drink you have consumed for a period of at least ______ day___. Recommendations and suggestions, if any, will constitute part of your treatment.

INSTRUCTIONS FOR THE USE OF THE FOOD DIARY

1. In the proper squares on the reverse side, immediately after each meal, record the time and all the food and drink you have consumed.
2. It is important that you continue your normal eating habits during the recording period.
3. Please list all the items in detail. Do not leave even the smallest item out (gum, colas, cakes, etc.)
4. Please use the following abbreviations:

T – tablespoonful	cn – canned	sm – small	gl – glass
t – teaspoonful	s – sugar	md – medium	bl – black
c – cup	sl – slice	lg – large	

5. Be sure to state the amount of each food eaten, such as:

INCORRECT	CORRECT
Juice	4 oz. Fresh Orance Juice
American Cheese Sandwich	American Cheese 2 sl., white bread 2 sl 1 leaf lettuce, ½ tomato, butter
Coffee	1 c coffee, 2 ts, with 2 T milk
Dessert	1 c peaches, cn
Vegetables	½ c peas, cn
Potato	1 md baked potato

6. **Please write clearly:**

Medications ______ Vitamins ______ Prescribed/Self ______ Height ______ Weight ______

Most recent weight gain or loss. Gain ______ Loss ______ lbs. Period of time ______

Meals: Regular ______ Irregular ______ Family ______ Alone ______

Appetite: Good ______ Bad ______ Cigarettes per day ______

Liquid intake glasses per day: Water ______ Coffee ______ Tea ______ Juice ______

Approximate meat consumption in lbs. per day: ______

Urinating frequency during the day ______ at night ______

Food dislikes: ______

Food allergies: ______

Food preferred: ______

General well being: Excellent ______ Good ______ Tired ______

Or use your own words in describing how you feel: ______

______

D Is your diet medically controlled? ______

Fig. 4–25 *continued.* *D*, 3-day food inventory (back side).

here has three main elements. First, it employs a multifactorial scoring system, based on written criteria, to note plaque level, stain and calculus, condition of the gingival tissues, and patient acceptance of preventive counseling. The criteria used to establish a numerical score are designed to provide uniformity among examiners, hence the limited number of categories. More importantly, the criteria are designed so that a score of "0" or "1" indicates optimal or good oral-health status, a score of "2" indicates a potential problem or early pathology, and a score of "3" in any category indicates serious problems of oral-health maintenance. There is nothing magical in the scoring system; it is simply a clinical evaluation that is standardized by the criteria. The criteria could easily be expanded if a wider range of numerical values was desired, or standardized systems of plaque and bleeding (plaque index, gingival bleeding index) could be used instead. This system opts for the relative simplicity of limited categories so that any auxiliary can carry out the scoring. Its main purpose is to differentiate between conditions that are not clinically dangerous and those that may be or are pathologic (Table 4–1).

Table 4–1. Criteria for Oral Health Progress Scoring

PLAQUE
- 0 Plaque free—no observable plaque with disclosant
- 1 Slight plaque—five teeth or less (is using floss)
- 2 Slight plaque—six teeth or more (generalized)
- 3 Moderate to heavy plaque (generalized)
- 4 Gross plaque and debris—no evidence of brushing or any oral-hygiene efforts

STAIN/CALCULUS
- 0 None
- 1 Very slight—lower linguals or upper buccals only
- 2 Moderate—requiring definite scaling and polishing
- 3 Heavy—requiring cavitron or multiple sittings

TISSUE (BLEEDING)
- 0 No observable inflammation or bleeding with probe or floss*
- 1 Slight inflammation, some bleeding with probe or floss*
- 2 Generalized inflammation, bleeding, with *pockets* measuring 3 mm or more
- 3 Periodontal disease

PROGRAM ACCEPTANCE
- 0 Patient is enthusiastic, volunteers information, uses disclosant at home
- 1 Receptive, interested, will respond to questions readily
- 2 Skeptical, but communicative
- 3 Disinterested—noncommittal or refuses preventive services

*Probe or floss interproximally five teeth: mesial interproximal nos. 3, 6, 13, 18, 27

The second element of the OHPR is its graphic depiction of subsequent evaluations over time. It is possible to see at a glance not only how the patient is faring in oral-health maintenance, but whether there has been improvement or decline with each succeeding visit or recall appointment. As the dentist-patient contact progresses over a number of years, it becomes exceedingly difficult to wade through all the treatment notes to determine the patient's progress or lack of it. The graphic nature of the OHPR greatly aids in this respect (Fig. 4–26 A).

The third element of the OHPR is the check-off system to indicate what preventive procedures were done and what types of instructions or counselling were given on each visit. Again, it is extremely helpful to see graphically and in one place what has been done in this regard, so as to avoid repetition of an instructional film, for example, or to see when the patient's flossing techniques were last reviewed and reinforced (Fig. 4–26 B).

The use of the OHPR is illustrated in the following sample, which is taken from an actual patient record. The first scoring represents the initial patient visit with the hygienist. The second scoring is following restorative dental treatment and the third at two follow-up recall visits. Subsequent scorings reflect periodic recalls over some time (Fig. 4–27).

This oral health progress record serves three main purposes. First, it is an excellent clinical tool both in evaluating and following the general oral health of the patient. Incipient problems can often be discovered with the OHPR when a score falls from "1" to "2" in a given category. Significant improvement can be noted and preventive efforts recorded in minimum space and time. Secondly, the OHPR can be used as a motivational tool for the patient. Many patients find it challenging to try to improve a numerical score and are motivated in their oral-health maintenance efforts. High praise is given whenever a score improves, thereby providing positive reinforcement for an accomplishment that the patient can see, perhaps more clearly than he sees the improvement in the clinical condition in the mouth. Thirdly, the OHPR positively documents the patient's level of maintenance and our efforts to improve or upgrade it. Legally, it demonstrates that the dentist has fulfilled his responsibility in the prevention of oral disease and that the patient has been informed of and instructed about his responsibilities. One hopes not to have need of such documentation, but having it gives a certain peace of mind, especially with those patients who cannot or will not maintain reasonable levels of health and hygiene.

date:										
PLAQUE	0 1 2 3 4	0 1 2 3 4	0 1 2 3 4	0 1 2 3 4	0 1 2 3 4	0 1 2 3 4	0 1 2 3 4	0 1 2 3 4	0 1 2 3 4	0 1 2 3 4
STAIN/ CALCULUS	0 1 2 3	0 1 2 3	0 1 2 3	0 1 2 3	0 1 2 3	0 1 2 3	0 1 2 3	0 1 2 3	0 1 2 3	0 1 2 3
TISSUE (BLEEDING)	0 1 2 3	0 1 2 3	0 1 2 3	0 1 2 3	0 1 2 3	0 1 2 3	0 1 2 3	0 1 2 3	0 1 2 3	0 1 2 3
PROGRAM ACCEPTANCE	0 1 2 3	0 1 2 3	0 1 2 3	0 1 2 3	0 1 2 3	0 1 2 3	0 1 2 3	0 1 2 3	0 1 2 3	0 1 2 3

A

NEW CARIES										
DISC										
P & P										
TBI										
FLS										
DIET										
FILM:										
KIT										
BRUSH										
"D" TABS										
COMMENTS										

B

Fig. 4–26. *A*, Oral Health Progress Record Scoring Graph. *B*, Oral Health Progress Record Check List.

date:	3-5-75	3-12-75	3-26-75	7-1-75	1-8-76	7-15-76	7-27-76			
PLAQUE	0 1 2 (3) 4	0 1 (2) 3 4	0 (1) 2 3 4	0 1 (2) 3 4	0 (1) 2 3 4	0 1 2 (3) 4	(0) 1 2 3 4	0 1 2 3 4	0 1 2 3 4	0 1 2 3 4
STAIN/ CALCULUS	0 1 2 (3)	(0) 1 2 3	(0) 1 2 3	0 (1) 2 3	0 (1) 2 3	0 1 (2) 3	(0) 1 2 3	0 1 2 3	0 1 2 3	0 1 2 3
TISSUE (BLEEDING)	0 1 (2) 3	0 (1) 2 3	(0) 1 2 3	0 (1) 2 3	0 (1) 2 3	0 1 (2) 3	(0) 1 2 3	0 1 2 3	0 1 2 3	0 1 2 3
PROGRAM ACCEPTANCE	0 1 (2) 3	0 (1) 2 3	0 (1) 2 3	0 (1) 2 3	0 (1) 2 3	0 (1) 2 3	(0) 1 2 3	0 1 2 3	0 1 2 3	0 1 2 3
NEW CARIES	YES	—	—	—	—	YES	—			
DISC	✓	✓	✓	✓	✓		✓			
P & P	✓					✓				
TBI	✓	REV	REV	✓	REV	✓	REV			
FLS	INTRO	✓	REV	✓	REV	✓	REV			
DIET		✓								
FILM:	P&P	TRIGGER FOODS								
KIT	✓					✓				
BRUSH				✓						
"D" TABS			✓				✓			
COMMENTS	ABILITY GOOD DIGEST REPRINT		MUCH IMPROVED			PT. HAS HAD PROBLEMS AT HOME— RE-EMPHASIZED PREV. SET UP FOR ADD'L APPT.				

Fig. 4–27. OHPR over 16 months. Again, it is easy to see at a glance how well the patient has been maintaining oral health and what the dental team has done on each preventive visit.

Legal Aspects of Dental Records

We live in an era of increasing litigation. As a result of mass-media reports about spectacular settlements in various types of liability actions, many people believe that lawsuits are the way to instant wealth; this has produced a climate of apprehension, if not fear, in the health professions. In this climate, it is important to maintain a sense of perspective. We should always remember that the standards by which we are judged (if we find ourselves being judged) are not found in legal texts or courtroom precedents: we are measured by our own standards. If we adhere to the high standard of dental practice that is taught in dental schools and practiced throughout the country, we need to do little else from a legal standpoint. I hasten to add that a high standard of dental practice does not only mean good technical performance; patient involvement, good communication, and good records are standards of dental practice that have value in dental treatment and can prevent the legal entanglements we all abhor. Therefore, I will discuss the legal aspects of dental records not from the standpoint of what one should do to prevent litigation or defend against it should it come, but rather how the dental records we develop for good patient treatment can also serve those ends. It is beyond the scope of this chapter to include all the legal ramifications of dental practice; entire texts have been written addressing the topic. However, dental records are highly significant in legal terms, because good record keeping is a standard of practice to which we can be held and because records document all our dealings with the dental patient.

With this in mind, I will discuss briefly some of the most important legal aspects of dental records:

1. *Have records.* As obvious as it may seem, there have been cases of litigation in which the dentist had no written record of his dealings with a patient. Whether the records were lost, misplaced, or never made in the first place, failure to keep records can pit your word (and memory) against that of a plaintiff patient's; since record keeping is an accepted standard of practice, the lack of records alone may be legally damning. In financial matters, lack of records may allow the Internal Revenue Service to make its own estimate of your income and to tax you accordingly. Now if one is doing something obviously illegal or unethical, written records might not be a good idea, but if errors of judgment or execution are made in the course of good-faith treatment, the patient should be told what has happened and the event should be immediately and accurately recorded.

In informing the patient of what has occurred, it is not necessary to admit negligence or to apologize; the disclosure should be phrased in neutral terms. Such candor with the patient is likely to prevent the initiation of most litigation. In the event that legal action ensues, the fact that disclosure was made immediately and the event recorded can be significant factors in the defense of the dentist. Any human being can make errors, but *covering up the error is often worse than the error itself.*

2. *Have good records.* If we are going to keep written records, they should be good ones. The criteria for dental records that were discussed previously in this chapter can be applied here.

An actual example of a situation in which accurate and complete records stopped a potential legal action involved an unpaid account that had been turned over to a collection agency. The patient retained an attorney and claimed that the fees charged were twice what had been estimated. The dental records included a complete treatment plan with estimated fees corresponding to the actual fees charged, a record of case presentation in which the total fee was presented, insurance coverage discussed, payments agreed upon, and a copy of a follow-up letter sent to the patient reviewing and reiterating the arrangement. When the patient's attorney received copies of the records (for which a reasonable fee was charged), the issue was dropped, the collection action proceeded uneventfully, and a judgment was rendered in favor of the dentist. The fact that the judgment has yet to be actually collected is interesting but immaterial. The point is that a potential countersuit was quickly eliminated simply on the basis of good records. Complete and accurate dental records provide the maximum protection to the dentist in legal proceedings, and one cannot wait for a subpoena to arrive before one develops good records.

A good means of evaluating one's records is to draw three or four patient's charts at random and pretend that copies of same have been subpoenaed for an impending legal action. Would they measure up? Would you care to testify using them as your memory? Would you be tempted to add to or alter them? If so, don't do it—altering records could result in criminal charges being brought against you. It is better to resolve that all future records will be up to standards and hope that you won't need those that aren't. If your records appear to be grossly lacking and they have not yet been subpoenaed, you may want to upgrade them as patients come in on recall visits.

3. *Retention and control.* It is generally accepted as a legal principle that medical and dental records are the property of the practitioner, not the patient. Fees paid by the patient for examination and x-rays are for the interpretation and diagnosis, not for the

physical records (films, charts, etc.) themselves. The dentist can always be required to produce originals or copies of records upon court order, such as a subpoena or a search warrant. Many states now have laws requiring that records be made available to a patient upon request without court order, based on the thinking that an individual has certain rights to his or her medical or dental records as a matter of course. Finally, in most cases, it is in the best interest of the patient to release copies of records to another dentist to permit more informed diagnoses and possibly reduce unnecessary radiation exposure. Guidelines for the release of dental records are simple and should be strictly adhered to:

(a) Release records only upon written request of the patient. This may be a letter, a form kept on file (authorizing release to insurance carriers, etc.), or even a handwritten note. Do not release records without the patient's signed authorization.

(b) Release only copies of records, never the originals themselves. Double film packs allow for duplicate radiographs, or simple radiograph-duplicating devices can be used. Charts can be duplicated easily if the office has a copier; local libraries or commercial printers may have copiers available at a nominal cost. While many dentists forward such records as a courtesy, a reasonable charge can and often should be made for the service.

An exception to the copy-only rule might be the submission of preoperative radiographs to a third party for predetermination of benefit, or to a specialist or another dentist for consultation or second opinion. In these cases, one would expect the radiographs to be returned prior to any treatment being rendered, and one would not want to lose diagnostic quality through duplication. If original records are released for any reason, when and where they were sent should be noted in the patient chart and logged again when they are returned. The release of copied records should also be noted in the patient chart, along with the signed authorization.

(c) Never release more than is authorized or requested.

The question of how long to retain dental records is sure to produce various answers. The safest policy, if space permits, is to retain them forever; for some dentists, this is possible but for most, it is a cumbersome solution at best and often impossible. Common sense suggests that, once the statute of limitations has run out on potential litigation arising from dental treatment, the dental record could be destroyed. The time involved here varies from state to state, and one must take care that while the statute for professional negligence (malpractice) may expire after 3 years, another statute covering willful injury may run longer. For the legally competent adult, dental records can be destroyed after the longer statute has expired. An attorney's advice in determining this length of time is generally advised for each state and locality. In the case of patients who have what are termed legal "disabilities"—that is, children, mentally retarded individuals, prisoners—the statutes do not begin to run until the disability is removed. In the case of children, this would be the age of 18. Therefore, if a patient was last seen at age 10 and the longest pertinent statute is 7 years, the records must be retained for at least 15 years—the 8 years between age 10 and the age of majority (at which time the legal "disability" is removed) and the 7 following years (assuming a statute of limitations on willful injuries of 7 years). Finally, if mentally retarded patients or people who are declared incompetent are treated, the legal disability might never be removed and those patients' records must be kept forever.

Retirement or even death of the dentist does not mean that records can be destroyed, since legal actions can be brought against the estate of the deceased. Provisions should always be made for the retention and control of original dental records, even if the practice changes hands or the dentist dies.

4. *The "magical signature."* It is often the impression among people not in the legal profession that a signature on some document makes that document more legally significant than it might otherwise be. For example, if questions arise about information gathered in a health history, having a patient's signature affixed to the history is probably a good idea. However, the existence of an unsigned written history, whether completed by the patient or taken orally and completed by the dentist is probably just as significant as one signed by the patient. Most lay people underestimate the weight of simple testimony. The dentist who can testify that he did take a health history from the patient in question, that it is his usual practice to do so, and that the unsigned written history in the patient's dental chart reflects the information elicited, need not worry that the patient's signature does not appear. Likewise, a signed health history that does not elicit information about allergies to drugs will be of little help if a patient develops an anaphylactic reaction to your prescription. Patient signatures are also in great demand on so-called "consent" statements. It should be helpful to discuss briefly the concept of "consent" or "informed consent," as it applies to the dental situation.

Consent

It is obviously true that a dentist cannot legally treat a patient without his consent. The image of a gowned dentist sneaking up behind an unsuspecting

Presented to patient 9-17-81. Patient agreed to proceed.

RBM

TENTATIVE TREATMENT

Systemic: PENICILLIN ALLERGY

Emergency/Investigative:

REMOVE CROWN UPPER RIGHT FIRST MOLAR, REMOVE DECAY, PLACE TEMPORARY RESTORATION $45

Preparatory: SCALING, PREVENTIVE INSTRUCTIONS COMPLETED

FOLLOW-UP SESSION TO POLISH AND REVIEW $25

REMOVE LOWER LEFT THIRD MOLAR (PARTIAL IMPACTION) $45

SILVER AMALGAM: 10 SURFACES ON 4 TEETH $115

COMPOSITE RESIN: 2 TEETH--UPPER FRONT $52

(POSSIBLE ROOT CANAL THERAPY UPPER RIGHT FIRST MOLAR, PENDING RESULT OF STEP 1 $225)

Corrective: PORCELAIN FUSED TO GOLD CROWN UPPER RIGHT FIRST MOLAR--PENDING RESOLUTION OF PULPAL STATUS $315

Maintenance: 6 MONTH RECALL VISITS

Fig. 4–28. Written treatment plan with notation of patient acceptance.

WILLIAM L. NEQUETTE AND ASSOCIATES, LTD.
PRACTICE OF DENTISTRY
14021 WEST GREENFIELD AVENUE
NEW BERLIN, WISCONSIN 53151
TELEPHONE (414) 782-4860

Dec. 1, 1982

WILLIAM L. NEQUETTE, D.D.S.
CHARLES W. McCAULEY, D.D.S.
ROBERT B. MORRIS, D.D.S.
THOMAS S. RYPEL, D.D.S.
KENNETH J. WALISZEWSKI, D.D.S., M.S.
JAMES C. HOVE, D.D.S.

REVIEW OF TREATMENT PLAN AND FEES: MRS. JANE DOE

Dear Jane,

This letter is to review and confirm the arrangements we discussed for your dental treatment. At your next visit we plan to remove the crown on the tooth which has been bothering you, remove the decay under it, and, if possible, place a temporary crown.

Following that, we plan to see you for a follow-up hygiene visit, and we hope to see continued improvement in the condition of your gum tissue.

The lower left third molar (wisdom tooth) must be removed to prevent future problems such as you had when we first saw you last month.

A total of six teeth (2 front, 4 back) will require fillings, composite resin (tooth colored) in front, silver amalgam in back.

Depending on the response of the upper right molar we may have to consider root canal treatment if the nerve has been affected. In either event a new crown (porcelain fused to gold) will be needed.

The total fee (not including root canal) will be approximately $600.

You indicated you would make an initial payment of $200, followed by $80/month payments for 5 months or until the balance is paid. If root canal becomes necessary on upper right molar you indicated you would pay that at the time of treatment. Would you kindly sign one copy of this review and bring it along next time, or send it with your initial payment.

Sincerely yours,

Robert B. Morris, D.D.S. ______________________ Patient signature

Fig. 4–29. Written review of treatment plan to be signed by patient.

citizen on the street, administering local anesthetic, and surreptitiously placing a restoration comes to mind and is rather far fetched. The patient's informed consent simply means that the patient understands what you are going to do and agrees to let you do it. The patient who calls your office and makes an appointment for cleaning, examination, and necessary radiographs has, in effect, consented to those procedures. This does not mean that a routine explanation of what is going to be done is not in order; it simply means that a written consent to perform those services is superfluous. One obvious exception to this statement is a case in which the patient is not a legally responsible adult. If you are dealing with a child, or any legally disabled individual, the consent of a parent or guardian is necessary. Again, the act bringing the child to your office for an examination/cleaning appointment is sufficient. If the child arrives for his first visit unaccompanied, at the very least, a phone call to parents confirming their consent for the proposed treatment is essential.

Beyond the initial diagnostic phase, a course of treatment might be outlined and proposed to the patient. A written record of the proposed course of treatment and its presentation to the patient is essential, along with a record of the patient's acceptance of the plan. If the treatment and its possible complications (those most likely to occur) have been explained to the patient and the patient elects to proceed, consent has been obtained.

While this is the minimal requirement, the patient-oriented dentist will explain at every appointment what is to be done and why and the possible common complications of treatment. This is the best and most rational way to ensure informed consent, as people do tend to forget what they are told rather quickly.

With this brief background on consent, we return to the "magical signature" and what it can and cannot do for us. If a treatment plan has been presented to the patient and it has been accepted and all of this information has been documented in the record, the patient's signature is probably not necessary (Fig. 4–28). On the other hand, if there were to be a question of consent raised in the future, having the patient's initial or signature in the record might be helpful. Even more helpful might be a copy of a letter or treatment plan signed by the patient, who has been given the original (Fig. 4–29). Finally, if one wishes to be fully protected in the consent department, a simple statement such as the one in Figure 4–30 can be employed. It should be emphasized that all such documentation, while potentially helpful, may not prevent a patient from claiming negligence and fraud if he wants to. If the patient did not understand what

WILLIAM L. NEQUETTE AND ASSOCIATES, LTD.

NAME Jane Doe DATE Dec 1, '82
ADDRESS 234 Pine St. PHONE 222-2222

At this time, the following services are to be performed:

[X] PREVENTIVE TREATMENT Follow-up hygiene session
[X] PERIODONTAL TREATMENT
[X] ORAL SURGERY Remove lower left wisdom tooth
[X] OPERATIVE DENTISTRY (fillings) 10 surfaces amalgam (4 teeth)
2 composite resins (front teeth)
[X] CROWNS/BRIDGES Porcelain/gold crown, upper right first molar
[ ] ORTHODONTICS
[X] OTHER Possible root canal upper right first molar
Removal of old crown and temporary restoration

At a total estimated fee of $600

INSURANCE:
Pre-estimate of coverage: NONE
Patient's portion (approximate)

The treatment summarized above and its possible complications have been discussed with me, and I have consented to proceed with it. I also agree to pay the fee (or my portion) on the following basis:

[ ] FULL AMOUNT (CASH OR CHECK) AS TREATMENT PROCEEDS WITH 5% DISCOUNT.
[ ] MASTERCHARGE/VISA, CHARGED AS TREATMENT PROCEEDS.
[ ] FULL AMOUNT ON MONTHLY STATEMENT WITHIN 10 DAYS OF RECEIPT.
[X] IN THE FOLLOWING INSTALLMENTS: $200 down, then $80/month for 5 months or until balance is paid. If root canal is required, will be paid in full at time of treatment.

There is no finance or interest charge to be paid provided the payment arrangement is adhered to. This arrangement is for the above treatment only and further treatment will be paid when rendered, or on the basis of future arrangements.

Signature of Dentist or Staff — Signature of Patient (or Parent if Patient is minor) — Dec 5, 1982 Date

Fig. 4–30. Treatment agreement with consent statement.

he was signing and can convince a judge or jury that he did not understand, the signature is worthless. For this reason, note that plain, simple English is used in the samples shown. All too often we hide behind a sea of "whereas's," "heretofore's," and "hereunder's" that certainly sound legal but may render the statement worthless. Consider the real worth of this consent statement:

> I, the undersigned, do hereby and forthwith consent, agree to, and subscribe in toto to the aforementioned stomatognathic procedures as listed in this document to which hereunder my signature is affixed.

and compare it to this statement:

> The treatment summarized above and its possible complications have been discussed with me and I have consented to proceed with it.

Neither statement is any more or less legally binding and either could be repudiated by a plaintiff patient. However, it would be more difficult to claim

I, the undersigned, hereby grant permission for diagnosis and or treatment in this dental office for myself or for the minor patient hereunder named. In consideration of acceptance for diagnosis and or treatment, I hereby release and forever discharge the dentists, their agents or employees of and from any claims of liability of any kind and nature arising out of dental services performed, or in any way connected with service or advice at this dental office. In regard to any and all claims on behalf of the hereunder named minor patient, I agree to release the above parties from all liability.

signatures, etc.

Fig. 4–31. An example, slightly paraphrased, of a "bad" consent form that is actually in use. Would you, as a patient, sign something like this?

the second statement was not understood, than the first. We should strive for clarity and simplicity in all our communications with patients.

This discussion concludes with a warning on what the "magical signature" cannot do for the dentist. Despite the advice given in some texts, the patient's signature under a legal-sounding statement cannot absolve the dentist or his staff of negligence and cannot prevent or deter the patient from exercising his legal rights. Any consent statement that releases the dentist from the responsibility that is his under the law or holds harmless the dentist and/or dental auxiliaries, isn't worth the paper it's printed on. No one can sign his legal rights away; indeed, anyone who knows what he is signing would not do so willingly. The consent cited in Figure 4–31 is an example of such a release and besides being cumbersome in its wording, it is useless both as a defense against negligence and a proof of informed consent. We would strongly urge dentists to avoid form legal statements, or at least those that include terms such as "hereunder affixed," and to opt instead for simply worded statements that anyone can understand (you may have your attorney review these statements to make sure that you have not unwittingly created more problems than you have solved). Clear and simple statements make for the best communication, and good communication provides for informed consent.

Today's legal climate requires that we do evaluate our dental records from the standpoint of their value in potential litigation. It is important, however, that we not become paranoid and do a lot of unnecessary things "to protect ourselves." Good dentistry, good records, good communication, and common sense add up to the best legal insurance we can have.

REFERENCES

1. Akerly, W.B.: Tripodal method of recording centric relation. J. Prosthet. Dent., *42*:461–465, 1979.
2. Antel, J., et al: Electrical pulp testing. J. Can. Dent. Assoc., *45*:597–600, 1979.
3. Bhaskar, S.N.: Radiographic Interpretation for the Dentist. 3rd Ed. St. Louis, C.V. Mosby, 1979.
4. Brown, W.T., and Bauer, J.C.: Today's approach to tomorrow's dentistry: Comprehensive oral health care. J. Acad. Gen. Dent., *27*(3):54–59, 1979.
5. Burket, L.W.: Oral Medicine, Diagnosis, and Treatment. 7th Ed. Philadelphia, J.B. Lippincott, 1977.
6. Chadha, J.M., and Rayson, J.H.: Diagnostic casts. *In* Clinical Dentistry. Vol. 1. Edited by J.W. Clark. Hagerstown, Harper and Row, 1979.
7. Clark, J.W., et al.: Clinical Dentistry. Hagerstown, Harper and Row, 1979.
8. Cohen, L.: Oral Diagnosis and Treatment Planning. Springfield, Charles C Thomas, 1973.
9. Davis, C.O.: The personal health history. *In* Clinical Dentistry. Vol. 1. Edited by J.W. Clark. Hagerstown, Harper and Row, 1979.
10. Dawson, P.E.: Evaluation, Diagnosis, and Treatment of Occlusal Problems. St. Louis, C.V. Mosby, 1974.
11. Freehe, C.L.: Clinical dental photography: Equipment and techniques. *In* Clinical Dentistry. Vol. 1. Edited by J.W. Clark. Hagerstown, Harper and Row, 1979.
12. Glickman, I.: Glickman's Clinical Periodontology: Prevention, Diagnosis, and Treatment of Periodontal Disease in the Practice of General Dentistry. 5th Ed., rev. Philadelphia, W.B. Saunders, 1979.
13. Goldman, H.M., and Cohen, D.W.: Periodontal Therapy. 6th Ed. St. Louis, C.V. Mosby, 1980.
14. Harper, P.L.: Laboratory values—normal, abnormal, and their significance. *In* Facial Trauma and Concomitant Problems, Evaluation and Treatment. Edited by W.B. Irby. St. Louis, C.V. Mosby, 1974.
15. Hirschfeld, L., and Wasserman, B.: A long-term study of tooth loss in 600 treated periodontal patients. J. Periodontol., *49*(5):225–237, 1978.
16. Kerr, D.A., Ash, M.M., and Millard, H.D.: Oral Diagnosis. 4th Ed. St. Louis, C.V. Mosby, 1974.
17. Knap, F. J., and Ziebert, G.J.: "Checkbite" technique in major oral reconstruction. J. Prosthet. Dent., *21*(4):458–465, 1969.
18. Komensky, A.M.: Ownership and maintenance of dental records. J.A.D.A., *97*:44–46, 1978.
19. Mesrobian, A.Z., and Barrett, R.: Laboratory diagnosis. *In* Clinical Dentistry. Vol. 1. Edited by J.W. Clark. Hagerstown, Harper and Row, 1979.
20. Mitchell, D.F., Standish, S.M., and Fast, T.B: Oral Diagnosis: Oral Medicine. 3rd Ed. Philadelphia, Lea & Febiger, 1978.
21. Ramfjord, S., and Ash, M.M.: Periodontology and Periodontics. Chicago, Yearbook Press, 1979.
22. Rieder, C.E.: Occlusal considerations in preventive care. J. Prosthet. Dent., *28*(5):462–468, 1972.
23. Rosenthal, D.S., and Maloney, W.C.: Hematology for the practicing dentist. *In* Symposium on Physical and Laboratory Diagnosis. Dent. Clin. North Am., *18*:171–186, 1974.
24. Segal, H., et al.: Informed consent in dentistry. J.A.D.A., *99*:957–958, 1979.
25. Shore, N.A.: Temporomandibular Joint Dysfunction and Occlusal Equilibration. 2nd Ed. Philadelphia, J.B. Lippincott, 1976.
26. Smith, G.T.: Caries prediction tests—new approaches and problems. Northwest Dent., *57*:309–312, 1978.
27. Updegrave, W.J.: Vertical interproximal radiography. Dent. Radiogr. Photogr., *51*(3):56–60, 1978.
28. Weine, E.: Endodontic Therapy. St. Louis, C.V. Mosby, 1972.

CHAPTER 5

Diagnosis

If you are not confused, you probably don't understand the situation . . . .

ANONYMOUS

The essence of diagnosis is identifying precisely what is happening and why; it is not, as is often thought, assigning a name to a clinical picture. Although we sometimes do assign names when making a diagnosis, the description of what is happening and the determination of a probable etiology will lead to effective treatment regardless of the label applied. For example, we could see a patient with pain on the right side of the face and make a tentative diagnosis of Costen's syndrome (an outdated term). This would not greatly aid us in selecting an appropriate course of treatment; neither, for that matter, would a diagnosis of temporomandibular joint pain dysfunction syndrome (a term preferred some years ago) or myofascial pain/dysfunction syndrome (a more current term, now likely to be superseded by the more general term "cranio-mandibular disorder"). None of these labels, even if accurate, provide a sound basis for a regimen of treatment. A brief description of major findings would be more likely to serve that end: "Pain in right TMJ area, recent in onset, worst in the A.M.; right-side muscles of mastication and TMJ area painful to palpation; distinct balancing-side function (polished facet) on gold crown recently placed on upper right second molar." Although it is more cumbersome, this approach tells us precisely what is happening and strongly suggests an etiologic factor to be investigated. In this respect, a description is more valuable than a label in treatment planning. Labels represent shorthand versions of the lengthier descriptions, but, because they are shorthand, may easily mislead us. Periodontitis, for example, has a very specific meaning, but unless we know a great deal more about the extent, severity, past history, and contributing factors, we are hard pressed to plan rational treatment. Compare this with appendicitis, which, if it is established as a diagnosis to explain abdominal pain, suggests logical treatment modes (antibiotic therapy, possible appendectomy).

Most dental texts outline the medical model of diagnosis and attempt to apply it to dental diagnosis and treatment planning. The application is sometimes pertinent, but often is not. In the medical model of diagnosis, the patient presents with certain signs and symptoms. The practitioner elicits the chief complaint, its history (present illness), and a general history. He carefully examines the patient and observes any pertinent signs. From the symptoms elicited and signs observed, he develops a clinical picture of the patient's problem and compares it with similar clinical pictures of various known disease states. Further tests can be selected to eliminate possibilities and/or identify which of those similar clinical pictures are present (differential diagnosis). The quality of the diagnosis is based on the examiner's ability to elicit information, his skill in observation, and his knowledge and experience in seeing and treating diseases. A skilled diagnostician can rapidly narrow the possibilities and thereby reduce the number (and cost) of tests required to make a positive diagnosis.

The medical model is pertinent in certain areas of dental diagnosis. Discrete soft-tissue lesions, for example, are diagnosed in this manner. The classic example is a burn of the oral mucosa that can appear clinically almost identical to a squamous cell carcinoma. The history and symptoms will differentiate the two, and observing the lesion in 7 to 10 days will positively verify whether it is a traumatic injury (in which case it will have healed) or a potential malignant lesion (in which case it will not have healed) biopsy can then be employed to make a positive diagnosis.

Acute pain in or around a tooth can be diagnosed in much the same manner. Signs, symptoms, and history are pieced together to form the clinical picture. The knowledgeable dentist might even be able to differentiate an acute serous pulpitis from an acute purulent pulpitis just from the symptoms.[21] In this case, however, the medical model may lose some of its usefulness. Knowing whether a patient is suffering from serous pulpitis or purulent pulpitis does not greatly aid in planning treatment. We know that the problem is irreversible and extraction or endodontic therapy must be performed. The choice of treatment, however, depends on a multitude of factors, such as the patient's general dental condition, attitude, ability to pay, and overall oral environment, the strategic value of the tooth in question, its periodontal status, and the status of the dentition as a whole. The medical model does not help us much in this situation; neither does it help in terms of etiologic determination. A pulpitis, whether serous or purulent, may have a demonstrable bacterial etiology (as shown by culture). If we look no further than this, our treatment plan may be doomed. How did the infective organism reach the pulp? If it was through a carious lesion, dental caries is the actual etiology. Remember, however, that caries is very much behavior-related, and, as such, the real etiology of the serous pulpitis may be plaque that has formed on tooth surfaces and that the patient is unable or unwilling to remove. The medical model of diagnosis does not lend itself to this kind of problem. It is most effective in discrete disease states of specific causation.

Most dental disease is chronic, diffuse, and behaviorally induced. We could easily envision a patient presenting with three painful teeth; using the medical model, the dentist could diagnose all three as having acute bacterial pulpitis. Yet the three could be vastly different in actual etiology. For example, a posterior molar might have been cariously invaded under an existing dental restoration; an upper first premolar in traumatic occlusion due to the absence or lack of guidance of a canine may have developed an infrabony periodontal defect that allowed bacterial invasion through accessory canals in the furcation; and a third tooth, an upper central incisor, might have been devitalized by a traumatic injury many years previous and invaded via the bloodstream during a transient bacteremia.

It is necessary to supplement the medical model of diagnosis with other intellectual approaches to determine not only what is happening in a given situation, but *why* it is happening. These approaches are designed for oral-health maintenance, rather than oral-disease management. They apply to the multifactorial disease states, which are often chronic and without noticeable symptoms, and represent a large part of the typical dental practice.

MULTIFACTORIAL DIAGNOSIS

The dentist often examines patients who present with no specific complaint or, more often, have one or more specific complaints that are not so severe as to demand immediate attention. These patients typically feel that a dental examination and cleaning is overdue, and the minor complaint (sensitive tooth, occasional bleeding gums, etc.) is the catalyst in finally making the appointment. Since they frequently request or readily agree to a general evaluation that will address the minor complaint in due course, the dentist is starting with a "clean slate." The task is to examine for and, if necessary, diagnose orofacial disorders that have produced few, if any, noticeable symptoms. This requires a routine systematic approach (outlined previously) in which the conditions observed are compared with standards of normality and health. This is the essence of diagnosis and requires that the following four processes occur, often simultaneously:

1. *Knowing the normal.* The clinician must have a good grasp of the clinical norm, both from textbook courses and from observation of many normal patients.
2. *Recognizing deviations from the norm.* Being able to recite the definition of normal for any given factor in oral diagnosis is of little value if one does not recognize abnormal findings when they appear. The careful observer is constantly on guard against complacency, which allows obvious abnormalities, and even gross pathology, to be overlooked.
3. *Describing the abnormality.* The clinician must be able to describe, in a few words, the deviation from the norm, so that a written diagnosis can be formulated.
4. *Analyzing the abnormality.* The clinician must ask himself questions regarding the findings to establish whether the abnormality is obviously benign and inconsequential, significant but not critical, potentially serious, or absolutely critical to the oral health (or systemic health) of the patient. Judgment should be withheld as to the exact nature, significance, and scientific name of the findings in question, but possibilities should be considered, both as to the nature of the abnormality and its etiology.

These processes are applied throughout each step of the routine systematic approach. What emerges is a multifactorial diagnosis—that is, abnormalities observed during the various steps of the routine systematic approach are grouped according to factors. The major factors considered can be broken down in a number of ways, five of which are discussed here: general systemic diagnosis; soft-tissue diagnosis; periodontal diagnosis; dental diagnosis; and functional diagnosis.

General Systemic Diagnosis

From our general appraisal and medical history, a thumbnail sketch should be made of the patient's general systemic condition. This general diagnosis should include any findings that may have significance in dental or oral conditions, or in dental treatment. The following are typical examples of general systemic diagnoses:

1. Normal, healthy, 30-year-old woman with an allergy to penicillin and gastric intolerance to aspirin
2. 18-year-old man, brittle diabetic on daily injectable insulin. He is rather obese; his diet is not well controlled. He seems apathetic, difficult to communicate with.
3. Severely debilitated 68-year-old man with a history of lymphatic cancer. He has had chemotherapy and irradiation of head/neck. He has a positive attitude and is concerned about appearance and function of teeth.
4. 53-year-old woman who is menopausal, on estrogen therapy, and who smokes heavily ($2^1/_2$ packs/day). She is rather defensive and emotional, has a history of frequent headaches for which there is no discoverable etiology.
5. Normal, healthy, 82-year-old woman with a history of arthritis that is fairly well controlled by aspirin (8–12 tabs/day). Blood pressure is 180/100, which is within normal limits for her age.

These thumbnail sketches summarize and highlight the comprehensive medical history and general appraisal and should capsulize those findings likely to be significant in dental treatment. In many cases, the general systemic findings may contain nothing that is significant to us and will therefore not be a factor in diagnosis. In other cases, the complexity and severity of a patient's systemic problems may preclude any or all but the most urgent dental treatment. In most cases, however, the general systemic findings will influence the dental situation in one of three ways:

1. *Indirect influence.* Findings that require precaution or premedication but may not directly affect the disease or treatment exert indirect influence on the dental situation. A history of rheumatic fever requiring prophylactic antibiotics or an allergy to a commonly used drug are examples of such influence.

2. *Direct influence.* General systemic findings that may be direct or indirect etiologic factors in dental disorders can have a direct influence on the dental situation. For example, diabetes may affect the severity of periodontal disease and loss of salivary flow may predispose directly to caries. Less obviously, severe arthritis may prevent plaque control, thereby aggravating most dental disease.

3. *Reverse influence.* General systemic findings that may turn out to be caused by the oral or dental disorder can have a reverse influence on the dental situation. Headaches, earaches, and associated head and neck symptoms may be related to occlusal or TMJ disorders. Sore throats may be secondary to pericoronitis of a partially impacted third molar.

The extent to which a systemic finding will influence dental treatment often depends on what type of dental treatment is contemplated. Bleeding disorders or hemophilia of various types may not be significant if one is going to do simple operative dentistry, but might be absolutely critical if multiple extractions are indicated. Since we probably will not establish a treatment plan until the diagnosis is fully developed, the systemic findings that we note in the general systemic diagnosis should include any or all that may potentially influence dental disorders or dental treatment. Finally, even though we draw a brief sketch for our multifactorial diagnosis, we do not preclude the possibility of returning to general systemic findings if other factors in the diagnosis or developing plan of treatment suggest we do so.

Soft-Tissue Diagnosis

From our examination of the external head and neck, lymph-node palpation, and the intraoral soft-tissue (oral cancer) examination, any significant findings can be listed briefly. These would include, but are not limited to, the following:

Lesions
Swellings or nodules
Asymmetry
Abnormal color or surface texture
Pain or tenderness on palpation

If the findings and their history are readily explainable and fairly innocuous—an ulcerated palatal lesion that the patient says is a result of hot pizza, for example—we may not even include them in our summary diagnosis. Findings that may be significant because of their clinical appearance and history—a unilateral swelling of the floor of the mouth, which the patient tells us comes and goes, for example—should be briefly summarized, thus becoming the soft-tissue diagnosis. The following are examples of common soft-tissue diagnoses:

1. Small (5-mm diameter), fibrous nodule on the

right buccal mucosa near commissure. A probable fibroma. Patient reports occasionally biting same.

2. Multiple petechiae spread over soft palate causing no pain or tenderness, of possible systemic origin. Patient had not been aware of them.

3. Small (2-mm diameter), painless, indurated ulcer on left lateral border of tongue; it is a possible neoplasm. Patient was not aware of it.

4. Swelling and tenderness in right submandibular lymph node of recent onset. It is probably associated with a toothache in the right mandibular molar region, which is the patient's chief complaint.

From the history and clinical picture, we may later elect to ignore the soft-tissue abnormality, to watch and evaluate it at some interval, or to perform a biopsy for a histologic diagnosis. Once again, keep in mind that the soft-tissue abnormality may be related to other aspects of our findings and to other factors in the diagnosis.

Periodontal Diagnosis

The periodontal diagnosis is intentionally separated from the rest of the soft-tissue findings because of its significance and high incidence in our patient population (this has already been addressed in Chap. 4). At its conclusion, the careful and exhaustive periodontal evaluation should produce a periodontal diagnosis that, like the other factors in the multifactorial diagnosis, gives a clear picture of the patient's status.

It is both possible and advisable in periodontal diagnosis to be very specific in our terminology so as to describe exactly the periodontal situation present. For example, the term "gingivitis" has a very definite meaning, especially as differentiated from "periodontitis." The former refers to an inflammatory condition involving soft tissues of the periodontium, but not the alveolar bone. The latter refers to a disease state that has resulted in destruction and loss of alveolar bone as determined through observation (probing) or radiographic evidence. These specific terms and others like them (e.g., juvenile periodontitis) can be modified to further refine the diagnosis. A periodontal condition can be acute or chronic in nature, localized or generalized in distribution, mild or severe in its apparent rate of progression, and incipient, frank, or advanced in its apparent state of progression. These are but a few of the modifiers that can be applied to a periodontal condition (Fig. 5–1). A few examples will illustrate:

1. Normal, healthy periodontium with local areas of recession—upper molars, lower canines

2. Acute gingivitis, generalized, with bleeding and hypertrophic tissue interproximally, 3- to 5-mm pockets posterior

3. Chronic advanced severe periodontitis, generalized with 50% or more bone loss, and Class III mobility throughout.

4. Periodontitis, generally incipient with localized severe lesions (5- to 8-mm pockets) between no. 2 and no. 3, mesial furca no. 5, and between no. 22 and no. 23

5. Chronic periodontitis, mild for age (70 years), less than 15% bone loss, slight mobility of lower anteriors

6. Acute necrotizing ulcerative gingivitis with loss of papillae, marked breath odor, and severe discomfort

It is also possible, and usually necessary if there are a number of periodontal pockets, to measure and record sulcus or pocket depths throughout the mouth, noting six points on every tooth.

It is appropriate to include in the periodontal diagnosis a brief evaluation of the patient's oral-hygiene status, as it is directly related to the etiology and treatment of the periodontal condition. Taking into account the levels of plaque, calculus, and stain observed on the teeth, we can roughly generalize oral hygiene as good, fair, or poor. Greater objectivity is possible using the criteria-based scoring system (the oral health progress record) described in Chapter 4 to indicate scores for plaque and stain/calculus. Finally, if a standardized scoring system such as the plaque index (PI) is employed, that figure could be included.

Dental Diagnosis

Dental diagnosis can be simplified greatly by considering that teeth that are not normal and healthy can be classed as *diseased* (generally caries), *dysfunctional* (with malformation, occlusal wear, erosion/abrasion, fractures, or faulty restoration), or *disfigured* (intrinsic or extrinsic stain, developmental defect, or discolored or nonesthetic restoration).

Disease

Diseased teeth may suffer hard-tissue lesions affecting enamel, dentin, and/or cementum, lesions of the pulpal tissue, or both. Caries is the most common dental disease and is produced by bacterial plaques. Contributing factors, particularly the availability of carbohydrate substrates, should also be considered in the diagnosis. It is fairly well established that dental caries is not a single-organism disease, but that different organisms may be active on different tooth surfaces. Thus, there are patients who have severe proximal lesions but few gingival caries, and vice

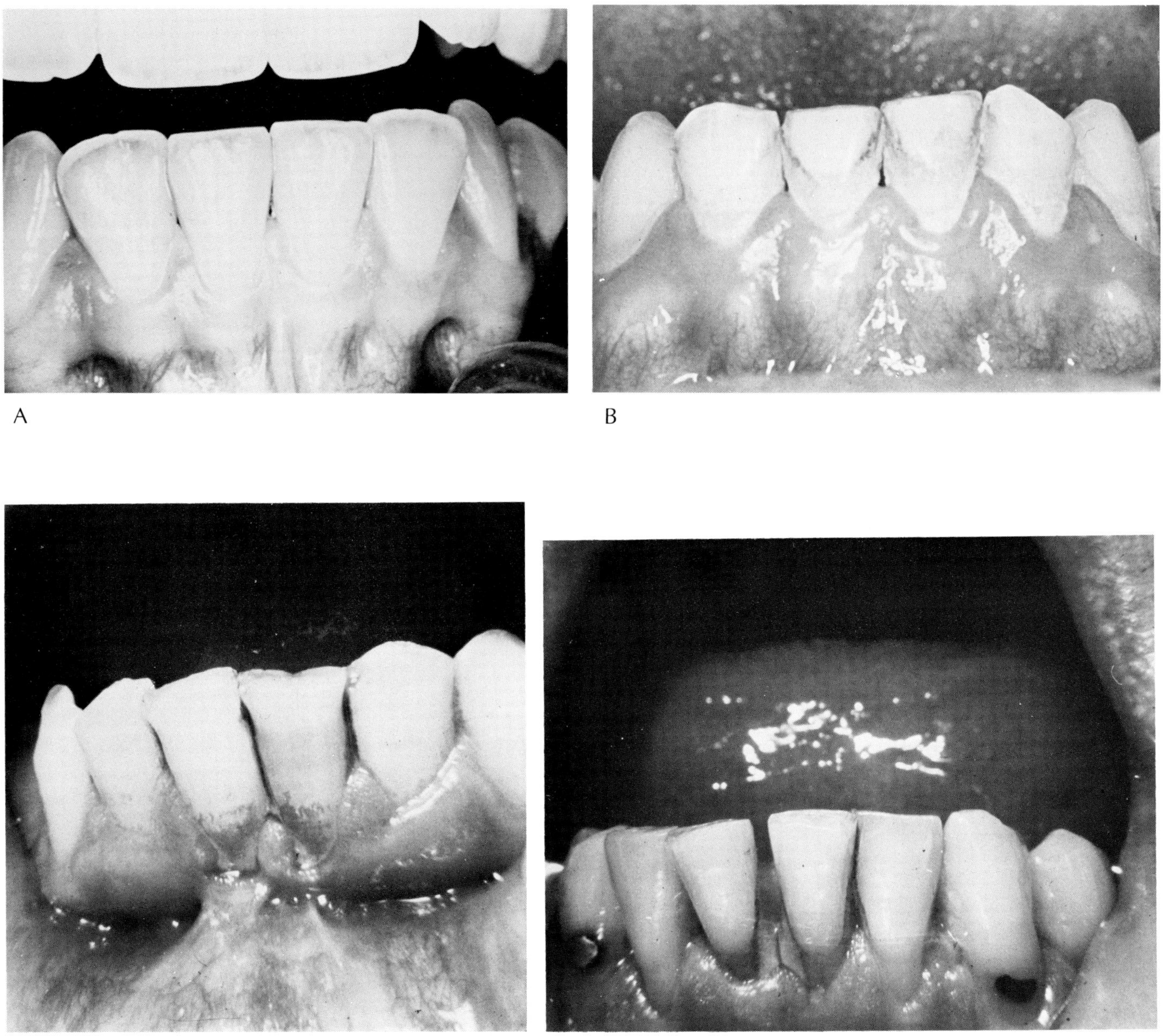

Fig. 5–1. Examples of fairly discrete periodontal conditions, and radiographic signs of periodontal disease., *A,* Normal, healthy gingiva. *B,* Gingivitis. *C,* Acute periodontitis that is localized and related to lower midline frenum pull. *D,* Chronic moderate periodontitis.

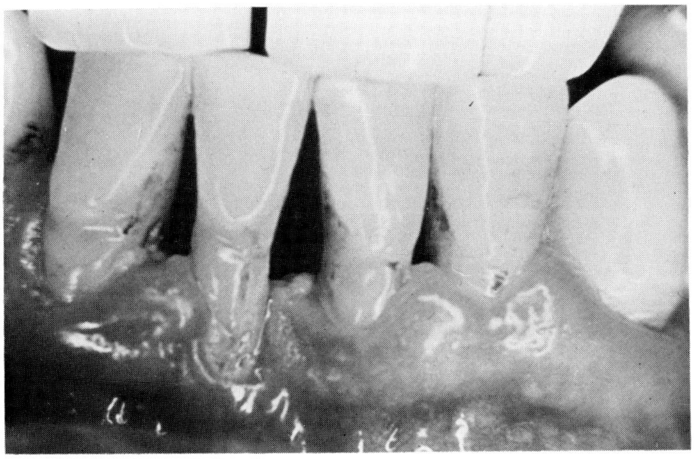

E

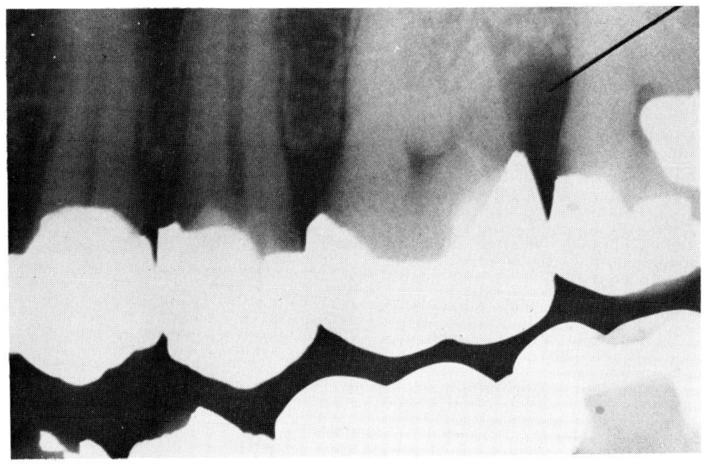

F

G

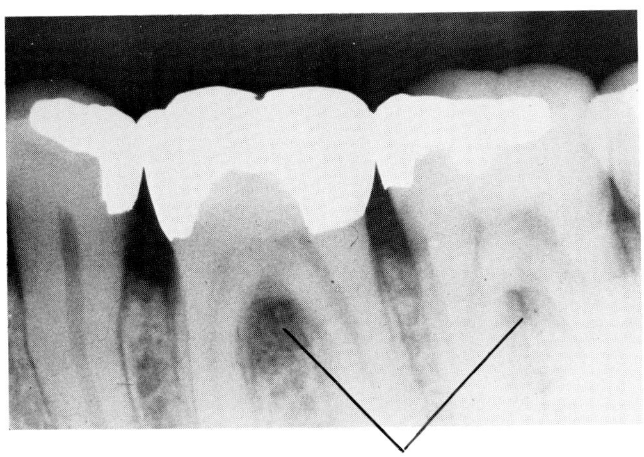

Fig. 5–1 *continued.* *E*, Acute severe periodontitis. *F*, Interproximal bone loss with possible early furcation involvement, distal furca of first molar. *G*, Frank furcation involvement, first and second molars.

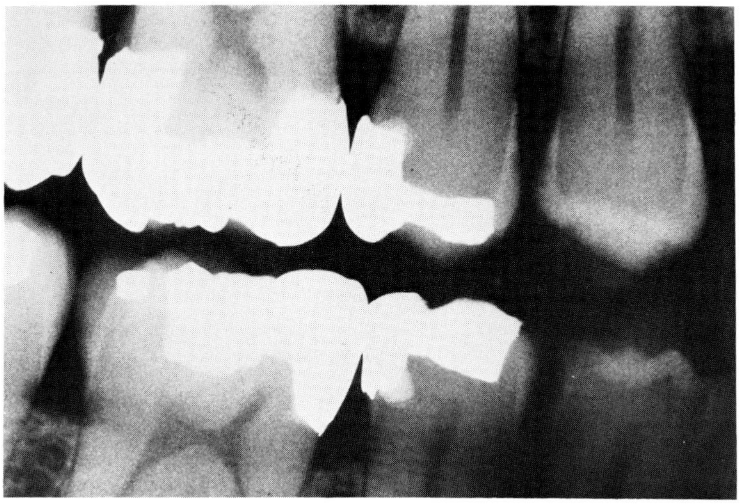

A

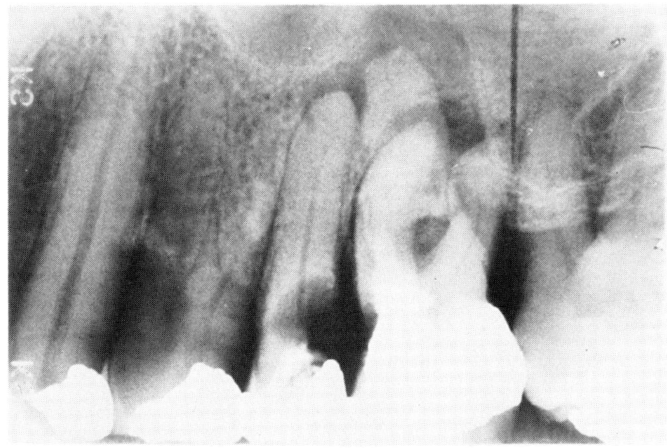

C

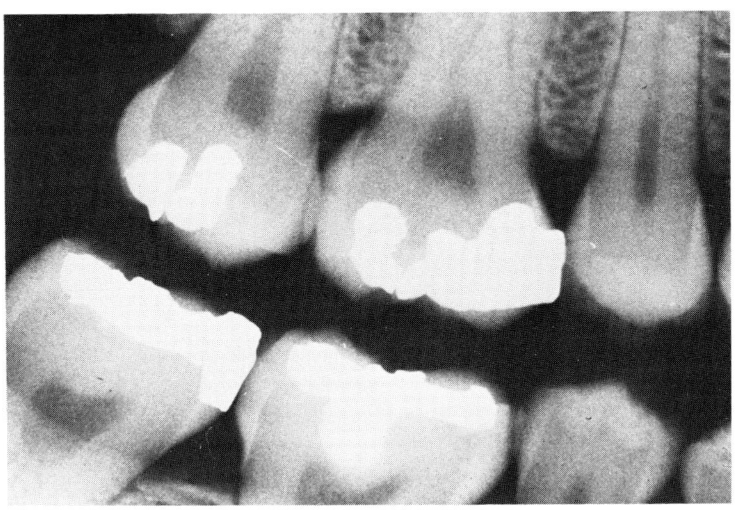

B

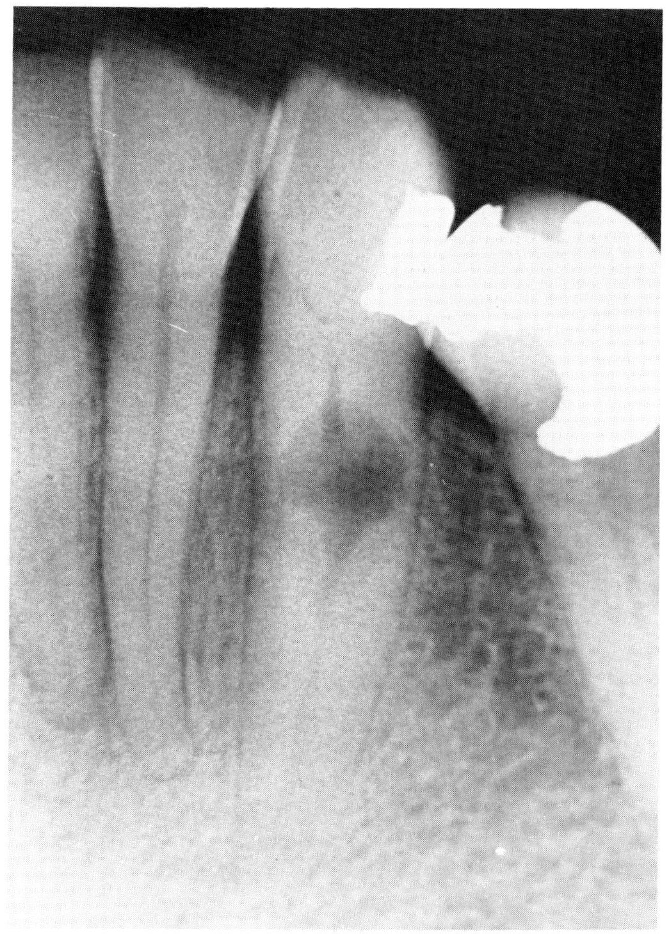

D

Fig. 5–2. *A,* Disruption of the enamel between upper first and second premolars may be incipient caries or arrested caries. In fact, the area has not changed in radiographic appearance in 12 years. *B,* Frank carious lesion distal of lower first molar, with radiolucent area into dentin. Distal of upper first molar incipient or arrrested. *C,* Rather severe caries, upper second premolar. *D,* Internal resorption.

versa. The incidence and distribution of the caries should be considered in the dental diagnosis (Fig. 5–2).

The only other common disease of dental hard tissue is resorption, either internal or external, which is a result of cellular modification and clastic activity. Resorption is understandable in some cases; for example, reimplanted, avulsed teeth commonly undergo severe root resorption, probably because they are no longer recognized as "self" by the body and are attacked as foreign objects. Various types of trauma (orthodontic movement, injury) have also triggered this resorptive process. Still other cases of internal or external resorption are unexplained (Fig. 5–2D).

Soft-tissue disease in teeth involves the pulp and is most commonly a bacterial invasion via caries or fracture. The blood supply and hence, the reparative potential of the pulp, is quite poor; thus, the pulp is also susceptible to sterile necrosis subsequent to trauma. That trauma may be a blow, long-term occlusal disharmony, or even the operative manipulations of dental restoration. There is a wide range of histologically discrete pulpal disease states; however, the clinical dentist need consider only two categories—the reversible and irreversible.

Transient pulpal hyperemia is a reversible state, and palliative treatment may relieve the symptoms. Frank pulpitis is irreversible; symptomatic relief is temporary at best, and pulpal death is the result. It is obvious that dental soft-tissue (pulpal) diagnosis must stress the difference between these states. As a rule, symptoms of pulpal hyperemia, such as sensitivity to heat and cold, percussion, and chewing, arise only when the stimulus is applied and are relieved when the stimulus is removed. Intensity of the sensation—that is, the degree of pain experienced—may not be a good diagnostic measure, since it is totally subjective. Extremely intense call-the-dentist-on-Saturday-night pain often indicates a more serious pulpal pathology than transient hyperemia; thus, pain or sensitivity that arises spontaneously, as well as in response to stimulus, and is not relieved when the stimulus is removed, usually indicates irreversible pulpitis or other pulpal pathology. Palliative treatments, such as application of sedative to dentin, placement of sedative temporary fillings, and the like, are of limited value and should be applied only when there is a reasonable doubt that the pulpal problem is irreversible. If there are signs of pulpal necrosis or infection, such as swelling, obvious exposure through fracture or caries, lymphadenopathy, or apical radiolucency, palliative treatment is contraindicated and more definitive treatment is necessary. This includes the following:

1. *Drainage.* Drain by opening the tooth coronally; drain it apically by incision; or drain it both ways.
2. *Pulpotomy.* This is useful as a temporary measure when there is still vital pulp tissue and initiation of endodontic therapy is not practical.
3. *Pulpectomy.* Pulpectomy is the removal of all pulpal tissues, and it usually leads to root-canal therapy.
4. *Extraction.* Extraction is necessary if the tooth is nonrestorable (fractures, gross caries) or nonfunctional (3rd molars, severely malposed teeth), or if the dentist and patient agree that removal is the best course of action under the circumstances. (Extractions as dental treatment will be discussed in more detail in Chap. 8.)

Soft-tissue (pulpal) disease can also be totally asymptomatic, and unless signs appear clinically or radiographically, it may remain undetected. In some cases, an acute episode of pain or sensitivity may have passed without treatment, or acute symptoms may never have arisen at all. Therefore, pulpal status is a critical aspect of both dental diagnosis and treatment planning, since an asymptomatic but nonvital tooth can potentially compromise a treatment plan. For this reason, any teeth that are suspected of having pulpal involvement should be carefully evaluated in the diagnosis. This includes teeth with deep carious lesions, a history of symptoms (although not currently present), discoloration, questionable radiographic appearance (slight radiolucency at or near the apex, or an increase in apparent bone density, which is called condensing osteitis), or large or deep dental restorations, especially those apparently without a protective base. Such teeth should be evaluated with an electronic pulp tester, percussion, thermal tests, and so forth for signs of pulpal involvement and should be kept under surveillance in the future should the findings be within normal limits.

It should be stressed that an apparently nonvital tooth does not always require definitive treatment. If the tooth is not directly involved in complex restorations, such as fixed or removable prosthetics, and has remained asymptomatic for many years, simple continued surveillance may be all that is indicated. Therefore, the dental diagnosis must take into consideration not only the status of a tooth, but its potential role in overall treatment. For example, a slightly discolored central incisor that is clinically asymptomatic and radiographically normal but does not respond to pulp testing, may be left alone if it is not a potential abutment tooth. It can also remain untreated if endodontic therapy will be possible should symptoms arise, and if prosthetic replacement appears possible should endodontics fail. On the other hand, if the same tooth is a potential abutment tooth for a fixed or removable prosthesis, it might require endodontic therapy to ensure the prosthetic result. While it is possible to perform endodontic therapy through a crown restoration, it is a more complicated procedure; if a dowel is indicated for retention and reinforcement, the procedure is even more difficult. The management of questionable teeth and alternative approaches to failed treatment will be covered in more detail in Chapter 9.

This discussion of asymptomatic pulpal pathology can be summarized by reiterating that not all abnormal pulps demand treatment. Teeth with nearly total calcification of the pulp chamber, teeth with overlarge pulp chambers, suggesting early pulpal death and therefore, the inability to produce secondary dentin, teeth with apparent large direct pulp caps, old pulpotomies, or apparently totally inadequate endodontic fills, and discolored, nonresponsive teeth have provided service for decades without need of treatment. In fact, attempting to treat such teeth is itself a risk, since failure of treatment or complications of treatment may result in the loss of a functional and asymptomatic tooth that seemed quite normal to the patient.

Relationship of Pulpal Disease to Periodontal Disease. Periodontal diagnosis and periodontal disease have been differentiated from dental soft-tissue or pulpal disease, but in fact, the two are often related. The pulp and the periodontal tissues communicate at the apex of the tooth, via accessory canals that can occur almost anywhere on the root surface, or from the pulp chamber into a furcation on multirooted teeth. Much attention has been given to the combination of endodontic and periodontal disease states, and the potential combinations, from the diagnostic view point, can be summarized as follows:

1. Pulpal disease can be present in combination with periodontal disease, with neither directly contributing to the other. Lesions are usually radiographically distinct from one another, with generalized periodontal lesions throughout the mouth. Treatment of either disease will not relieve the other; however, periodontal treatment may be compromised if pulpal disease is not addressed.

2. Pulpal disease arising from bacterial invasion from a periodontal lesion through a lateral or accessory canal is impossible to ascertain with certainty, but is a likely etiology if no other reasonable cause is present. Treatment of the periodontal lesion will not correct pulpal pathology, as any frank pulpitis is irreversible, and the periodontal treatment may be compromised if pulpal disease is not treated. The significant factor here is in the potential for periodontal lesions to lead to future pulpal pathology,

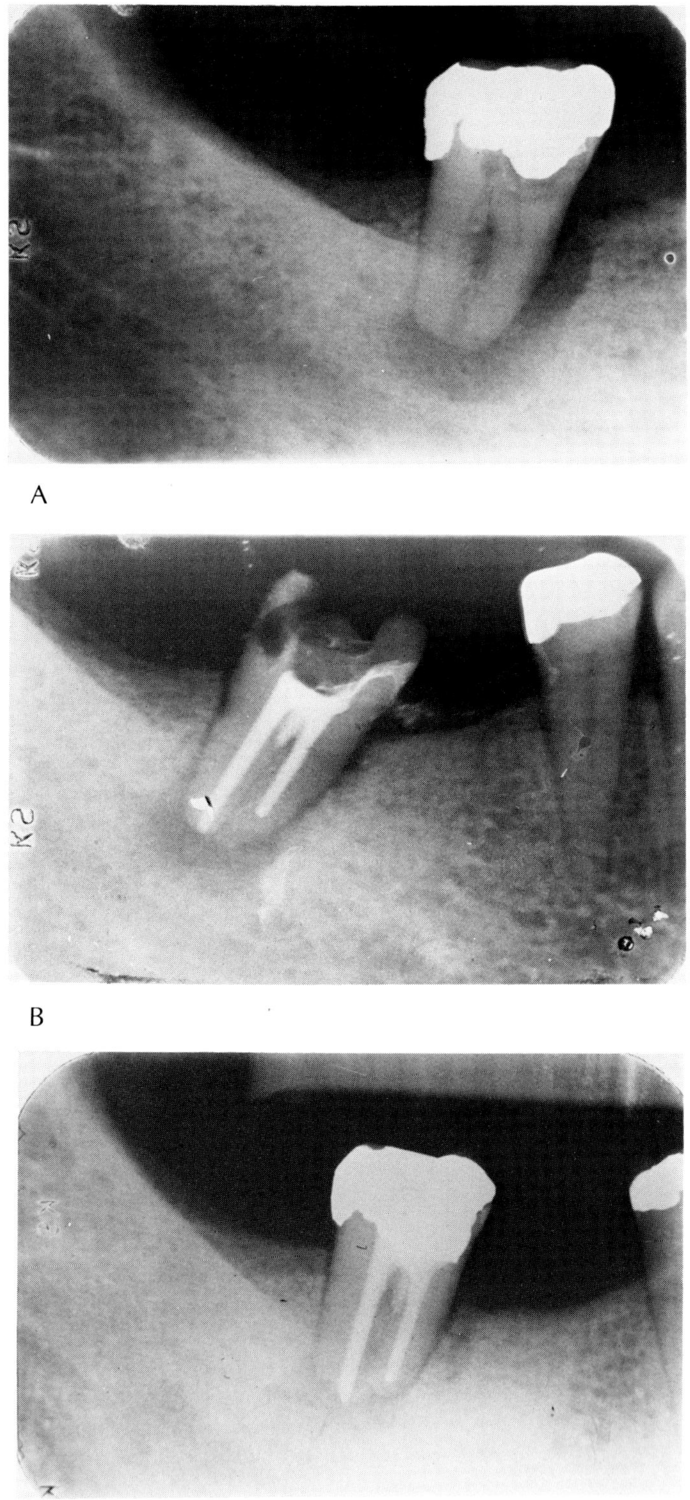

A

B

C

Fig. 5–3. *A*, Severe bone loss, Class III mobility, and mesial periodontal defect that could be probed to apex of tooth. *B*, Approximately 6 months after endodontic treatment, mobility is lessened, and mesial periodontal defect has resolved and is no longer probeable. *C*, Five years after endodontic treatment, tooth is completely stable endodontically and periodontally.

which must be considered whenever periodontal lesions are advanced (as in deep, infrabony pockets) or involve a furcation.

3. Periodontal lesions arising from pulpal pathology is the most significant combination, in that endodontic therapy can result in remission of the periodontal lesion, resolution of bony defects, and restoration of the gingival attachment (Fig. 5–3). In such cases, the periodontal lesion may be an isolated defect, unusually severe in relation to the rest of the mouth, with angular bony defect(s).

In some cases, the periodontal pocket may lead all the way to the apex (gutta-percha points may be employed to demonstrate this radiographically). An unmistakable sign of this condition is a radiographically observed periodontal lesion, or a furcation bone loss that is *not* clinically detectable with the periodontal probe. We can be nearly certain that the periodontal lesion is secondary to the pulpal pathology and that endodontic therapy will resolve the periodontal problem in such situations.

It is not understood at this time how bony defects and pockets arising from pulpal pathology will resolve completely, while true periodontal lesions seldom resolve through repair and require excisional treatment to arrest them. Discovery of the mechanisms involved may well lead to more effective periodontal therapy. In the meantime, the dentist must deal with the situation as it is presently understood, no matter how poor that understanding may be.

In our dental diagnosis, we must consider the possibility of the pulpally induced periodontal lesion. Periodontally involved teeth with severe bone loss and infrabony pockets might easily be condemned and extracted prior to definitive periodontal therapy; yet, if the lesion was pulpally induced, the tooth might well be retained and have an excellent prognosis. Unfortunately, the true test for this condition is the performance of endodontic therapy, a fairly involved and costly test if the severe periodontal lesion does not resolve. In cases in which pulpal/periodontal lesions are a likelihood, such as the loss of bone in a furcation without a probeable periodontal pocket, endodontic therapy is advisable if it would otherwise be indicated. When a pulpally involved tooth is also seriously involved periodontally, the decision is less clear. In such cases, overall treatment goals, treatment options, cost-effectiveness, and patient desires have to be weighed before multiroot endodontics are employed as a diagnostic procedure. The strategic value of the tooth in question is significant, and this concept will be discussed further in Chapter 8.

Dysfunction

Dysfunctional teeth are those that are not able to perform their normal physiologic function due to defects in formation or insults suffered following eruption. Malposed teeth are excluded from this category and will be dealt with in this chapter's discussion of the functional diagnosis.

Malformation. Poorly formed teeth that are dysfunctional include the following characteristics:

1. Enamel defects, poorly formed or "chalky," that do not provide the structural strength required in occlusion or are overly susceptible to carious breakdown

2. Abnormal crown morphology that does not provide function and occlusal support (dwarfing) or that, due to severe anatomic anomalies, predisposes to caries and/or makes restoration difficult or impossible (accessory cusps, deep developmental grooves, "twinning")

3. Abnormal root morphology that does not provide support for occlusal forces (short, blunted roots) or that predisposes to caries and/or periodontal lesions (deep axial grooves, furcations close to cemento-enamel junction)

Poorly formed teeth may have mild problems that bear watching (slight enamel defects) or severe problems that may so jeopardize the tooth as to preclude any long-term treatment planning. Often the patient may not be aware of such dysfunctional teeth unless they are also visibly disfigured. Nevertheless, the effects of severe malformation on the prognosis of the tooth can be considerable, and they must be considered in the dental diagnosis.

Occlusal Wear. Occlusal wear represents a form of dysfunction that is based on the nature and severity of the wear in relation to the age of the patient. Types of wear patterns to consider include the following:

1. Faceting, circumscribed wear spots in the enamel involving few teeth, may be an accommodation to the overall occlusion and within normal limits, or it may be indicative of occlusal traumatism, which can produce mobility, tenderness, and severe localized bony defects in the presence of periodontal inflammation.

2. Faceting seen throughout the arches may also be an accommodation to the occlusion, particularly in older individuals, or it may indicate a bruxing or clenching habit that can lead to serious dental and periodontal damage.

3. Severe wear resulting in loss of enamel and exposure of dentin is serious in all but the old patient, because dentin is susceptible to rapid wear as well

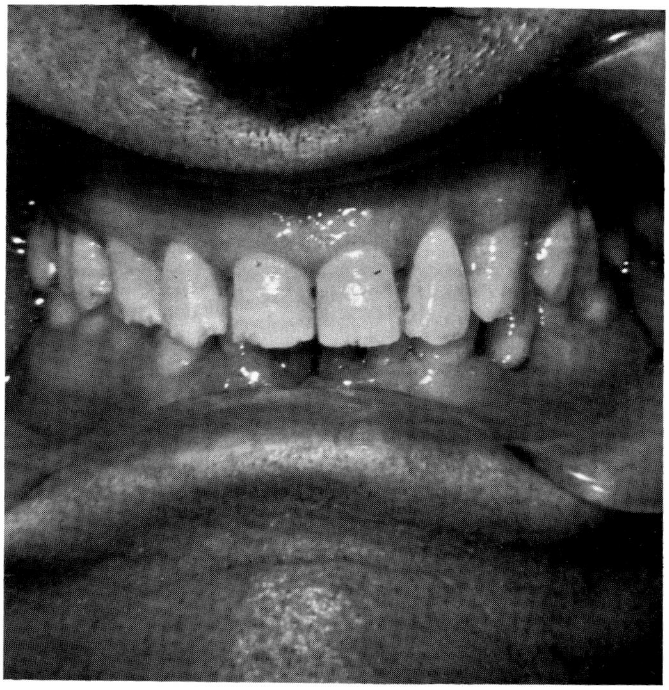

A

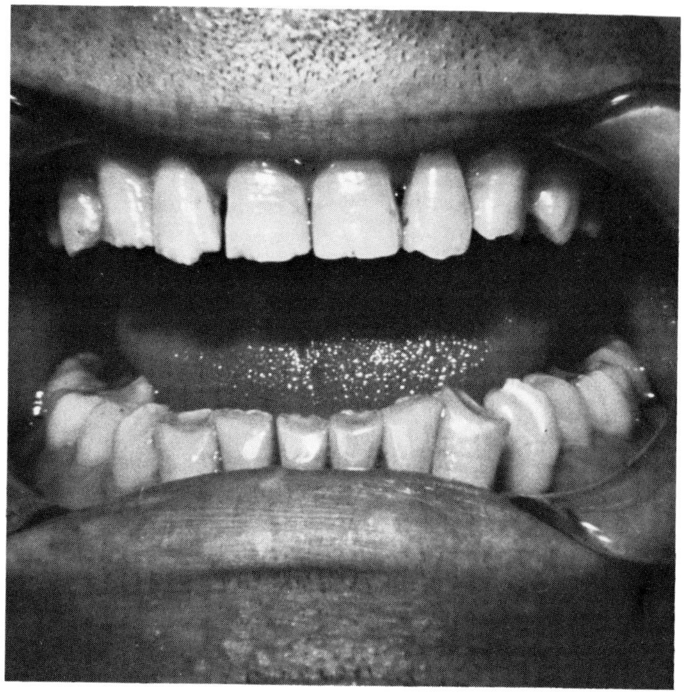

B

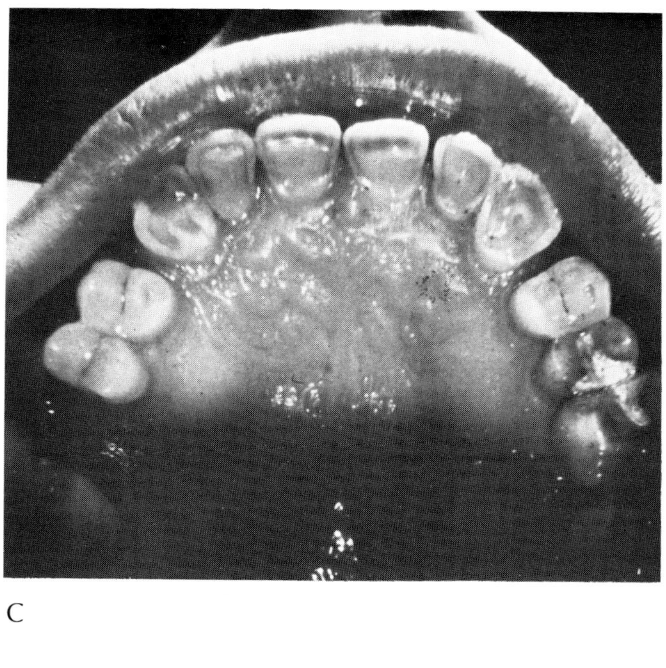

C

Fig. 5–4. *A,B,C,* This 40-year-old man admitted to nocturnal bruxism and clenching during the day. His masseter muscles were massive, and, in addition to the tremendous abrasion and loss of enamel depicted, he had generalized severe periodontitis with 20 to 50% bone loss throughout.

as to caries. The situation is often worst when enamel is lost in one arch but remains in the other, in which case the remaining enamel may not wear further, but devastate the opposing dentin. Although most often seen in individuals who exhibit bruxism, other factors may also predispose an individual to severe wear: end-to-end occlusion, occupational environment (masons, quarry workers, anyone working with abrasives), or faulty selection of dental restorative materials, placement of porcelain dentures or full porcelain crowns against the natural dentition, or, worse yet, against an already worn natural dentition.

Worn teeth may be a normal finding as the occlusion functions over a span of time. Unusual or severe wear may suggest functional or psychologic problems and can greatly complicate dental treatment planning, since restoration of severe wear often requires extensive use of castings. Care must be taken when diagnosing wear as a dysfunction that its probable etiology is established and corrected, or provided for in planning treatment. For example, if we are planning restorative dentistry for a patient with large masseter muscles and a long history of nocturnal bruxing (Fig. 5–4), it may influence our choice of materials (gold castings or silver amalgam), our design (onlay or inlay), and our execution (removing more tooth structure occlusally to provide for greater thickness in the restoration). We may even wish to take steps to protect the new restoration, such as night guards, to prevent abnormal wear from jeopardizing the treatment.

Whenever possible, the likely etiologic factor of occlusal wear should be identified and eliminated.

Abrasion and Erosion. Abrasion and erosion can cause severe loss of tooth structure and are, therefore, dysfunctional. Abrasion produced by mechanical means is the analog to severe occlusal wear in that the enamel or cementum is lost and the exposed dentin is highly susceptible to further attrition. Toothbrushing is the most common etiologic factor; stiff-bristle brushes usually are considered the primary culprits when employed in a back-and-forth brushing technique. Even soft nylon brushes can aggravate existing abrasions if used in a sawing motion, since the V-groove most often created at the gingiva of the tooth directs the bristles into the same pattern that originally produced the abrasion (Fig. 5–5).

This situation makes effective plaque control difficult and leads to further abrasion, suggesting that restoration of this type of defect may be indicated even if caries are not present and the area is asymptomatic. On the other hand, many abraded areas can remain unrestored and progress no further if they are carefully maintained with a soft toothbrush and nonabrasive brushing techniques.

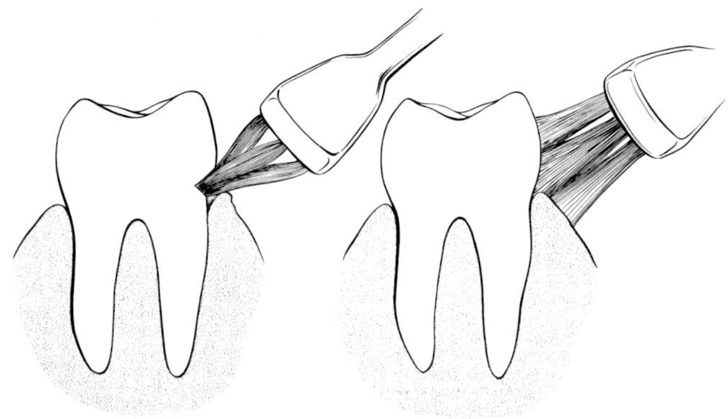

Fig. 5–5. Once a gingival groove has been established, (left), bristles will tend to concentrate in the groove, rather than to spread out as in a normal gingival crevice (right).

Abrasion at its worst can decimate the teeth and result in such gross defects that full crown coverage is required to adequately restore them.

Erosion is generally considered to be a chemically induced loss of tooth structure that is often related to unusual dietary patterns such as lemon sucking. The presence of citrus fruits and other highly acidic foods in the mouth seldom results in loss of tooth structure by itself, so erosion is generally seen and treated in combination with mechanical abrasion. Occupational environment may also produce acidity in the mouth and should be considered in the diagnosis. Another less obvious cause of erosion is self-induced vomiting as seen in the condition known as bulimia. Bulimics indulge in extreme overeating followed by use of laxatives, emetics, or self-induced

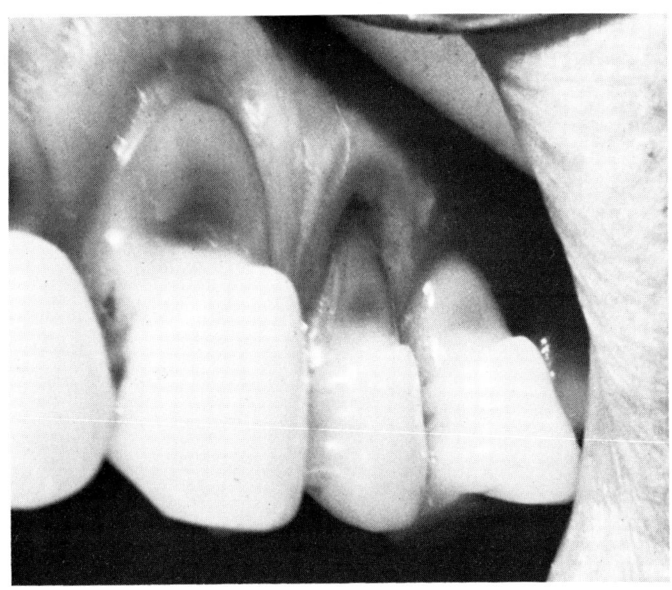

Fig. 5–6. Severe gingival abrasion.

vomiting. Related to anorexia nervosa, the condition may be more common than one might imagine and can produce striking erosion of teeth in a relatively short time.

Finally, it should be noted that abrasion is generally found along the gingiva of a tooth and often does not involve the enamel, which is hard and resistant to wear. Instead, the cementum is usually violated and the loss of tooth structure is dentinal, occurring on the root surface. For this to occur, there generally must be some amount of gingival recession; therefore, there is a relationship between periodontal status (gingival height) and dental dysfunction (Fig. 5–6).

Fracture. Fracture of tooth structure can create dysfunction depending on the type and severity of the fracture. The diagnosis of fractures can be categorized into two main groups: one in which the fracture is complete and the fractured piece separates and one in which the tooth remains intact (the so-called "cracked" tooth).

In the separation fracture, the diagnosis concentrates on the severity of the condition to decide the indicated treatment. A slight chip that is entirely in the enamel can often be ignored, or smoothed and polished. If an esthetic problem is created by the separation fracture, it is even possible to create a matching situation in the contralateral tooth in order to avoid placing a restoration. Enamel fractures of greater size or those exposing a small bit of dentin may also be smoothed and polished, but should restoration of esthetic contour and dentinal protection be required, the acid-etch bonded composite resin restoration can play a vital role. Even if esthetics is not a consideration, this approach should be considered if the exposed dentin is sensitive to temperature, probing, etc.

Major fractures involving extensive dentinal exposure, loss of a cusp on a posterior tooth, pulp-horn exposure, or frank pulpal involvement require definitive treatment. Endodontic therapy might be planned or at least allowed for in the future should it become necessary, and cast restorations are usually indicated for adequate restoration of form and function. Acid-etch bonded composite restorations can be employed as interim restorations on immature anterior teeth, and polycarbonate crowns can likewise be used if there is insufficient tooth structure to hold a restoration. Posterior fractured teeth can be restored with amalgam cores, pin-retained if necessary, prior to definitive restoration. Dysfunctional fractured teeth are often treated with interim types of restorations and no further treatment is pursued. Many such restorations hold up for long periods of time and provide good service at low cost. The patient, however, must be made aware of the shortcomings of such restorations, including the risk of early failure, of pulpal damage from further trauma, and of axial fractures resulting in tooth loss. On the other hand, these risks are often minimal, and a fractured tooth might be restored with interim restorations and left to function for as long as the restoration serves.

In the nonseparation fracture, or "cracked" tooth, the dentin has been violated and fluids can penetrate the enamel, but the tooth apparently remains intact. The diagnosis of this condition can be very difficult, and treatment is dependent upon the severity of the fracture once the existence of the fracture has been established.

"Cracked" teeth usually present first with symptoms: sensitivity to temperature (especially cold), sweets, and chewing (especially resistant or substantial foods). The symptoms may be localized to the offending tooth, but are often diffuse, making the differential diagnosis difficult. Other possible sources of these symptoms such as deep caries, leaking restorations, pulpal death, or periodontal disease must be considered and either ruled out or dealt with (temporary restorations, etc.). If symptoms persist after other likely causes have been addressed, a fracture must be suspected. Sometimes waiting and watching will result in a fracture becoming complete thus confirming the diagnosis. More often, further diagnostic measures are necessary. The patient may be asked to bite on wooden wedges or pieshaped wedges cut from $^5/_8$ in. knife-edge rubber discs (dental floss may be passed through the center hole to prevent swallowing or aspiration), or a lead shot may be placed between two pieces of cellophane tape. Placed on one tooth at a time, such objects may elicit the pain response that identifies the cracked tooth. Removal of all old restorations and placement of a sedative temporary-filling material is often advisable. It is not uncommon to see fractured tooth walls simply fall off when old restorations are excavated. Once excavated, the suspected tooth can be inspected for signs of fracture lines in the pulpal floor (disclosing solution or other vital stains can be employed to assist in this). A fiber-optic light source can also be used to detect fracture lines through transillumination. Pressure can be applied to each cusp from inside the cavity preparation to precipitate, if possible, actual separation of the fractured segment. It is sometimes necessary to apply considerable force, and as a last resort, a mallet and chisel might be employed to locate a fracture prior to pursuing endodontic therapy, if such therapy is the only remaining alternative. If the fracture is not axial and does not involve the pulp, endodontics may be averted. If applying heavy force reveals a fracture running down the long axis of the tooth, endodontic treatment is probably doomed to failure. If the cracked segment can be separated from the rest of the tooth, the diagnosis is confirmed and treatment planning is based on the severity of the fracture and the involvement or noninvolvement of the dental pulp.

Although the nonseparation fracture is often difficult to diagnose, it is apparently quite common and should be suspected in the following situations:

1. Sharp, deeply interdigitating dental anatomy in which the cusps can act as wedges
2. Any tooth with a restoration in it, especially MOD restorations, restorations leaving fairly thin walls of tooth buccal and/or lingual, and cast intracoronal restorations (inlays) that may have been driven into the prepared tooth creating stresses
3. Any endodontically treated tooth with recurrent apical, lateral or furcal lesion, or any endodontically treated tooth with a post (especially a screw-type post) that could have been driven into the tooth, thereby creating stresses

Early detection of an axial fracture can avoid much frustration on the part the dental team and patient in attempting to treat a hopeless tooth. On the other hand, detection of a highly symptomatic but non-pulpally involved fracture may avert unnecessary endodontic treatment. It is even possible, if symptoms are not chronic and severe, to preserve a cracked tooth with a cast crown restoration, which "binds" the tooth and removes the wedging forces producing the symptoms. This might be done when replacing the tooth would be impossible (second molar), impractical (first molar with no second, making a removable partial necessary), or undesirable (a young patient with virgin teeth on either side of the cracked tooth). Generally, such a restoration should be only extracoronal and may be cemented temporarily with a highly sedative cement. Not only is this kind to the pulp, but it will assist in further diagnosis. If symptoms persist even with the tooth bound and a sedative cement employed, endodontic treatment (or extraction) is the only logical alternative. Temporary cementation then allows for removal of the crown to facilitate the endodontic opening.

Defective Restoration. A defective restoration is one of the most common dental dysfunctions and is not necessarily a reflection on the dentist who originally placed the restoration, although it all too often is just that (Fig. 5–7). Defective restorations are considered here in three main categories: marginal integrity, morphology, and occlusion. The most common critical defect in dental restorations is probably the lack of or failure of the marginal seal. If a clinically detectable open margin is not corrected, macroleakage will likely lead to caries that are often deep in the tooth and in close proximity to the pulp. Occasionally, it is possible to correct such a condition conservatively by "patching" the offending margin. This presumes good accessibility and little or no caries, such as in the case of an enamel fracture adjacent to a sound restoration. In many cases, however, a failure in the marginal seal has already allowed penetration of fluids and bacteria, and conservative repair is difficult, if not impossible. For example, an open margin on a cast restoration that is due to incomplete seating means that the entire casting has been cemented short of the prepared margin; patching one or two accessible openings may prolong the useable life of the casting but may also create a false sense of well-being, since leakage and caries can also be occurring elsewhere around the restoration and remain clinically undetected until it is too late.

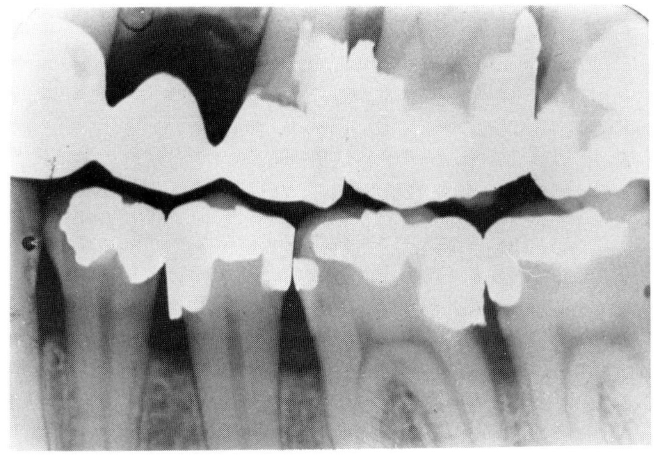

Fig. 5–7. This radiograph speaks for itself. I might only add that the bridge depicted was just over a year old and an esthetic disaster as well.

The diagnosis of an open margin must be made with a good deal of clinical judgment, since, in theory at least, virtually all margins are open to some degree. When viewed microscopically, and especially when analyzed ultramicroscopically (electron micrographs), the finest clinical margins resemble the Grand Canyon. We must take these microscopic findings not as an excuse for poor work, but as a challenge to improve. We must also consider that the criteria that have evolved for clinically acceptable restorations are based on generations of clinical experience. We know that a restoration that is sealed well upon clinical and radiographic examination will provide long and dependable service as compared to a margin that is not sealed well. The microscopic and ultramicroscopic appearance of the clinically acceptable margin is of interest, but may not be of great clinical significance.

To carry the point to the other extreme, even restorations with less than clinically acceptable marginal integrity may provide years of service without jeopardizing the teeth restored. Good clinical judgment again demands a pragmatic approach in the diagnosis of open margins. For example, to condemn every amalgam restoration with slight ditching around the margin is to condemn nearly every amalgam restoration after 1 to 3 years of service. The dentist must then diagnose lack or failure of marginal seal using a number of judgmental factors that include the following:

1. *Caries.* If definite, visible, probeable (soft, tacky), or radiographic caries are on a margin, the margin is defective, whether the open margin allowed carious invasion, or if caries developed and created the defect. Likewise, if an open margin is probed with a diagnostic explorer and resistance to withdrawal is encountered, as is characteristic of caries, it should be treated as caries and repaired or replaced.

2. *Caries rate and oral-hygiene status.* A restoration having a less-than-acceptable marginal seal may hold up and provide years of service in a well-maintained, nearly caries-free mouth, but may fail quickly in a more hostile environment.

3. *Age of the restoration.* A less-than-ideal marginal seal that is noncarious after 3 to 5 years of service might simply be watched and noted, while a deteriorating margin on a restoration that is 15- to 20-years old may indicate the end of a long and useful term of service.

4. *Cost/benefit considerations.* Does the benefit to be gained in replacing or repairing the less-than-ideal margin justify the cost of the procedure? This decision must be made by the dentist and the party responsible for the fee.

Improper morphology is a defect that can be found in nearly all dental restorations if evaluated closely enough. It is less often a critical defect, however, in that long-term clinical success is often seen despite poor or improper morphology. Some defects are critical in that they can result in failure of the restoration, or more often, can create or contribute to pathology of the periodontium and thereby require repair or replacement. The following are some of the factors to be considered in the diagnosis of improper morphology:

1. *Axial contours.* Improper contour can include all deviations from natural tooth contour, but the most common critical fault is overbulking of restorations in the gingival third, resulting in a protected area for plaque formation and unhealthy gingival tissues, especially where this overcontour is subgingival.

Recently, some excellent work has been done on natural contours in the gingival third, and the results have shown that many earlier texts have depicted that area of dental anatomy incorrectly, much to the detriment of periodontal health.[2,34,35]

2. *Contacts.* Faulty contacts in dental restorations include open contacts, which permit food impaction and subsequent gingival irritation, and broad, rough, tight contacts, which are not readily cleansed with floss. Either situation presents the potential for periodontal damage. Diagnosis of faulty contacts should consider the severity of the problem, the status of the affected periodontal tissues, and the potential for conservative correction of the contact discrepancy.

3. *Overhangs.* As opposed to overcontour, overhangs are inadvertent extrusions of restorative material, usually at gingival margins, that are due to poor matrix adaptation or failure to check the margin immediately upon placement. While usually a feature of amalgam restorations, overhangs may also be found with composite resin and other anterior materials, and occasionally in cast restorations in which poor impressions or laboratory techniques produce a casting that does not adapt closely to the tooth at the gingival margin.

4. *Surface smoothness.* Defects in surface smoothness range from a smooth but unpolished amalgam restoration, to gross pits, pockmarks, and corrosion that is due to improper handling and placement of materials or the great age of the restoration. Because surface roughness contributes to the formation of plaque and complicates its removal, it can be a critical defect over a period of time.

Good subjective clinical judgment is required in assessing the significance of improper morphology in the diagnosis of defective restorations. The severity of the defect, the visible evidence of pathology stemming from it, the potential for future pathology, the possible options for conservative correction or total replacement, and the cost/benefit picture must all be considered in the diagnosis.Thus, a restoration with improper morphology may be ignored, watched, repaired, or discarded entirely, and a new restoration proposed once the factors have been evaluated. The dentist should not hesitate to indicate the need for treatment, even if there are no caries, should frank pathology be diagnosed as stemming from the morphologic defect.

Occlusion and the occlusal diagnosis will be discussed as a separate entity later in this chapter. Faulty occlusion, as it applies to defective restorations, falls into two categories: the hyperoccluding, or high restoration, and the hypo- or nonoccluding restoration. The most noticeable occlusal defect in restorations is the high spot, in which occlusal contact in full closure is made primarily on the restoration rather than in harmony with the entire dentition. The patient will usually be aware of this discrepancy and request treatment. If the discrepancy is slight or the patient's tolerance great, the hyperoccluding restoration can lead to pulpal pathology, periodontal destruction in the presence of inflammation, fractured restorations, fractured teeth, or alterations in the functioning occlusion so as to avoid the high spot, which in turn may affect other teeth or the TMJ. For this reason, recently placed restorations should be evaluated in terms of their comfort and compatibility, and any signs of hyperocclusion noted in the diagnosis.

A restoration can also be hyperoccluding in excursive strokes, and this situation is often more subtle in its clinical appearance. Although the restoration may feel comfortable in full closure, excursive interferences can produce the same harmful sequelae as the simple high spot. Wear facets or "skid" marks may aid the diagnosis, as well as mobility and tenderness to percussion or chewing. Because of their subtlety, excursive occlusal discrepancies may prove to be more serious restorative defects than those in full closure and are often more difficult to eliminate. An improperly placed cusp or groove that creates a major excursive disharmony may not be adjustable, but require another restoration entirely. Other minor occlusal discrepancies might be adjusted and repolished with minimal time and effort. The diagnosis of faulty occlusion in a restoration should consider both the need for correction and the potential for conservative adjustment vs. replacement.

A subtle problem and one that is least often considered when discussing defective restorations is the hypo- or nonoccluding restoration. Such restorations do not support the occlusion and provide less function than those that make contact in full closure. If a contacting point (centric stop) is removed in preparation for a restoration and is not replaced, the opposing tooth may shift its relationship and both the restored tooth and its opponent may drift, tip, or supererupt, depending on the number of contacts that have been lost and their importance in maintaining stability of the occlusion. These observations hold true not only for the full occlusal cast restoration, but for silver amalgams as well. Indeed, while a "short" full-cast crown may successfully and uneventfully supererupt into an acceptable occlusion, overcarved, "short" silver amalgams may supererupt into deeper intercuspation of already weakened cusps, with greater potential for fracturing. While it is postulated that silver amalgam cannot support the occlusion, it is absolutely certain that overcarved and nonoccluding amalgams that fail to replace lost centric-stop contacts haven't a chance of even trying to support it. Such restorations are just as defective (relatively) as those placed in hyperocclusion. Once again, the significance of faulty occlusion in determining whether a restoration is defective is judgmental, and similar criteria can be applied, as outlined for defective margins and improper morphology.

Disfigurement

Disfigured teeth are those that present an unnatural and displeasing appearance due to stains, developmental defects, or nonesthetic dental restorations. There is certainly an overlap between this classification and that of dysfunction, as many developmental defects are both dysfunctional and disfiguring. The same is true of many defective restorations. Disfigurement is considered separately for two reasons: First, in a great many situations, a tooth or restoration is perfectly functional, but looks hideous. Second, the criteria for what is disfigured, or unesthetic, are determined by the patient as well as the dentist. The dentist should refrain from making an esthetic judgment regarding his patient's teeth; rather, he should discover the patient's feeling about his teeth before he diagnoses a disfigurement. Disfigured teeth fall into three general categories: stained teeth, misshapen teeth, and teeth with discolored or nonesthetic restorations.

Stained teeth may be extrinsically stained, due to poor hygiene, dietary factors (coffee, tea), habits (smoking, chewing tobacco), or other unexplained factors. Extrinsic stains are often removable, although considerable effort may be required. More effective home care may reduce such stains, but unless the apparent etiologic factor is eliminated, it may provide only temporary improvement. If possible, the diagnosis of extrinsic stain should include the probable staining agent.

Stained teeth may also be intrinsically stained, due to alterations in enamel formation resulting from systemic disease states (high fevers, etc.) or ingested substances incorporated into the enamel (fluorosis, tetracycline stains, etc.). Nonvital or pulpally damaged teeth may become discolored because of the breakdown of vital tissues, and this discoloration may permeate the tooth. Intrinsic stains are difficult to remove, and the bleaching and masking techniques

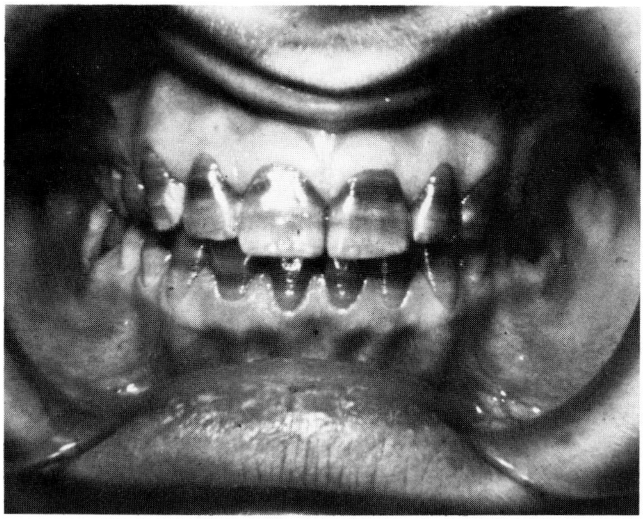

A

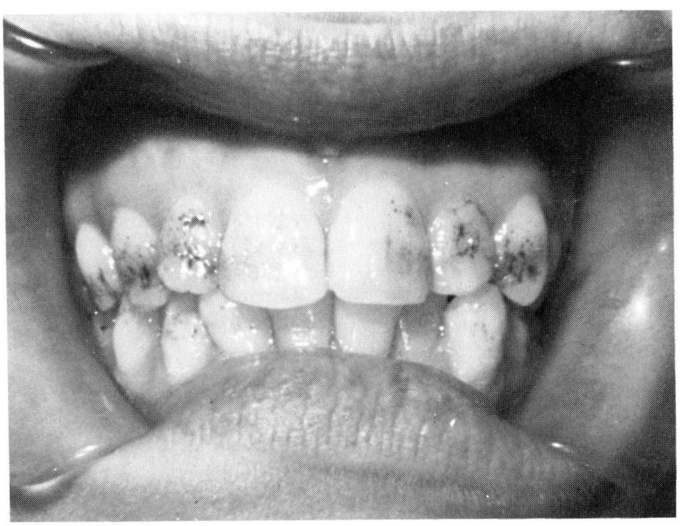

B

Fig. 5–8. *A,* Tetracycline staining. *B,* Severe congenital pitting that accumulated extrinsic stain.

currently available are not uniformly successful in application or predictable in long-term use (Fig. 5–8).

Misshapen teeth have an abnormal size, shape, or appearance because of fracture or developmental defect. This assessment is highly subjective and should be left primarily to the patient. For example, one patient may find his pegged lateral incisors quite acceptable—even a visual plus—while another patient may detest them. The dentist should seek the patient's assessment of all such teeth, since many patients may be unhappy with their appearance but be unaware that simple and low-cost treatment is available. The advent of the acid-etch bonded composite resin has made possible many small cosmetic repairs or cover-ups at reasonable cost without reduction of tooth structure. Patients who are unaware of that potential and/or who have been told that nothing can be done short of full coverage crowns, may not mention their displeasure regarding a misshapen tooth, but may deeply appreciate the dentist's concern for them, especially if a simple solution can be offered.

Discolored or nonesthetic restorations should be noted in the dental diagnosis. These are dental restorations that have an unnatural or unpleasant visual appearance but function adequately and have an acceptable marginal seal. Nonesthetic restorations must be judged in relative terms, because what is acceptable to one patient may seem grossly disfiguring to another. At the same time, practicality must be considered, since many tooth-colored, esthetic restorative materials are unsuitable for use in certain areas and situations. We have too often seen the extensive use of resins in large, Class II posterior restorations with disastrous results. The same might be said about many full porcelain occlusal crowns and bridges in the posterior segments, due to their abrasiveness. On the other hand, there are many situations in which esthetics can be enhanced by choices of technique or material without compromising functional requirements; a consideration of discolored or nonesthetic restorations should be made in the dental diagnosis.

Because the teeth are fairly accessible to visual and radiographic examination, it is customary to diagnose each tooth individually. Dental record systems must provide for the documentation of status for each tooth, as well as for an indication of missing teeth. This is usually done through a graphic or written chart listing the 32 permanent teeth (and 20 deciduous teeth, when applicable) and allowing for indications of the presence or absence and status of each tooth.

This detailed listing serves as the basis for the dental diagnosis, and in many cases, is the diagnosis itself. A detailed description of individual tooth status may not satisfy our criterion for diagnosis, which is the identification of what is happening and why. It tells us in detail what is happening to individual teeth, but the etiologic factor may not be clear. For this reason, the dental diagnosis should also consider the teeth as a whole as well as overall patterns of disease and dysfunction in the dentition. Figure 5–9 is an example of a written record of a dental diagnosis; the findings are abbreviated or encoded in order to save time and space (Fig. 5–9).

A brief summary of the detailed findings may better serve to identify potential etiologies; the following examples illustrate this:

DENTAL AND RADIOGRAPHIC FINDINGS

TOOTH #	EXISTING REST.	CL. CAR.	RADIOGRAPHIC: BW car. oh con	RADIOGRAPHIC: PERIAPICAL bone & root end pathology	VITALITY	MOBILITY	SUMMATION: SURFACES	SUMMATION: PROCEDURE
1	X							
2	MO/A							
3	MO/A	O	D					
4	MOD/A	FRACTURED						
5					4			
6	M/R				5			
7	D/R	DISCOLORED						
8	M/R							
9	M/R		D					
10			M		3			
11					3			
12	MOD/A	O		P.A. LUCENCY	10 (N.V.)			
13	MO/A	D			4			
14	X							
15	MO/A	M(OH)		MESIAL TIPPING		2		
16	—	—	—	IMPACTED				
17	—	—	—	IMPACTED				
18	FCC	B(G)	OH	THICKENED PDL		1		
19	MODB/A	MARGINAL		DITCHING				
20	DO/A							
21	DO/R		DO?					
22								
23				}		1		
24				} BONE LOSS		2		
25				}		2		
26				}		1		
27								
28			OPEN	CONTACT				
29	X							
30	X							
31	MOL/A	B	M	MESIAL TIPPING		1		
32	X							

NAME JANE DOE DATE 11-20-82

OD 103

Fig. 5–9. Completed dental chart, the basis for the dental diagnosis.

1. Teeth are heavily restored and have generalized new and recurrent caries; patient is missing lower first permanent molars due to caries-related abscesses.

2. Patient has generalized occlusal wear, and his dentin is exposed throughout posterior; he has a low caries rate and few restorations.

3. Patient's dentition is fairly sound, but many existing alloy restorations are old and show marked marginal breakdown with several overhangs and open contacts.

4. Teeth have moderate to severe discoloration, probably due to tetracycline therapy; there is abnormal enamel formation on molars.

Functional Diagnosis

Based on the findings of the examination of the occlusion and the temporomandibular joint, and the myofunctional analysis of tongue, lips, and cheeks, the dentist can address the last factor in the multifactorial approach to diagnosis.

In many respects, the functional diagnosis is the most important factor, since it considers how and whether the entire stomatognathic system, teeth, periodontium, temporomandibular joint, and the neuromuscular components surrounding and supplying them serve their intended purpose. Does the system provide efficient function in mastication, deglutition, and speech? Do the components of the system function in comfort and harmony with one another? How does the system relate to the general health and well being of the individual patient?

The functional diagnosis is the most difficult factor in the multifactorial approach, since it is more difficult to evaluate and analyze a system than a tooth or a soft-tissue lesion, for example. Likewise, relationships of teeth and bone to muscles and joints are more difficult to identify than the relationship of a periodontal lesion to an overhanging restoration. Finally, our knowledge and understanding of these functional relationships are not yet standardized by definitive research and documentation. We must work primarily with empirical principles, which rely on subjective clinical impressions of experienced clinicians, and temper them with our own results and observations.

The absence of hard scientific data should not discourage the dentist from dealing with functional problems, since there is a growing body of clinical experience suggesting considerable consensus in many areas. Given a clinical approach that has proven consistently effective in treating functional problems, the dentist can certainly utilize that approach to help patients despite a lack of scientific evidence to support it. For example, zinc oxide and eugenol was being used as a sedative treatment in deep cavities with good results long before definitive histologic and biochemical studies confirmed its effectiveness. Today, we routinely utilize bite-plane therapy in the diagnosis and treatment of myofascial pain/dysfunction syndromes, but we do so without a clear, scientific understanding of the nature and causes of the problem and without definitive proof of the mechanism of action of the bite-plane therapy. We do, however, have a consensus of clinical opinion about the efficacy of the approach, which is supported by our own good clinical results.

In this way, we go about the task of analyzing and evaluating the function of the stomatognathic system, using the knowledge that is currently available, some of which is definitive but much of which is empirical. In so doing, we must be prepared to adjust to new data that may support or disprove the theories upon which we operate. Flexibility in thinking and the ability to adjust to new information and scientific evidence are crucial in this area of dental diagnosis. All too often, practitioners cling to outdated, discredited theories and concepts and are less effective clinicians as a result.

With this background, we approach the functional diagnosis. Diagnosis generally involves comparing a set of findings to scientifically documented norms. A histologic comparison of normal, healthy epithelium to a suspected lesion that shows many abnormal mitotic figures and other signs of malignant growth provides a definitive diagnosis. In the functioning of the stomatognathic system, certain norms also exist, but they are more empirically derived, and hence, less dependable as diagnostic criteria. While comparing our findings with these norms, we must also utilize a more pragmatic approach—that is, despite apparent deviations from normal, does the patient have a real problem? Does the patient perceive any difficulties in mastication, deglutition, or speech? Does the fact that an occlusal arrangement varies from our textbook description of normal (Class I Angle) really make it a malocclusion?

It has been postulated that, in the absence of pathology, whatever occlusion, TMJ function, lip, cheek, or tongue function the patient may have is normal for that patient. This definition of the normal, healthy stomatognathic system should be considered at all times in the functional diagnosis. It emphasizes that not all edentulous spaces demand fixed bridges, not all Class II occlusions need to be Class I's, and not all noisy TMJs require bite-plane therapy and occlusal equilibration. Unless pathology (disease or dysfunction) can be identified as arising from the

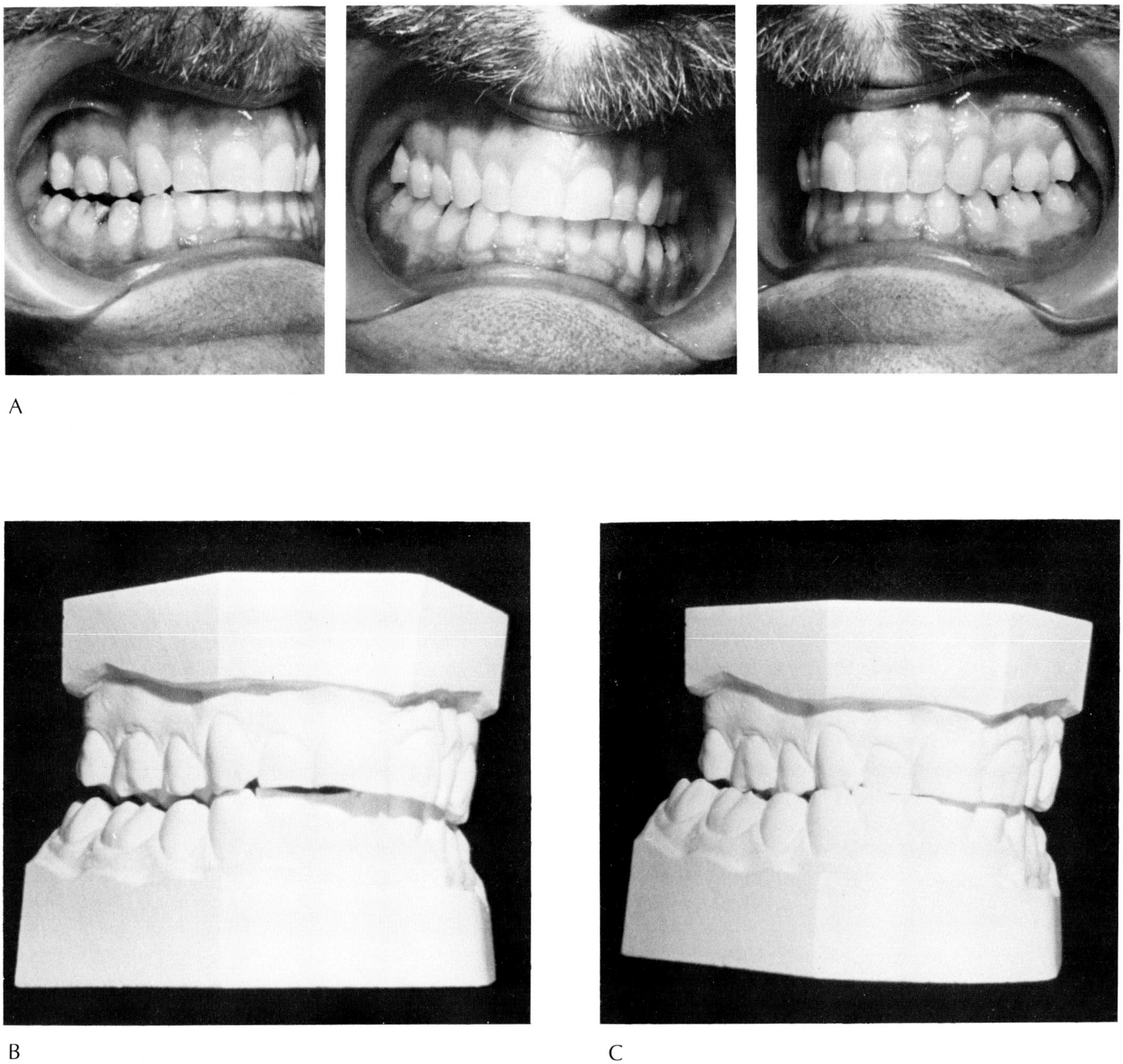

Fig. 5–10. *A*, Clinical view of a "healthy, abnormal" occlusion. *B*, Diagnostic casts demonstrating anterior-posterior open bite. *C*, Probable habitual centric position producing incisal wear.

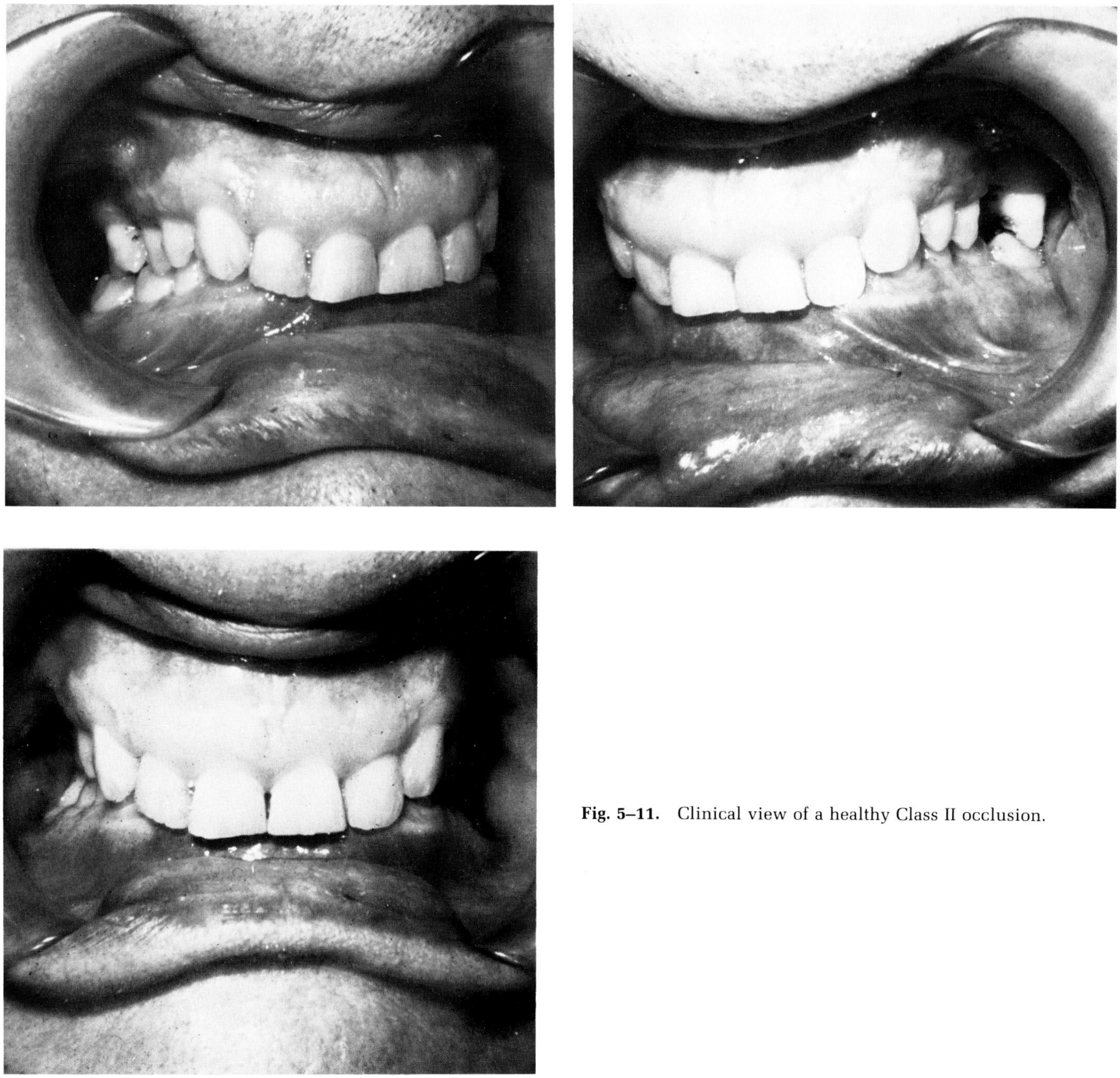

Fig. 5–11. Clinical view of a healthy Class II occlusion.

apparent abnormality, it may not be abnormal for that patient. Indeed, we have all observed gross occlusal disharmonies that require extreme accommodation of the TMJ and that are coupled with unusual lip and tongue habits; these disharmonies are present without any noticeable symptoms or signs of pathology. Figure 5–10 illustrates this point through the brief case history of a 35-year-old physician, whose progress has been followed during periodic recall visits for 10 years.

From the outset, severe occlusal abnormalities were present, including severe, anterior open bite (horizontal) (Fig. 5–10B), CO-CR discrepancy of more than 2 mm, no cusp-fossa relationships in the posterior, and consistent interposition of the tongue between anterior teeth on swallowing. At no time did the patient experience pain or discomfort, difficulty in mastication, deglutition, or speech, or any other noticeable symptom.

His treatment to date has been confined to regular preventive counselling and prophylaxis and minor operative dentistry. At this time, however, incisal wear is becoming a concern. The nature of the wear would suggest that it is the result of fairly striking excursive movements that the patient is unaware of; hence, the movements are probably nocturnal (Fig. 5–10C). Conservative treatment is still contemplated, however, since wear is the only observable sign and the patient remains free of symptoms. Fabrication of a night guard is potentially the next step should the wear continue.

Describing maxillomandibular relationships other than Class I as malocclusions may also be misleading. Figure 5–11 illustrates this point with the case history of a 46-year-old engineer, whose progress has been followed during periodic recall visits for 6 years.

Despite his striking Class II relationship and deep anterior overbite, the patient's periodontal health is excellent; he has only normal occlusal wear, and is perfectly comfortable and functional. The missing upper left first molar may be replaced with a fixed bridge at some future date, but the second molar appears stable (no observable tipping or drifting in 6 years).

The concept of treating as normal any state or condition that is not frankly pathologic has much to recommend it, especially when our understanding of the norm derives from empirical observation and clinical experience. To diagnose a 5-mm discrepancy between CO and CR (IP and RCP) as abnormal presupposes that the more distal position is a physiologic standard, but most dentists will agree it is not. Therefore, the functional diagnosis should concern itself with actual signs and symptoms of pathology.

The absence of pathology, however, must not be assumed simply because the patient does not appear incapacitated. Pathology (disease or dysfunction in the stomatognathic system) can be subtle and diffuse. Functional disturbances, moreover, can arise in any of the components of the system and be reflected in various ways throughout. A disharmony between occlusion and the TMJ, for example, may lead to pulpal involvement from traumatic occlusion, severe occlusal wear in the attempt to accommodate, extensive periodontal destruction in the presence of inflammation, TMJ disturbances from accommodation attempts, myofascial pain, muscle spasms, or even headaches and neck pains. One cannot dismiss the potential of pathology arising in the system unless an exhaustive evaluation of the entire system is done.

Symptoms of pathology in the system can arise so gradually over such a period of time that the patient may not be aware of them. If you have never had a harmonious occlusion, you may not know that yours is compromised. As with most oral and dental problems, acute pain is seldom present in the early stages. Finally, many patients possess high levels of tolerance to insults and injuries that would be immediately noticed and attended to by others. Pathology that is well tolerated by the patient is still pathology, and it must not be considered normal.

With this general concept of normality in mind, I will briefly describe present clinical concepts of normality in occlusion, TMJ, and myofunctional environment. I will also discuss what signs/symptoms are considered potentially pathologic and some examples of frank pathology in those areas.

Occlusion

1. *Array*. The normal adult complement of 32 teeth is desirable, if not functionally necessary, and requires sufficient room in the arch to accommodate them and allow effective plaque removal. This is not commonly seen, however, and for most people, 28 teeth seems to be the norm. Furthermore, clinical experience would suggest that adequate function and support is obtainable with first-molar occlusion—that is, 24 permanent teeth.

Potential pathology in the array ranges from too many teeth to too few. Third molars that are distal to the available attached gingiva, surrounded in full or in part by mucosa, have partial flaps of tissue around or over them, and deep, pocket-like crevices around them are potentially pathologic. Unerupted third molars that can be probed—that is, molars whose coronal surface and periocoronal space communicates with the oral cavity—are potential sites for periocoronal infection. Unerupted third molars or unerupted supernumerary teeth that do not communicate with the oral cavity and are full bony impactions, or at the least, fully enclosed by intact soft tissue, are potential sites for cyst formation. An array of less than 28 permanent teeth due to extraction or congenital partial anodontia is potentially pathologic from two standpoints: first, missing teeth within the array (not the distalmost teeth) may lead to tipping and/or drifting of teeth adjacent to the space, especially those distal to it, and/or supereruption of opposing teeth; second, missing posterior teeth may increase the functional load of remaining teeth, compromising them physically, periodontally, or orthodontically.

Frank pathology in the array is seen when any of the potential situations just described are present. Presence of inflammation or infection around third molars, radiographic evidence of cyst formation around unerupted teeth, tipping, drifting, or supereruption that jeopardizes the teeth involved or compromises function, or evidence of occlusal traumatism in the anterior, where posterior support is lacking, are some of the possible pathologic findings. As a general rule, an array that does not have first molar occlusion at least on one side will not provide normal support and function, and may therefore be pathologic.

It should be noted here that we are discussing occlusal arrays that have not been prosthetically restored. Obviously, if missing teeth have been adequately replaced with fixed and/or removable appliances to approximate the normal, healthy array, the pathology has been arrested.

2. *Alignment.* Alignment refers to the mesiodistal relationships of the teeth, the overall arch form in mesiodistal, facial-lingual dimensions, the occlusal plane, and the axial orientation of the teeth. Normal alignment would entail snug contacts between all teeth, which prevent food impaction but are readily cleansible with dental floss. A line envisioned passing through the center of each tooth should describe a smooth arch form, more or less symmetrical left and right. All teeth should fall approximately into the same occlusal plane vertically, so that marginal ridge height is fairly even from tooth to tooth. Teeth should be oriented axially so that forces are directed approximately along the long axis.

Potential pathology in the alignment arises when deviations from the norm are present. It is obvious that most normal, healthy occlusions deviate from the "dentoform" model we have just described. Taking any or all of the alignment factors listed, we can easily cite clinical examples in which open contact areas, irregular and asymmetrical arch form, unusual occlusal plane arrangements, and tipped teeth were present without any sign of pathology. The degree of potential pathology seen in deviations from the norm depends on the severity of the deviation as well as the individual's tolerance to the deviation.

Frank pathology must be diagnosed on the basis that the alignment has produced other pathologic processes or contributed to them. An open contact area that shows signs of periodontal inflammation, particularly if there is pocket formation and/or bone loss, is a pathologic finding. A tooth that is positioned at an angle divergent from the applied functional forces and exhibits mobility and/or periodontal pathology is in a pathologic alignment. A tooth (or teeth) that is crowded in an irregular arch form that makes effective plaque removal impossible (or unlikely, given the human factor) constitutes pathology in alignment.

3. *Maxillomandibular relationship.* The essential element in occlusion is precisely that—how the teeth occlude. Indeed, it is quite possible to have a sufficient array in terms of numbers of teeth, with each arch having reasonably normal form and alignment, but with such disharmony between maxillary and mandibular teeth that the patient is dentally disabled. Furthermore, it is not possible to discuss interarch relationships without considering the source of that relationship—the TMJ. The normal interarch relationship can be summarized as follows: maxillary and mandibular teeth meshing together comfortably and in harmony with the TMJ, with freedom in all excursive movements. This general description can be detailed in terms of static occlusal relationships and dynamic occlusal relationships.

In the static occlusion, or full closure of the teeth, posterior teeth should interdigitate so as to provide efficient mastication and, ideally, occlusal stability. Occlusal stability is gained by multiple point contacts (tripodization or some approximation of it), which serve to prevent the teeth from tipping or drifting. Anterior teeth should contact lightly in full closure, preferably with some vertical and horizontal overlap of upper teeth over the lowers. These conditions may be met even with molar relationships other than Class I (Angle classification), and many so-called malocclusions are comfortable, functional, esthetically satisfactory, and free of pathology. In the full-closure position (CO, IP), the mandibular condyles should be comfortably seated in the glenoid fossae, neither forcibly retruded, nor significantly protruded down the eminence. The question of what is significant deserves discussion and requires consideration of the retruded or centric relation position.

Centric Relation Position. Centric relation position: That position of the mandible created by the prosthodontist only to be hopelessly confused by the periodontist and totally ignored by the orthodontist. This tongue-in-cheek definition serves to illustrate some of the controversy involving the position. Centric relation is defined as the most retruded position of the mandible from which lateral movements can be made. It has been described as that position in which the condyles of the mandible are in the uppermost, rearmost position in the glenoid fossae. It is further described as that position in which slight opening and closing movements are purely hinge motions, without translation of the condyle. The confusion that exists regarding centric relation centers around its clinical and physiologic significance.

Clinically, the centric relation position is highly significant in that it is fairly stable, readily reproducible, and predictably functional. Although long-term changes, such as condylar-head remodeling, may affect the exact location, the retruded position generally can be consistently located without change before, during, and after most clinical procedures. Different operators using similar methods will most often agree on its location. Therefore, unlike most mandibular movements and positions that have infinite and random variations, centric relation remains stable on repeated observations. Centric relation is also readily reproducible through the process of hinge-axis location and transfer, thus allowing the dentist to duplicate on an articulator the exact arc of closure and maxillomandibular relationship in retruded position. Finally, clinical experience has demonstrated that occlusions equilibrated to or restored in the centric relation position will be stable, well tolerated, and functional. This predictability of success is the key to the clinical significance of the retruded position.

Because centric relation is stable, reproducible, and functional, it has been inferred that it is a physiologic norm. No evidence presently available suggests that this is true. Indeed, while a clinical impression exists that deviations from centric relation in full closure (centric occlusion) produce or contribute to occlusal or TMJ pathology, we see many normal, healthy, functional individuals with gross discrepancies and many severely dysfunctional individuals with very slight or no discrepancies. Studies done on asymptomatic, normal individuals suggest that rather than viewing centric relation as a physiologic norm, it should be viewed as a reference point for a range of normality. These studies suggest that most normal individuals reach full intercuspation (centric occlusion) within 1 to 1.5 mm of their fully retruded (centric relation) position.[5,12,24,27]

For condylar positioning in the static occlusion, centric occlusion should occur within 1 to 2 mm of centric relation in a normal model—that is, the condyles should not translate down the eminence a great distance to accommodate intercuspation. There is a wide range of normality here, however, and the individual patient's physiology and tolerance must be considered in the diagnosis.

Potential pathology in the static occlusion may be evidenced by any of the following:

1. Lack of interdigitation in the posterior due to open bite, cusp-to-cusp alignment, or discrepancies in arch size or form between maxilla and mandible
2. Lack of stability in posterior occlusion evidenced by cuspless teeth (congenital, flat-plane anatomy, worn teeth, or iatrogenic flattening due to nonanatomic restorations or irrational equilibration), or by intercuspal contacts limited to inclined planes (slope-to-slope contact, rather than cusp-fossa or cusp-marginal ridge)
3. Anterior open bite, or severe anterior overlap, either of which may compromise the function and health of the anterior teeth and the dentition as a whole
4. Deviation in full closure from centric relation of more than 2 mm, discrepancies between CO and CR that require lateral movements to achieve intercuspation, or static occlusions that tend to forcibly retrude the mandible beyond its centric relation position

Dynamic occlusal relationships are those that occur in any excursion from full closure and are guided by the teeth and the condylar heads of the TMJ functioning in the glenoid fossae. They are influenced by the neuromuscular components and, inasmuch as the mandible is virtually free floating, can present infinite variety to the observer. This variability must be understood and appreciated when attempting to diagnose the occlusion.

To understand the range of normality in dynamic occlusal relationships, we must briefly review the guidance factors and their possible combinations. Teeth, either singly or in groups, act as one factor in the guidance system. Tooth guidance patterns include the following:

1. Pure canine guidance (cuspid rise), in which lateral excursive contacts occur only on upper and lower canine teeth on the working side, causing all other teeth to disocclude in lateral or lateroprotrusive movements.
2. Anterior group function, in which canine, lateral, and central incisors act in concert or in sequence to disocclude posterior teeth in excursions. This situation might be considered an ideal norm, in that it

is the most common pattern in protrusive guidance and seems to have many advantages in lateral and lateroprotrusive function. Specifically, lateral stresses, which are generally considered deleterious to teeth, are applied at the furthest point from the TMJ, or fulcrum of the lever system, and are minimized. Secondly, these forces are applied to teeth whose root structure and length seem able to tolerate them. Finally, teeth acting in concert or in smooth sequence share the load applied and thus minimize both stress and wear factors.

3. Anteroposterior group function, working side, in which posterior teeth also contact in excursive movements. This could involve the first premolar only or may extend to upper buccal cusps against lower buccal cusps of every tooth on the working side.

4. Balancing-side contact. Any contact of teeth on the side opposite the excursive movement is a balancing-side contact. Such contacts may range from momentary contact in the initial movement, which is very common, to the balanced occlusion of a well-worn dentition, or to sole guidance of a balancing-side tooth in which teeth on the working side do not contact. The clinician should not be influenced by terminology in the diagnosis of the occlusion. The term balancing side "interference" should be avoided unless the contact in question is interfering with something.

Just as significant in the dynamic occlusion is the guidance of the TMJ, which acts in concert with tooth guidance. Viewed from the starting point of static occlusion, the condyle heads move in a variety of ways in the glenoid fossa, dictated by the cartilage and ligaments associated with the joints. Movement is caused by the muscle groups associated with the TMJ and the tonus of these muscles may also influence mandibular movements. While mandibular movements can occur in nearly infinite variety in three dimensions, they can be grouped as protrusions or lateroprotrusive excursions.

Protrusion, or a simple opening beyond the hinge range, requires the condylar head to move downward and forward on the eminentia. The angle of this downward incline in relation to the plane of occlusion and cuspal height influences the degree of anterior tooth guidance in protrusion. In other words, a steep angle may tend to disocclude posterior teeth and result in total anterior tooth guidance, while a flatter angle may allow posterior cusps to contact in protrusion. Conversely, deep, severe, anterior overbites and the resultant anterior guidance may disocclude posterior teeth even with a flat condylar angle, while anterior open bites result in posterior guidance no matter how steep the condylar incline. This relationship between condyles and tooth guidance should be kept in mind throughout the diagnosis of the dynamic occlusion (Fig. 5–12).

Lateral excursion, or lateroprotrusive excursions, involve a number of condylar guidance factors:

1. The balancing-side condyle moves downward, forward, and inward in the fossa. This is the result of a rotation around the working-side condyle and may result in a steeper angle than straight protrusion.

2. The working-side condyle, while essentially in simple rotation, moves slightly upward and backward.

3. The entire mandible may shift to the working side (Bennett shift), and this shifting may occur immediately in the excursion (immediate side shift) or as the excursion progresses. This side shift may be highly significant in relation to tooth guidance in that a relatively rapid and distinct mandibular shift may produce posterior lateral interferences even with apparently adequate anterior guidance and steep condylar angles.

While highly significant, the movements of the condylar heads in the dynamic occlusion are difficult to diagnose without sophisticated and time-consuming procedures. Pantographic tracings may be made in three dimensions and duplicated with fully adjustable articulators. When study casts (see Chap. 4) are mounted using the hinge-axis and centric-relation bites, we can see the relation of condylar guidance and tooth guidance in dynamic occlusion. Another gnathologic technique can produce molded analogs of the glenoid fossa, demonstrating graphically the factors just discussed. In most cases, however, such sophisticated approaches are not indicated. While the information they may provide is interesting and significant, it may not be necessary, unless one contemplates total reconstruction of a dentition. Just as important, the guidance of the TMJ in dynamic occlusion cannot be altered effectively and therefore, must be accepted as a constant—that is, while we can possibly alter the plane of occlusion, the transverse and anteroposterior curves of Wilson and Spee, and the tooth guidance through occlusal adjustment or restoration, the condylar guidance remains relatively unchanged. One exception to this statement is TMJ dysfunction, which, when relieved, may allow fuller retrusion of the condyles and lateral movements free of spasm. In such a case, the condylar guidance seen initially may change somewhat as the pathology is eliminated. Conversely, TMJ dysfunction arising after careful analysis of condylar

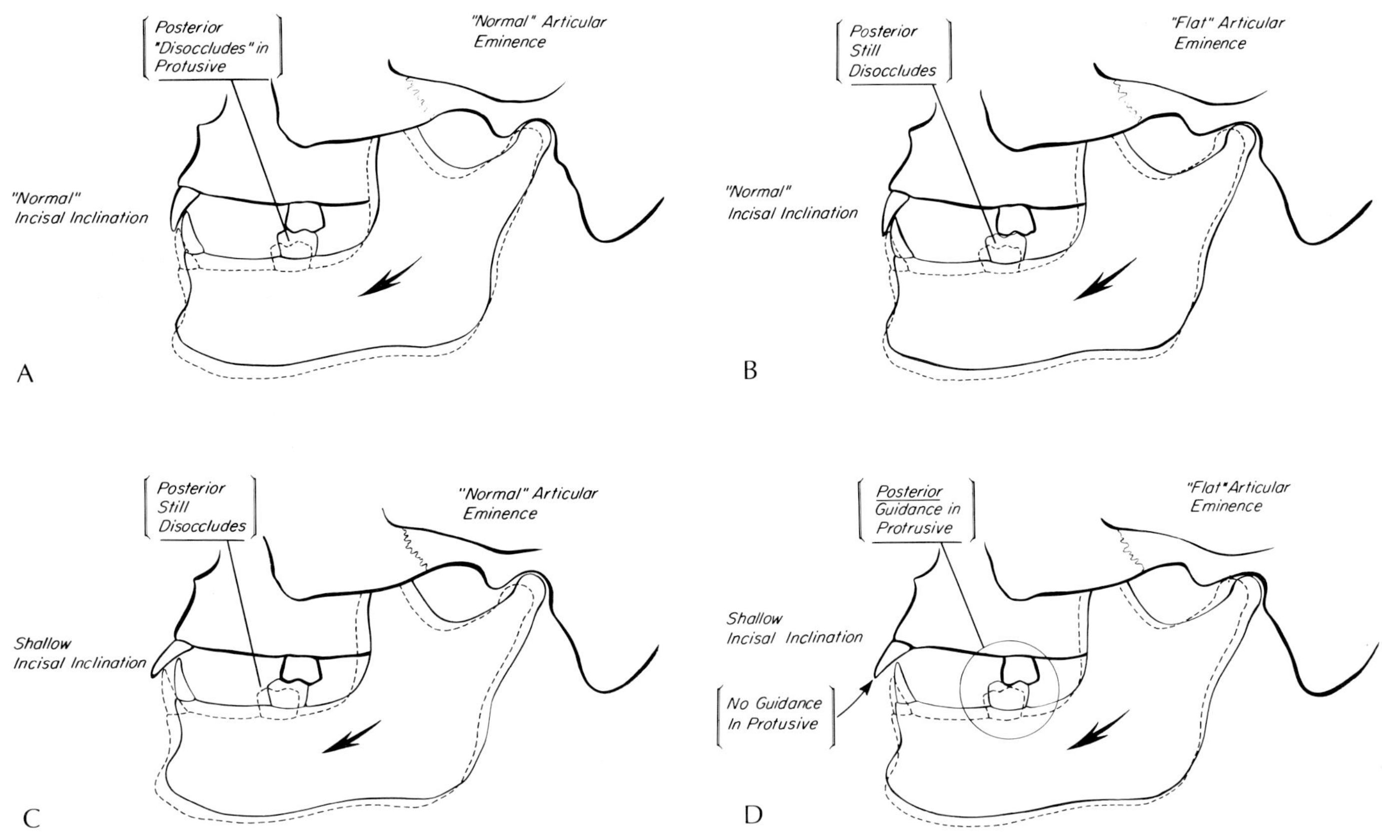

Fig. 5–12. Hypothetical combinations of tooth and condylar guidance in protrusive excursions. *A*, With relatively "normal" articular and incisal inclinations, posterior teeth disocclude in protrusive stroke. *B*, A "flat" articular inclination combined with normal incisal guidance still allows posterior clearance. *C*, Conversely, relatively shallow incisal guidance may be overcome by normal articular inclination in disoccluding posteriors. *D*, An anterior open bite, however, or shallow inclines of anterior teeth and joint create posterior guidance in protrusive excursions.

guidance may produce changes in the guidance that affect the dynamic occlusion. The following example may illustrate this point.

A healthy 24-year-old man was seen for restorative dentistry that involved cast occlusal restorations on all eight molar teeth and Class II restorations on premolars (four of which had been removed to facilitate orthodontics some time previously). Anterior teeth were sound, and provided very adequate guidance (disocclusion) in all lateral movements. Centric occlusion related well to centric relation, and when the molar restorations were made all at one time, a hinge axis was located and utilized to refine the coincidence of CO and CR. Restorations were designed to be free of any contact in excursions on working or balancing sides. The restorations were placed, and checked at 1 week, 6 weeks, and 3 months. On each of these occasions, occlusion was stable, with tripodization of cuspal contacts, coincidence of CO and CR, and no posterior contact in excursions.

Approximately 7 months following insertion, the patient called complaining of TMJ tenderness upon awakening. He was observed that day, and two findings were evident: first, an apparent CO-CR discrepancy of more than 1 mm was present; and second, a distinct balancing side interference was detectable in left lateral excursion. The right TMJ was symptomatic, and associated muscles were tender to palpation. Resisting the temptation to adjust the occlusion, which only a few months previously had been carefully analyzed and meticulously restored, I took a history that revealed considerable stress in the patient's life. A wife who was seriously (and, it was later found, terminally) ill, small children to be cared for, occupational stresses, and the recent development of a gum-chewing habit (albeit sugarless gum) were considered possible contributing factors.

The patient was asked to stop chewing gum and to use a mild sedative at bedtime (Scotch whiskey being the sedative of the patient's choice). Within 2 days, the symptoms had abated. Upon examination 4 days later, CO and CR were found to coincide exactly, and no balancing contact could be detected in lateral excursions.

It is clear from this and similar clinical experiences that, while the anatomy of the TMJ is relatively stable, the neuromuscular components greatly influence condylar guidance in the dynamic occlusion. Therefore, if one is attempting to analyze this guidance in diagnosis, that influence must be considered. Centric relation records, lateral checkbites, and even pantographic tracings may be altered by neuromuscular dysfunction, and as the problems are alleviated, further analysis is necessary to obtain a truer picture of TMJ guidance. Unlike occlusal modification, such changes are neither predictable nor controllable by the clinician.

Keeping these guidance factors in mind, we can consider the following as potential pathologic findings in the dynamic occlusion:

1. Posterior tooth guidance in protrusive movement, due to anterior open bite, a tipped or supererupted posterior tooth (or teeth), or exceedingly flat condylar angles. This can lead to excessive stresses on the teeth or the TMJ, but if well tolerated, should not be considered pathologic in itself.

2. Posterior tooth guidance in lateral excursions, especially seen on molars without group function, throughout the working side. Another potentially deleterious situation is that of lateral guidance involving only first premolars, as their root systems generally are ill-suited for lateral forces; periodontal inflammation can be exacerbated by the lateral occlusal trauma. Root morphology of upper first premolars, moreover, lends itself to incomplete plaque removal and resultant inflammation. Mobility of premolars involved in lateral excursions should be evaluated in this light.

Related to this is any lateral excursive guidance that pairs a strong tooth against a weak tooth in the opposing arch, such as upper canine/lower lateral incisor guidance or upper first premolar/lower canine guidance.

3. Balancing-side contacts in lateral excursion. While this finding may be completely normal and healthy in many, if not most, patients, it can predispose to TMJ problems or serve as a trigger mechanism in bruxism. Such contacts fall into four general categories: (1) Balancing-side contacts in immediate excursion, due to lack of immediate anterior disocclusion or the Bennett shift. These contacts are significant because they are subtle and may be missed in the examination. (2) Balancing-side contacts in combination with working-side guidance in frank excursion, that is, from 1 mm into lateral excursion to a cusp-to-cusp working side relationship. (3) Balancing-side contacts in the range just described that cause disocclusion on the entire working side. This is generally seen where missing, tipped, or supererupted teeth have disrupted the normal plane of occlusion. It is the contact most likely to have pathologic consequences. (4) Balancing-side contacts without working-side guidance that occur beyond the normal, functional range of motion—that is, beyond a cusp-to-cusp relation. Such contacts are quite common if a patient can move that far laterally, but are of little significance in most cases because they occur far out of the range of normal movement.

4. Wear patterns on teeth indicative of parafunctional activity (clenching, grinding) in excursive positions. The significance of wear produced in excursive positions is related to the amount and severity of the wear, the age of the patient, and whether the wear process is ongoing or has stopped. Minor, isolated facets on tooth enamel may represent a healthy accommodation for function. Multiple facets, especially if the enamel is lost or nearly lost and the dentin is exposed, are more likely to represent occlusal pathology. Exposure of dentin may be less significant in an otherwise healthy patient of 70 than in a much younger individual. Finally, the history of the wear must be established. If the patient is conscious of a clenching or grinding habit (or if others have verified a nocturnal habit), wear is a sign of pathology. It may also be a contributing etiologic factor in bruxism, as flatter, broader occlusal contacts seem to provide reflex stimulation for the bruxism. The clinician must also consider the possibility that the wear facets represent scars of some past habit or dysfunction and are no longer significant.

Actual movement of the teeth can sometimes be observed or palpated in clenching or in slight lateral excursive movements. This movement is referred to as fremitus. While all teeth exhibit some mobility, excessive mobility in these situations or isolated mobility may be indicative of occlusal pathology. This finding is not uncommon with teeth that have had cast restorations placed on them that, while not "high" in centric occlusion, may not allow for disocclusion in excursive movements, or may occlude on inclined planes in centric occlusion and thus produce lateral stresses.

Often related to occlusal pathology is a pattern of periodontal involvement. Severe, isolated infrabony pockets, angular bony defects, furcation involvements, and "funneling" of the alveolar crest may all be suggestive of occlusal pathology influencing the course of periodontal disease. Two categories of occlusal influence on periodontal disease can be distinguished: primary occlusal traumatism and secondary occlusal traumatism.

Primary occlusal traumatism includes any of the

potential pathologies just discussed that would be considered abnormal function—that is, that produce occlusal stresses beyond those of normal function. Primary occlusal traumatism can influence and contribute to periodontal disease, producing the typical pattern described previously.

Secondary occlusal traumatism arises after periodontal disease has compromised the supporting structures of the tooth or teeth in question and renders them incapable of withstanding normal occlusal function. In other words, in the absence of any potential occlusal pathology, the periodontium cannot withstand the normal functions of chewing and swallowing contacts, and teeth remain mobile. This is seen following periodontal therapy in which many teeth are missing, placing greater than normal stress on remaining teeth, and where much bone has been lost both to disease and in the osseous surgery necessary to eradicate defects and restore physiologic form to the periodontium.

Symptoms appearing in and around the TMJ may be reflective of occlusal pathology and must be evaluated in that light. An occlusal interference in lateral excursion may produce severe tooth wear with loss of enamel and pulpal irritation in one case, extreme mobility and periodontal destruction in the presence of inflammation in another, or pain and muscle spasm in yet another—all resulting from the attempt to accommodate to the interference. Indeed, in a highly resistant and tolerant individual, that same occlusal interference may be well tolerated and, in the absence of pathology, be considered normal for that patient. Thus, the relationship of the component parts in the system must be considered, including the potential influence of occlusal pathology on TMJ disorders.

Temporomandibular Joint

Evaluation and diagnosis of the temporomandibular joint and associated musculature is done primarily through observation of the function and palpation of the joint and its associated musculature. Recent work using myomonitors which record and detect electrical activity in selected muscles, may prove helpful in TMJ evaluation. Radiographs have long been employed in TMJ evaluation and are essential in diagnosing many gross disorders. Fractures, missing condyles, dislocations, severe arthritic changes, cysts, or tumor masses in the joint area can be demonstrated with TMJ radiographs, panoramic views, or tomograms.

Less striking pathologies, however, are less evident on radiographs; for example, even sophisticated techniques have failed to demonstrate radiographic evidence of myofascial pain syndromes. Furthermore, radiographic changes evident with these techniques often have not been reflected clinically. Recently, arthrography of the TMJ, in which a radio-opaque medium is injected into the joint, has been used to demonstrate displacements of the articular disc, primarily anterior and medial, and herniations of the disc. The procedure is not without risk, however, and its invasiveness may limit its use in TMJ diagnosis. The normal radiographic appearance of the TMJ should reveal condylar heads on the distal aspect of the eminence without any of the gross conditions mentioned previously.

The normal, healthy TMJ should be symmetrical upon observation, and straight opening and/or protrusive movements should be free of lateral deviations or noises. Palpation of the condylar heads during opening/closing and lateral excursive movements should reveal smooth and quiet joint operation in the functional range. Palpation of the associated musculature usually includes masseter, temporalis, internal and external pterygoids, but can also include palpation of the digastric and sternocleidomastoid muscles as well as the hyoid area, occipital area, and shoulder area. The musculature palpated should be free of tension and should not be tender to palpation.

The brief patient history should reveal no symptoms and no difficulties in chewing, yawning, or other functional movements. Indeed, most normal, healthy patients are remarkably unaware of the joint and its function and hope to remain that way.

Significant abnormalities in the TMJ that are potentially pathologic include the following:

1. *Pain.* Any report of pain in or around the TMJ, especially if associated with functional movements such as chewing or wide opening, should be evaluated as an indication of possible pathology, This includes symptoms such as headache, earache, and stiff neck or shoulder.
2. *Tenderness to palpation.* Tenderness to palpation directly over the joint or in the associated musculature is a significant abnormality.
3. *Limitation of motion.* Inability to open the mouth normally or great difficulty in lateral excursive movements is suggestive of TMJ problems.
4. *Deviation.* Asymmetrical function of the joints, which produces deviation in opening and/or protrusion, is a significant finding and should be investigated further.
5. *Noises during functional movements.* Noise from the TMJ during functional movements is not a rare finding. In the absence of any other signs or symptoms, it can be assumed to represent simple arthroidal crepitus, and as such, is a normal, benign sign.

Such noises may derive from the anatomy of the joint itself, or may be sequelae to trauma from a blow or accident.

Should the noise be accompanied by other signs/symptoms, it may be a significant abnormality. Indeed, the sudden onset of joint noise (as opposed to a long-standing crepitus) or an increase in the frequency or amplitude of the joint sound should be investigated. A greater awareness of joint sounds can be gained from the use of a stethoscope over the joint during movements. The clarity and variety of the sounds are striking. Unfortunately, there are presently no established standards by which to assess such joint sounds.

One promising area of clinical study suggests that joint clicks may indicate an internal derangement of the TMJ, in which the articular disc has been displaced anterior to the condylar head. The click then occurs when the condylar head moves downard and forward in opening and, in effect, "recaptures" the disc. Further work in this area is necessary and is likely to be of great significance in TMJ diagnosis and treatment.

6. *Roughness in condylar movements.* Deviations from a normal, smooth joint function can be described in a number of ways. Crepitus (a crackling sensation), clicking, and popping describe potentially significant abnormalities. These should be distinguished from actual subluxation, a "clunking" sensation, resulting when the condylar head actually slips anterior to the eminence or to the articular disc. Some individuals have TMJs that allow this to occur without pain or dysfunction, while most individuals would find such a maneuver quite unpleasant—what we would call a dislocation. As with joint sounds, roughness on palpation is neither rare nor pathologic in itself, but must be evaluated in the light of other findings.

This brief discussion of TMJ diagnosis does not attempt to delve into the question in its entirety and the reader is referred to the many excellent works available on the subject. Indeed, frank pathology associated with the TMJ and the so-called myofascial pain/dysfunction syndrome is one of the most difficult diagnostic problems in dentistry. Given a clinical picture that includes pain, tenderness in associated musculature, myospasm, or limitation of movement, it is very simple to apply the label MFPD syndrome and thereby, make a brilliant diagnosis. Unfortunately, our limited knowledge prevents us from answering "why" the condition is present; at best, we have empirical solutions to the problem. For this reason, early signs of TMJ pathology should not be overlooked when dealing with the normal, healthy patient and care might be advised when manipulating the occlusion through prophylactic equilibration (seldom indicated) or through careful execution of the occlusion if restorations are placed (always indicated).

The clinician must also inform the patient if significant findings are discovered, even if no pathology is established and treatment is not contemplated. Should symptoms arise in the future, considerable suffering (not to mention the expense of time and money) might be avoided if the patient seeks appropriate care. Clinical experience has demonstrated a number of patients with apparent occlusally induced MFPD syndromes who underwent months of medical treatment for nonexistent ear infections, who had multiple diagnostic radiographs (all negative), or who had long-term antibiotic therapy—all at considerable cost and to no avail. Had these patients been informed of potential bite-related problems prior to their onset, unnecessary and ineffective treatment might have been avoided.

Myofunctional Status

The diagnosis of abnormalities in lip, cheek, and tongue function depends greatly on careful observation and the dentist's skill in obtaining patient histories. As with many of the factors in the functional diagnosis, deviations from the clinical norm may or may not be harmful to the system, but we must be aware of the deviations (whether we attempt to correct them or not) if we are to deal effectively with the patient. Indeed, the correction of myofunctional abnormalities presents a greater challenge to the dentist than most of the problems we have heretofore discussed. A carious lesion can be excavated and restored, a periodontal pocket surgically eliminated, a Class II malocclusion corrected. An unconscious habit is generally more difficult to approach, and the clinician's tendency is to ignore it, having no treatment modality readily available. Such practice is an invitation to disaster, because the myofunctional environment can drastically affect the course of oral health and disease. Available treatment modalities can be applied to correct or alleviate myofunctional problems; failing that, the clinician must at least be acutely aware of how the problem is likely to affect the prognosis of dental treatment.[1,10,13]

A standard of clinical normality in the myofunctional environment can be expressed in general terms. The lips, cheek, tongue, and associated musculature of the stomatognathic system should perform comfortably and efficiently during normal function—that is, during mastication, swallowing, and speech. Muscle tension should be minimal when the system is at rest. Parafunctional movements and habits that are conscious (e.g., pipe smoking, gum chewing) or unconscious (e.g., lip sucking, bruxism) should not be present. More specific descriptions of clinical normality include the following:

1. Lips should have normal anatomical form, normal surface tissue characteristics, good muscle tone (not flaccid) and should be closed when at rest.
2. Cheeks should have normal masseter activity, with mucosal tissues having no keratinization other than a slight linea alba.
3. Tongue should be of normal size and shape, with freedom to move in all directions and the ability to reach the upper lip easily (not ankyloglottic).
4. Comfortable mastication without pain or fatigue should be possible on either side, although most patients will tend to have a preference.
5. Swallowing should be comfortable and performed without difficulty. The tip of the tongue should contact the palate posterior to the upper anterior teeth (usually the rugae area), the middle third rising to the palate, and the posterior third dropping down. Speech should be normal and free of defects.

Potential problems in the myofunctional environment arise with any deviation from the norm. While abnormalities are not all pathologic (requiring treatment), they should be considered significant findings, and their relationships to each other and the overall function of the system examined. The following are indications of clinical abnormalities:

1. Lips that have an unusual anatomic form, are asymmetrical, are notably short, exhibit changes in surface tissue suggestive of sucking or lip-biting habits, have poor muscle tone, flaccidity, or are kept apart in rest position (i.e., mouth breathing)
2. Cheeks that have hyperactivity of the masseter, which is often combined with overdevelopment of the muscle, a heavy linea alba, or obvious tissue changes, which are indicative of parafunctional activity involving the cheek
3. A tongue of abnormal size or configuration, surface features suggesting parafunctional movements (e.g., serrations on anterior border mirroring linguals of upper anterior teeth), and decreased range of motion due to ankyloglossia, a short lingual frenum, or other factors, especially if the result is an inability to reach the palate effectively with the tip and the middle third of the tongue
4. Assuming that a sufficient number of teeth are present in the array, reported difficulties in chewing and/or swallowing food must be considered highly significant, as they suggest incompetence in a vital function of the stomatognathic system.
5. In the postadolescent patient, a swallow in which the tongue tip does not rest against the anterior palate may represent pathology. Common associated signs are a pursing of the perioral muscles, contraction of the mentalis muscle in the chin, and the interposition of the tongue between the teeth during the swallow. This may occur anteriorly or posteriorly, unilaterally or bilaterally. Related findings are mouth breathing and habitual tongue postures between teeth. This abnormal tongue function may play a significant role in malocclusions and their treatment, in mobility and migration of periodontally involved teeth, and in the stability of fixed and removable prostheses and must be considered in the functional diagnosis.
6. Abnormal speech patterns may be significant both in terms of muscle function and tooth position. Lisping, sibilant, or hissing "s," sounds, or other apparent speech defects should be evaluated as potential oral-myofunctional problems. Cooperation with a speech therapist may be essential.

Existing Prostheses or Appliances

Obviously, the functional evaluation is incomplete without considering the status of existing appliances. The patient's assessment of his comfort and function is of primary importance, since it is the patient's comfort and function that the dentist must serve. In the absence of pathology, even the loosest, most poorly designed partial prosthesis may be successful for the patient who likes it and functions well with it; thus, our diagnosis of previously placed appliances rests on two factors: Is the appliance or prosthesis creating pathology? If not, is the patient satisfied with its comfort and function?

Once the factors in the functional diagnosis have been considered, a brief, capsulized diagnosis, such as the following examples, can be drawn:

1. Class II occlusion with moderate anterior overbite, moderate faceting suggestive of bruxism, which the patient admits to, TMJ and myofunction appear within normal limits.
2. Class I occlusion with anterior open bite, balancing contacts in both excursions, tongue-thrust swallow with noticeable hissing in "s" sounds during speech
3. Class I occlusion with group function bilateral; balancing contacts on right side in left lateral excursion; crepitus of right TMJ; patient admits occasional pain and difficulty in chewing, primarily on his right side; buccal mucosa heavily keratinized and abraded on the left side
4. Class III occlusion, end-to-end anterior relationship; patient has had lower, removable, partial denture but has not been able to wear it.

MULTIFACTORIAL DIAGNOSIS:

23-YEAR-OLD FEMALE STUDENT

CHIEF COMPLAINT: LEFT CENTRAL INCISOR IS TURNING DARK; IT WAS TRAUMATIZED ABOUT 4 YEARS PREVIOUS.

DENTAL GOAL: TO HAVE FRONT TOOTH "FIXED" AND ANY OTHER NECESSARY WORK DONE.

1. MARGINAL GINGIVITIS, GENERALIZED; HOME CARE IS REGULAR BUT NOT HIGHLY EFFECTIVE
2. PERICORONAL INFLAMMATION ASSOCIATED WITH MESIOANGULAR, PARTIALLY IMPACTED LOWER THIRD MOLARS
3. NUMEROUS PROXIMAL CARIES, UPPER AND LOWER POSTERIOR
4. NONVITAL, DARKENED MAXILLARY LEFT CENTRAL INCISOR (SOURCE OF CHIEF COMPLAINT)

FACTORS GENERALLY UNRELATED, BUT ALL REQUIRE TREATMENT

A

52-YEAR-OLD MALE POSTAL EMPLOYEE

CHIEF COMPLAINT: SHARP EDGE ON LOWER RIGHT MOLAR

DENTAL GOAL: "GET TEETH 'IN SHAPE'—WOULD LIKE TO KEEP TEETH."

1. GENERALIZED CHRONIC PERIODONTITIS; LOCALLY SEVERE BONE LOSS (UPPER RIGHT POSTERIOR, LOWER ANTERIOR)
2. PARTIAL EDENTULISM, NOT REPLACED, WITH SOME TIPPING AND SUPERERUPTION
3. SOME CARIES; SLIGHT, BUT EXTENSIVE WEAR OF TEETH; BREAKDOWN OF OLD RESTORATIONS; AND SOME CHIPPING OR FRACTURE (SOURCE OF CHIEF COMPLAINT)
4. PROBABLE LOSS OF VERTICAL DIMENSION, CO ≠ CR; SLIGHT CLICKING IN TMJ (BILATERAL)

ALL FACTORS PROBABLY INTERRELATED TO SOME DEGREE

B

Fig. 5–13. Two examples of brief multifactoral diagnoses. Note the chief complaint, the dental goal, and the list of problems to be solved. *A*, This is a fairly simple case, and the problems are generally unrelated to one another. *B*, This is more complex, and the problems are most likely interrelated.

Establishment of Multifactorial Diagnosis

Once all the pertinent factors in the diagnosis have been considered, two processes must occur. The first process, which should be occurring during each step but which must be addressed formally after all the information is gathered, is the possible correlation of factors in the diagnosis. Relationships of malocclusion to periodontal problems, of dental wear to myofunctional disorders, of general systemic health to the oral factors, and vice versa can be considered once the individual factors have been delineated. These relationships are often the key to effective treatment planning, since some problems must be addressed simultaneously to correct them; other problems respond better if they are dealt with in sequence. The sequence itself is often critical, since problems addressed in the wrong sequence may lead to failure of treatment.

In addition to establishing possible relationships among the factors in the diagnosis, the diagnosis itself must be finalized. The multifactorial diagnosis can be considered a list of problems seen in the examination that must be addressed in the treatment plan. In contrast to the medical model, which attempts to narrow the range of possibilities to a single disease state (or syndrome), this approach allows the consideration and treatment of all pathology within the system, not only that which produced the chief complaint. In this sense, the goal is to establish a healthy oral environment, rather than to eliminate a specific disease state. All problems and potential problems, including the chief complaint, are identified and addressed; contributing factors and any concurrent but unrelated pathology that threatens the long-term health and function of the stomatognathic system are addressed as well. From this list of problems, some of which are interrelated or isolated, a treatment plan can be devised that will address each and every aspect. The development of that plan is the subject of the following chapter (Fig. 5–13).

REFERENCES

1. Barrett, R.H., and Hanson, M.L.: Oral Myofunctional Disorders. 2nd ed. St. Louis, C.V. Mosby, 1978.
2. Becker, C.M., and Kaldahl, W.B.: Crown contour, margin placement, pontic design. J. Prosthet. Dent., *453*:268–277, 1981.
3. Bell, W.E.: Orofacial Pains; Differential Diagnosis. 2nd Ed. Chicago, Yearbook Publishers, 1979.
4. Bhaskar, S.N.: Radiographic Interpretation for the Dentist. 3rd ed. St. Louis, C.V. Mosby, 1979.
5. Brill, N. and Tryde, G.: Physiology of mandibular positions. Front. Oral Physiol., *1*:199–237, 1974.
6. Brisman, A.S.: Esthetics: A comparison of dentists' and patients' concepts. J.A.D.A., *100*(3):345–352, 1980.
7. Burket, L.W.: Oral Medicine, Diagnosis, and Treatment. 7th ed. Philadelphia, J.B. Lippincott, 1977.
8. Carlsson, G.E.: Mandibular dysfunction and temporomandibular joint pathosis. J. Prosthet. Dent., *43*:658–662, 1980.
9. Christen, A.G.: Suspected factors in tooth erosion and abrasion. Texas Dent. J., *94:10*, 1976.
10. Cole, R.M., and Cole, J.E.: Myofunctional therapy in tongue-thrust, swallowing, and related problems. *In* Clinical Dentistry. Vol. 2. Edited by J.W. Clark. Hagerstown, Harper and Row, 1979.

11. Comar, M.D., Kollar, J.A., and Garjiulo, A.W.: Local irritation and occlusal trauma as co-factors in the periodontal disease process. J. Periodontol., *40*:193–200, 1969.
12. Dawson, P.G.: Centric relation: Its effect on occluso-muscle harmony. Dent. Clin. North Am., *23*(2): 169–180, 1979.
13. Garliner, D.: Myofunctional Therapy. Philadelphia, W.B. Saunders, 1976.
14. Glickman, I.: Glickman's Clinical Periodontology: Prevention, Diagnosis, and Treatment of Periodontal Disease in the Practice of General Dentistry. 5th ed., rev. Philadelphia, W.B. Saunders, 1979.
15. Goldman, H.M., and Cohen, D.W.: Periodontal Therapy. 6th Ed. St. Louis, C.V. Mosby, 1980.
16. Haddad, A.W.: Physiology of occlusion: A scientific rationale. J. Ala. Dent. Assoc., *62*:27–42, 1978.
17. Hirschfeld, L., and Wasserman, B.: A long-term study of tooth loss in 600 treated periodontal patients. J. Periodontol., *49* (5): 225–237, 1978.
18. Issa, H.: The relationship of erosion and attrition in extensive tooth tissue loss. Br. Dent. J., *135*:519, 1973.
19. Karlsen, K.: Traumatic occlusion as a factor in the propagation of periodontal disease. Int. Dent. J., *22*:387–393, 1972.
20. Kerr, D.A., Ash, M.M., and Millard, H.D.: Oral Diagnosis. 4th Ed. St. Louis, C.V. Mosby, 1974.
21. Lawson, B.F.: Odontalgia, diagnosis and emergency treatment. Dent. Clin. North Am., (March):15–29, 1968.
22. Mitchell, D.F., Standish, S.M., and Fast, T.B.: Oral Diagnosis: Oral Medicine. 2nd Ed. Philadelphia, Lea & Febiger, 1971.
23. Pindborg, J.I.: Pathology of the Dental Hard Tissues. Philadelphia, W.B. Saunders, 1979.
24. Posselt, U.: Physiology of Occlusion and Rehabilitation, 2nd ed. Philadelphia, F.A. Davis, 1968.
25. Ramfjord, S., and Ash, M.M.: Periodontology and Periodontics. Chicago, Yearbook Press, 1979.
26. Rieder, C.E.: Occlusal considerations in preventive care. J. Prosthet. Dent., *28*(5):462—468, 1972.
27. Rieder, C.E.: The prevalence and magnitude of mandibular displacement in a survey population. J. Prosthet. Dent., *39*(3):324–329, 1978.
28. Rosenberg, M.M., et al.: Management of osseous defects, furcation involvements and periodontal pulpal lesions. *In* Clinical Dentistry. Vol. 3. Edited by J.W. Clark. Hagerstown, Harper and Row, 1979.
29. Sarnat, B.G., and Laskin, D.M. (eds.): The Temporomandibular Joint: A Biologic Basis for Clinical Practice. 3rd ed. Springfield, Charles C Thomas, 1980.
30. Schwartz, L.: Diagnosis and treatment planning in disorders of the temporomandibular joint. Dent. Clin. North Am., Philadelphia, W.B. Saunders, 1963.
31. Sessle, B.J., and Hannam, A.G.: Mastication and swallowing. Toronto, University of Toronto Press, 1976.
32. Shore, N.A.: Temporomandibular Joint Dysfunction and Occlusal Equilibration. 2nd ed. Philadelphia, J.B. Lippincott, 1976.
33. Solberg, W.K., and Berke, F.A.: Myofascial pain and dysfunction. *In* Clinical Dentistry. Vol. 2. Edited by J.W. Clark. Hagerstown, Harper and Row, 1979.
34. Stein, R.S., and Kuwata, M.: A dentist and dental technologist analyze current ceramo-metal procedures. Dent. Clin. North Am., *21*:729, 1977.
35. Tjan, A., Freed, H., and Miller, G.: Current controversies in axial contour design. J. Prosthet. Dent., *44*:536, 1980.
36. Tyldesley, W.R., and Mumford, J.J.: Dental pain and the histological condition of the pulp. Dent. Pract. Dent. Rec., *20*:333, 1970.
37. Weine, F.: Endodontic Therapy. St. Louis, C.V. Mosby, 1972.
38. Woda, A., et al.: Nonfunctional and functional occlusal contacts: A review of the literature. J. Prosthet. Dent., *42*(3):335–341, 1979.
39. Zarb, G.,P., and Carlsson, G.E. (eds.): Temporomandibular Joint Function and Dysfunction. St. Louis, C.V. Mosby, 1979.

CHAPTER 6

Synthesis of the Treatment Plan

Are you sure you know what you're doing?

FIVE-YEAR-OLD PATIENT TO AUTHOR ON "ONE OF THOSE DAYS"

We can now reiterate the essential steps in the treatment-planning process:

1. Gather all relevant information
2. Arrive at a diagnosis or set of diagnoses
3. Develop a treatment plan that
   a. Addresses all known problems
   b. Deals with etiologic factors
   c. Relates effectively to the patient

These steps must be followed in sequence in order to arrive at a rational and effective plan of treatment, since the quality of the treatment plan is dependent upon accurate diagnoses, which demand comprehensive and correct information. The prudent clinician will not attempt comprehensive treatment planning until all preliminary steps have been completed. The product of these steps is essentially a list of problems to be addressed that deal with those problems. Two processes must occur in the synthesis of the plan for it to be effective. First, the general procedures addressing the problems must be arranged in an effective *sequence*. Second, the general procedures must be analyzed and broken into distinct and *specific procedures* with time and cost estimates. These two processes will be discussed in turn.

SEQUENCE

The arrangement of procedures into an effective sequence is based on two main criteria: urgency and efficiency in achieving the treatment goal. The treatment sequence may be determined by an urgent need felt by the patient, clinical urgency, or practicality; these may or may not coincide. One can look at urgency-based treatment as being problem-oriented, addressing the immediate needs of the patient. Efficiency-based treatment, on the other hand, is more goal-oriented and works towards the long-term goals established by the dentist and patient. Both concepts are valid and should be addressed in dental treatment planning.

Urgency-Based Treatment

The patient's most common felt need is relief of pain or discomfort. More often than not, it is this stimulus that prompts the patient to seek dental treatment. Procedures to alleviate or eliminate the patient's pain or discomfort will nearly always take precedence in the treatment plan. This is also true when more serious problems are present but remain unknown to the patient. Unless those other problems are an immediate threat to the patient's health and well-being, the felt needs should be addressed first.

Another common felt need on the part of the patient is loss of esthetics. A chipped anterior tooth, lost restoration, or caries may prompt the patient to seek dental treatment. Again, that problem should be addressed first, even if we risk having the patient fail to return for treatment that is more urgent from the clinical viewpoint. We must certainly *inform* the patient of other problems that are apparent to us. It is the patient's decision whether or not to deal with those problems.

The type of treatment procedure selected in meeting the patient's immediate felt need must be based on the overall treatment plan. For example, the patient presenting with pain diagnosed as irreversible pulpitis may be treated in a number of ways. If the patient is new to the dentist and is seen after office hours on an emergency basis, opening the tooth to allow drainage and relieving pressure with appropriate medication (analgesics, possibly antibiotics) will address the felt need without a commitment to a specific, definitive procedure. Indeed, depending upon periodontal and overall treatment considerations, such a tooth may be extracted on some subsequent visit. Should other problems need to be addressed in the meantime, vital pulpotomy or pulpectomy, as indicated, may relieve the patient's symptoms and allow weeks or months to pass before further definitive treatment is necessary. On the other hand, a regular patient who is under control and well-restored and who develops a pulpitis might be treated immediately with definitive endodontic procedures that are followed by definitive restoration. The clinician must consider all the available options in dealing with the patient's felt need and not consider symptomatic relief an inferior treatment; instead, he must consider it an interim measure in the overall plan.

The following examples further illustrate this point. A patient presenting with an esthetic problem as the primary felt need can be dealt with in a variety of ways, depending upon the circumstances. For example, a lost anterior facing, while obviously requiring fabrication of a new fixed bridge, might be treated with some soft, white wax if the patient is a distraught mother-of-the-bride on her way to the church. In another instance, in which the patient expresses a concern about the appearance of a tooth, composite resin can be quickly adapted to restore esthetic competence even if the tooth in question is periodontally condemned and slated for extraction at some later date. Dealing with the patient's felt need does not necessarily require interim types of treatment. An anterior jacket placed to correct an esthetic problem need not wait until posterior periodontal pockets are eliminated and bridges placed. If the patient is fully aware of the scope of his dental condition and the treatment necessary to attain good oral health and function, but would like an esthetic improvement first, the esthetic improvement should get precedence.

While considering the patient's felt needs in establishing a sequence of treatment, effective communication is essential for the patient to elicit those feelings. In the communication process, the dentist's assessment of clinical needs can be conveyed to the patient. Once aware of other problems, the patient's immediate complaint may become less critical and be given a more appropriate place in the overall sequence.

Clinical urgency is based on the following criteria (in order of their importance):

1. *Systemic threats*. These are conditions that affect or threaten the general systemic health of the patient. Virtually any general systemic conditions that affect or threaten health will take immediate precedence in the treatment plan. Indeed, in certain situations, any dental treatment is contraindicated pending medical attention; such situations must be addressed with care and tact, since the patient's felt need in coming to the dentist may be totally unrelated to the systemic problem. While some patients are grateful that such problems have been identified by the dentist and understand their significance, other patients, due to fear or ignorance, may resist referral to a physician and insist that their perceived dental needs be taken care of. Conflict in these cases is nonproductive and generally unnecessary. A gentle, caring explanation of the potential import of the systemic discovery is essential. Occasionally, it is necessary to compromise, and one may find oneself replacing a missing anterior restoration for a patient with a highly suspicious (malignant?) oral lesion. This need not jeopardize life and health if biopsy and/or referral is also carried out. On the other hand, the patient presenting for dental treatment whose blood pressure is extremely elevated (200/110) presents the dentist with the risk of a medical emergency. Patients presenting with dental problems who also exhibit signs and symptoms of contagious systemic diseases (mononucleosis, hepatitis, venereal diseases) threaten not only their own health, but the health of the dental team as well.

2. *Dental or oral threats*. These are dental or oral conditions that are presently producing pain or discomfort, or that, in the dentist's judgment, threaten the vitality of dental pulp or the integrity of the periodontium. This criterion is the most likely to coincide with the felt need of the dental patient presenting for treatment, for relief of acute symptoms nearly always takes precedence in treatment sequencing if systemic factors are not involved. Secondary to relief of acute symptoms is the treatment of potentially acute situations, such as excavation of deep carious lesions or removal of gross periodontal insults. Addressing such potential problems often takes precedence over what are apparently more serious conditions, such as terminally involved, periodontally condemned teeth or nonvital teeth with periapical lesions that are visible radiographically. The reason for this is twofold: First, the likelihood of painful symptoms arising in a long-standing chronic periodontal or pulpal infection is less than in the more immediate situation. More importantly, quick action may save a cariously involved tooth from irreversible pulpal damage, while the nonvital, apically involved tooth has already lost its battle.

The treatment indicated for these urgent conditions may be merely palliative, or at the most, preliminary. Indeed, definitive treatment is often contraindicated from the standpoint of clinical success (better to place a sedative temporary restoration over a large excavation than to subject the tooth and pulp to the greater insult of complete preparation and placement of a metallic restoration); it is also contraindicated by the urgency principle, since other problems may demand rapid attention prior to completion of the definitive treatment in question. Excavations and sedative temporary restorations, pulpotomy, or pulpectomy, and temporary restorations, immediate relief of gross occlusal interferences, and local curettage of an acute periodontal lesion—all are examples of priority measures in treatment to relieve acute symptoms or to address a threat to pulpal vitality or periodontal integrity.

While they relieve symptoms and intercept potential acute problems, these types of treatment are often *investigative;* that is, they may help determine much of the treatment plan and sequence. A deep excavation, for example, may prove uneventful and allow simple restoration of the tooth in question, or it may reveal a large carious exposure, indicating the need for endodontic therapy that is followed by dowel and core and crown restoration. Indeed, should pulpectomy be attempted and the root-canal system prove impassable, extraction and replacement with fixed bridgework may be the treatment of choice, which is a far cry from the simple restoration first mentioned. Many procedures, even some we consider definitive treatment (such as periodontal surgery), are also investigative or exploratory and should be carried out prior to other procedures, which might be affected by their outcome. This concept will be developed later in this chapter.

3. *Asymptomatic, potential oral threats.* These are dental conditions that, although asymptomatic, have the potential for acute involvement. This level of clinical urgency includes treatment of apically involved, nonvital teeth, extraction of hopelessly involved teeth (caries, periodontal disease, severe malposition), and possibly, the removal of partially erupted but asymptomatic third molars (potential sites for pericoronitis). The degree of urgency in dealing with these conditions depends on the clinical picture and the logistics of the specific patient's treatment plan. For example, the partially erupted third molar might be left alone if the patient is proceeding with other treatment and can be monitored well, but should probably be removed if the patient is leaving for 2 years of service in the Peace Corps. The likelihood of acute flare-up as it relates to the patient's accessibility to care is of prime importance in assessing this level of clinical urgency. The clinical picture is also important. Using the example of a partially erupted third molar, we can imagine ignoring a situation in which the pericoronal tissues are clean, pink, and firm even though a pocket exists, but assigning some urgency to a similar situation showing inflammation, puffy or spongy tissue, plaque, debris, and a so-called "hungry-looking" partial impaction.

Using an asymptomatic, periapical lesion as an example, the small well-circumscribed lesion that does not encroach on important anatomic structures may be far less urgent than a large lesion possibly involving more than one tooth or encroaching upon the maxillary sinus, the floor of the nose, or the mandibular canal. The degree of urgency should be carefully considered, especially in view of the asymptomatic nature of these conditions. Indeed, we can easily envision indefinite postponement of treatment in certain situations. For example, an asymptomatic, periodontally condemned tooth that does not interfere with the overall treatment may be left alone, especially if the patient does not wish to have it removed until symptoms develop. The same might be true of an impacted third molar. If the patient has been informed of the problem and its potential risks, he may opt for watchful waiting. The clinician is often advised to agree to such an arrangement, since treatment of an asymptomatic condition will often produce symptoms and entail complications. The patient may end up with more and greater problems than he started with—a situation that does not enhance the patient-dentist relationship (a mandibular paresthesia following extraction of an asymptomatic, impacted lower third molar is a typical example). Another pitfall often encountered is the severe exacerbation of a long-standing periapical lesion, the so-called "Phoenix abscess," during the course of endodontic therapy.

Another common situation is the discovery of a radiographically insufficient endodontic treatment, the old vital pulpotomy, the "short" endodontic fill, or the apparent failure to fill one or more canals in a multirooted tooth. Obviously, if such teeth are to be used strategically in a treatment plan (for abutments or crowns, for example), retreatment is probably indicated, although not immediately urgent. Retreatment of such teeth is fraught with peril, however, because the canal systems may have become impassable; not only may new symptoms associated with treatment arise, but the tooth may be lost in the process.

While treatment of such teeth is justifiable if the teeth are directly involved in an overall treatment plan, they are often better left alone if no such involvement is contemplated. In this case, the patient should be informed of the possible endodontic insufficiency, and asked to watch for symptoms. Periodic radiographic examination is certainly indicated in such cases.

In summary, the treatment of asymptomatic, but potentially urgent, pathologies or abnormalities that do not threaten the systemic health and well-being of the patient, do not involve strategic teeth or areas in the overall treatment plan, and do not threaten other teeth or oral structures can often be postponed indefinitely. In this situation, the risk-vs.-benefit principle must be applied (this principle will be examined more closely later in this chapter). The patient must always be involved in the decision to treat or to postpone treatment of such conditions.

Once a sequence of treatment steps has been established based on need or urgency, the balance of the treatment sequence can be established. It may be necessary to actually carry out some or all of the urgency-based treatment prior to planning the balance of treatment This is true when life-threatening conditions are discovered, when the patient requires immediate relief of symptoms, or when the investigative nature of the immediate treatment will provide necessary information for planning and sequencing later treatment.

The urgency-based treatment sequence is not goal-oriented, but problem-oriented. Indeed, until the patient's immediate felt needs are addressed, it is often difficult or impossible to discuss long-term goals. How a toothache relates to the patient's oral status 20 years hence is irrevelant as long as the pain is present. The dentist may also be unable to consider long-term goals pending the results of investigatory, urgency-based treatment. It makes little sense to establish a goal of keeping teeth only to find, following scaling/curettage, full radiographs, and periodontal evaluation, that the dentition is hopelessly involved. At some point, however, the dentist and patient must progress from the urgency-based sequence to a sequence based on efficiency in achieving treatment goals.

Sadly, many patients and dentists never make this transition; instead, they choose to go from crisis to crisis, treating only what hurts, and in the long run, fail to reach any goal at all. The dental patient who, having been given the opportunity, rejects goal-oriented treatment, has made his decision and must live with it. It is not productive or appropriate to criticize that choice or to engage in verbal conflict, which only serves to harden attitudes on both sides. The charitable dentist will express concern for the patient's oral and general health and well-being and keep the door open if the patient changes his mind. On the other hand, the dentist who fails to make goal-oriented treatment available to a patient, who tacitly treats the patient in crisis after crisis without attempting to break the cycle, does gross disservice to himself and his patient. Assuming that the dentist and patient can agree on some long-term goals (see Chap. 2), a treatment sequence can be established based on efficiency in achieving treatment goals.

Efficiency in Goal-Oriented Treatment

Simply stated, efficiency means that the desired goal is attained in the fewest possible steps, that treatment is carried out with as little redundancy as possible, and that care is taken not to perform treatment early in the sequence that might be undone later.

An example of reducing steps in treatment is to remove both upper and lower third molars instead of only the lower when the upper is likely to require extraction in the future. Performing operative dentistry in quadrants reduces the total number of visits and anesthetic administrations necessary. Indeed, an experienced clinician may carry out multiple procedures in an anesthetized quadrant under the same rubber dam doing, for example, root-canal procedures, followed by some minor operative dentistry, or minor periodontal surgery along with an extraction.

Redundancy can be avoided, for example, by not treating small to moderate carious lesions on teeth slated as abutments requiring crowns, except when excavations are indicated due to possible pulpal encroachment or when an amalgam or composite resin core build-up is indicated for crown retention. Redundancy can also be avoided by refraining from operative or endodontic treatment on periodontally questionable teeth pending the outcome of periodontal treatment. Such teeth may be extracted later or, if they are retained, require a different restoration design due to the altered periodontal tissues or modifications in the overall treatment plan. Finally, one can avoid redundancy by not placing restorations on teeth that may later be extracted in an orthodontic treatment plan.

Because it is not always easy to see the entire treatment picture at the outset, the goal-oriented treatment should be broken down into three major sequential stages. If treatment is carried out within this framework, it will generally be in an efficient sequence:

1. Establishment of a healthy oral environment
2. Restoration of form, function, and esthetics
3. Maintenance of the environment and its restorations

A healthy environment is critical to and must precede definitive restoration, and effective maintenance is essential in achieving any long-term treatment goal following restoration.

Establishment of a Healthy Oral Environment

The concept of the mouth as an environment rather than as a complex mechanical device is a key in goal-oriented treatment planning. Both dentists and the public have likened the mouth to a pop-up toaster that, if it isn't working, can be taken to a repairman (the dentist) who will putter around a bit, replace a few springs and wires, and all will be as good as new. This mechanistic approach is responsible for much of the failure in dental treatment. The environmental model of the oral cavity better reflects the actual situation, for in this model, we have an ecosystem (living organs, teeth, living tissue, and numerous and diverse bacterial flora) with most of the problems of our own macroenvironment. Pollution, blight, mismanagement, and even crime are problems in the oral environment. Also, individuals have vastly different patterns in their oral environments; for example, one person may have great hereditary resistance to insult, while another might have a very delicate balance between health and disease. There are racial and cultural differences as well. The critical fact is that teeth and the restorative appendages applied by dentists cannot survive in an unhealthy environment. Any treatment sequence that does not begin with the establishment of basic oral health is irrational. Assuming that immediate needs (urgency) have been addressed, the types of treatment that serve this end can be described.

1. *Control of etiology*. Preventive measures, as they relate to the prevention of future dental disease, have been discussed previously. The term "prevention," then, is somewhat misleading in this context, because the disease is already present and must first be controlled and arrested before it can really be prevented. In order to achieve a healthy oral environment that can be maintained by prevention, one must apply the so-called "preventive procedures" described in Chapter 3 in this step of the sequence. Direct and early involvement of the patient (as discussed in Chap. 2) is imperative, because most of these procedures relate to and depend upon patient cooperation and commitment.

2. *Control of periodontal pathology*. The periodontium is the foundation upon which teeth and all dental restorations are built. A healthy oral environment demands a healthy periodontium at the outset. Indeed, deep pockets and calculus deposits (especially those that are subgingival) may render the most ardent preventive efforts ineffectual. Preliminary periodontal therapy (complete and thorough calculus removal—combined with curettage when indicated) must occur early in the treatment sequence to establish a healthy oral environment.

Definitive periodontal therapy may be more effective, however, if it is carried out over a longer period of time, thus allowing as much natural healing and repair as possible through the patient's efforts and our scaling and curettage. Therefore, while initiation of periodontal therapy generally takes precedence in the establishment of a healthy environment, other procedures may be performed concurrently.

3. *Surgical procedures (excisional and reparative.)* Oral surgical procedures ranging from necessary extractions to edentulous ridge reductions or augmentations, removal of cysts, foreign bodies, root tips, or impacted teeth generally will be performed early in the establishment of a healthy oral environment. While often considered primarily excisional, some reparative procedures (such as vestibular extensions and gingival grafts) directly enhance the oral environment. These procedures include not only the typical oral-surgical procedures that might be performed by a dentist or oral surgeon, but also those procedures involved in periodontal and endodontic surgery. Efficiency may call for minor surgical procedures of several types to be carried out in a single sitting, under one anesthetic. A typical example of this might be the extraction of a hopeless molar tooth combined with a flap or free-graft procedure re-establishing attached gingiva on a second premolar (now a potential abutment). Indeed, the donor site might well be from the tooth to be extracted.

A word of caution is in order regarding the sequencing of surgical procedures. One must take care not to negate efforts in preventive procedures by creating difficult surgical sequelae; that is, having established the need for effective plaque control and painstakingly instructed the patient in how to achieve it, we should not perform or have performed, surgical procedures that, for some time afterward, cause tenderness and swelling and prevent the patient from effectively using a toothbrush or dental floss.

Minor surgical procedures that are local and heal quickly may not present a problem in this area. More extensive procedures (complex third-molar impactions, for example) should precede preventive therapy or be postponed until the patient has had ample time to develop and perfect his preventive skills. Even then, it is often necessary to repeat and review the techniques following an interruption in the home-care routine. This is especially true following periodontal procedures, such as a simple graft or full flaps and osseous surgery, since these procedures not only interrupt the patient's new regimen, but often change the architecture of the periodontium in the treated areas. Such changes may call for drastic modifications in plaque-removal techniques, or at the very least, minor corrections in technique when the topography of the mouth has been altered.

4. *Caries elimination.* Assuming that preventive measures have already been instituted to control the etiology (plaque control, reduction, elimination, or substitution of refined carbohydrates in diet) and that appropriate fluoride therapy has been instituted when necessary, caries control will involve the actual elimination of carious lesions and appropriate restoration. The actual placement of caries elimination in the treatment sequence depends on the severity of individual lesions and the overall caries rate. Large or deep lesions might be dealt with early in the sequence on an individual basis. A high caries rate (many active lesions of significant size and depth) might also indicate early treatment. In both cases, however, care should be taken in the choice of restoration. The use of temporary or interim sedative materials can be an effective tool in eliminating the carious lesions without committing to a specific, definitive, restorative material. Until the high caries environment is modified, relatively definitive restorative materials (silver amalgam, composite resins) should be used with caution; cast restorations are usually contraindicated.

If, on the other hand, caries are neither severe nor rampant, caries elimination can be performed and definitive restorations placed as a step in establishing a healthy oral environment. Efficiency in this case suggests that the procedures be done in clusters, or quadrants, thus reducing the number of visits and anesthetic administrations as well as the total time required for all the procedures. This will benefit both patient and dentist.

Finally, there will be situations in which caries are incipient, indicating re-evaluation over time rather than immediate restoration, or in which caries are not immediately pressing and can best be addressed concurrently with another procedure. An example of this might be a small proximal lesion on a potential bridge abutment that can be readily excavated when the tooth is prepared as a retainer. In these cases, caries elimination might be safely postponed for extended periods of time (6 months to 1 year), provided the patient is well informed. Postponement might also be indicated in cases in which periodontal surgery is involved, since operative procedures might be less complicated (less bleeding, better access) after pocket elimination and preparations more appropriately designed in a postperiodontal environment.

5. *Elimination of endodontic and apical pathology.* Definitive endodontic therapy may be a priority in some cases, but can generally be postponed if the tooth is asymptomatic, or if pulpotomy or pulpectomy procedures performed in the urgency sequence have proven effective. The rationale for such temporary postponement is that caries elimination often reveals pulpal involvement that was not apparent in the initial diagnosis. Caries under old, large restorations may involve the pulp, or lesions that look uncomplicated radiographically may involve a pulp horn. We must also accept that our best efforts at careful but thorough caries removal may occasionally produce pulpal exposures requiring endodontic treatment. Therefore, until the full extent of endodontic involvement is established, definitive therapy might be postponed. A specific example might involve three anterior teeth—one with a periapical lesion, another with very deep caries, and a third with a large, old, and apparently leaking acrylic restoration. To perform definitive endodontic therapy on the apically involved tooth before determining the pulpal status of the other two might necessitate two or three series of endodontic appointments (or referrals) when the same procedures could have been combined.

Obviously, there are numerous cases in which isolated endodontic therapy can and should be instituted early in the sequence, particularly when there are no other likely candidates for endodontic therapy in the area. This may also apply to suspected endoperio lesions, in which case, endodontic therapy is necessary prior to or in combination with periodontal treatment.

6. *Correction of functional disorders.* Functional disorders involving the occlusion, TMJ, or neuromuscular components that directly compromise the health of the oral environment are generally dealt with after preventive, periodontal, surgical, caries-elimination, and endodontic procedures have been performed or at least begun. This is due to the often diffuse nature of such disorders and the occasional difficulty in accurate diagnosis. By eliminating or controlling intraoral disease states, we may alleviate symptoms mistaken for functional disorders. At the very least, we eliminate other possible causes and ensure more accurate diagnosis. In addition, it is usually more efficient to deal with functional disorders last. For example, caries removal and restoration can be done with orthodontic bands in place, but it is not easy. Equilibration carried out prior to excavation and interim restoration may have to be redone after the occlusal anatomy has been altered. Appliance therapy of any kind may be complicated if extensive periodontal, surgical, or restorative procedures are

not performed first. The obvious exception to this is occlusal therapy (equilibration) that is carried out for periodontal reasons.

Taking precedence in the sequence are those procedures that address functional disorders that are actually producing symptoms or those that are identifiably contributing to an unhealthy environment. Such functional disorders include severe malocclusions, lost vertical dimensions caused by severe wear, anterior collapses caused by loss of posterior support, myofascial pain/dysfunction symptoms, or obviously deleterious lip, cheek tongue or speech abnormalities.

Of lower priority are functional disorders that, while not immediately compromising oral health, must be corrected prior to definitive restoration to ensure good, long-term clinical results. Thus, a CO-CR discrepancy, which by itself is not immediately threatening, may require correction prior to multiple posterior bridges.

The completion of the first sequential stage should see the establishment of a healthy oral environment that is free of infection, active disease, and potentially pathologic conditions. The patient should be free of major symptoms and in control of his mouth. What teeth are present should be pulpally (if not endodontically treated) and periodontally viable; this is the foundation for all further treatment and must be well-established if that treatment is to succeed. Should financial concerns or other matters inhibit the patient from proceeding with more definitive treatment, this healthy environment can often preserve the dentition for some time and allow definitive treatment in the future. On the other hand, failure to establish a healthy oral environment prior to definitive treatment may compromise the future of the patient's dentition (Fig. 6–1).

Restoration of Form, Function, and Esthetics

Definitive restorations, be they amalgam, composite, or cast metal, and prosthetic appliances, either fixed or removable, constitute the second stage in goal-oriented treatment. The sequencing of the steps within the restorative stage must be based on urgency and efficiency. In this instance, the urgency factor is not one of immediate relief from an existing problem, but rather the avoidance of potential crises. The prime example of this is the endodontically treated tooth. If the tooth in question is a molar and subject to occlusal forces, there is a high risk of fracture, which can easily result in tooth loss. Therefore, definitive restoration is called for early in the sequence. The urgency also exists in endodontically treated premolars, but may be somewhat less critical due to the lesser forces and narrower occlusal tables generally seen in premolar teeth. Anterior teeth are perhaps more susceptible to lateral stress fractures following endodontic treatment, and definitive restoration generally calls for reinforcement of the root through dowel or dowel and core (an approach that is often appropriate in the posterior teeth as well). An endodontically treated anterior tooth that is virtually

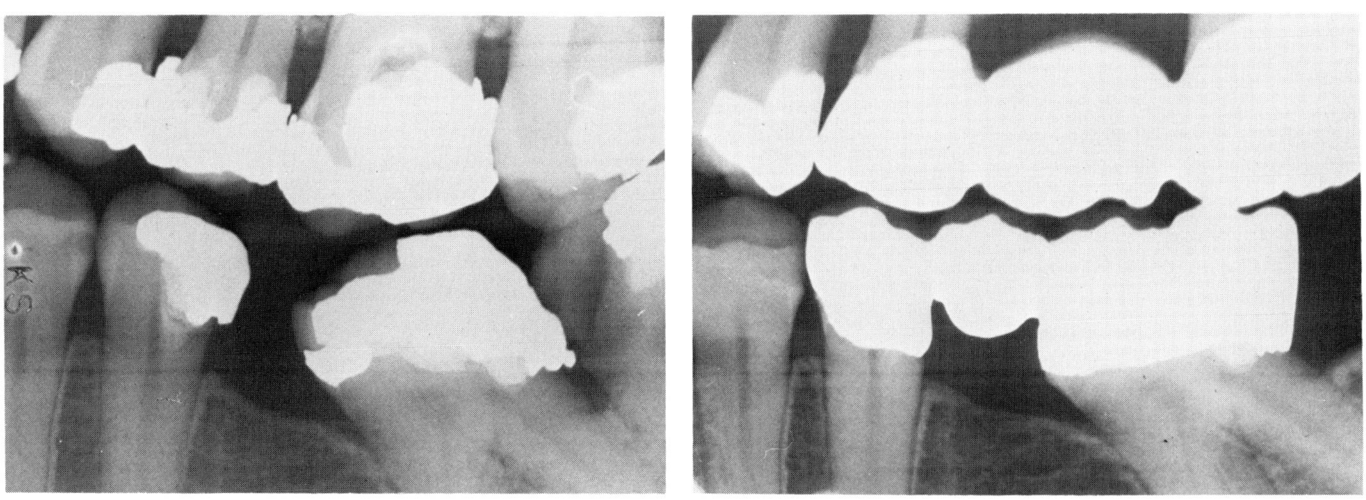

A

Fig. 6–1. Establishment of a healthy oral environment. *A*, These radiographs depict the left side dentition of a 42-year-old male engineer. The film on the left bespeaks a steadily deteriorating oral environment. The patient had experienced continual dental disease all his life, and recurrent caries, failed restorations, and a sense of frustration and dental fatalism colored his attitude toward his teeth and dentistry in general. The film on the right depicts the same area 5 years after a course of treatment stressed the establishment of a healthy oral environment.

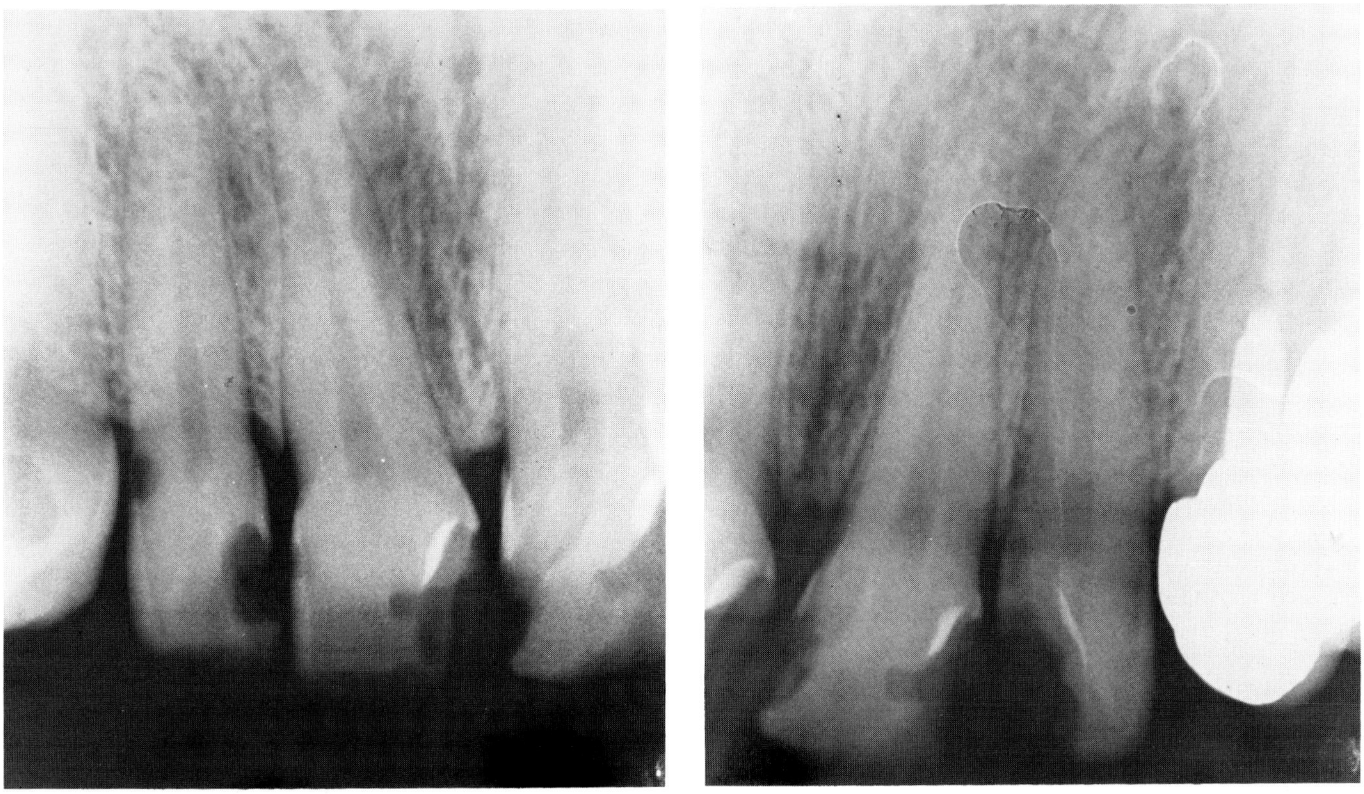

B

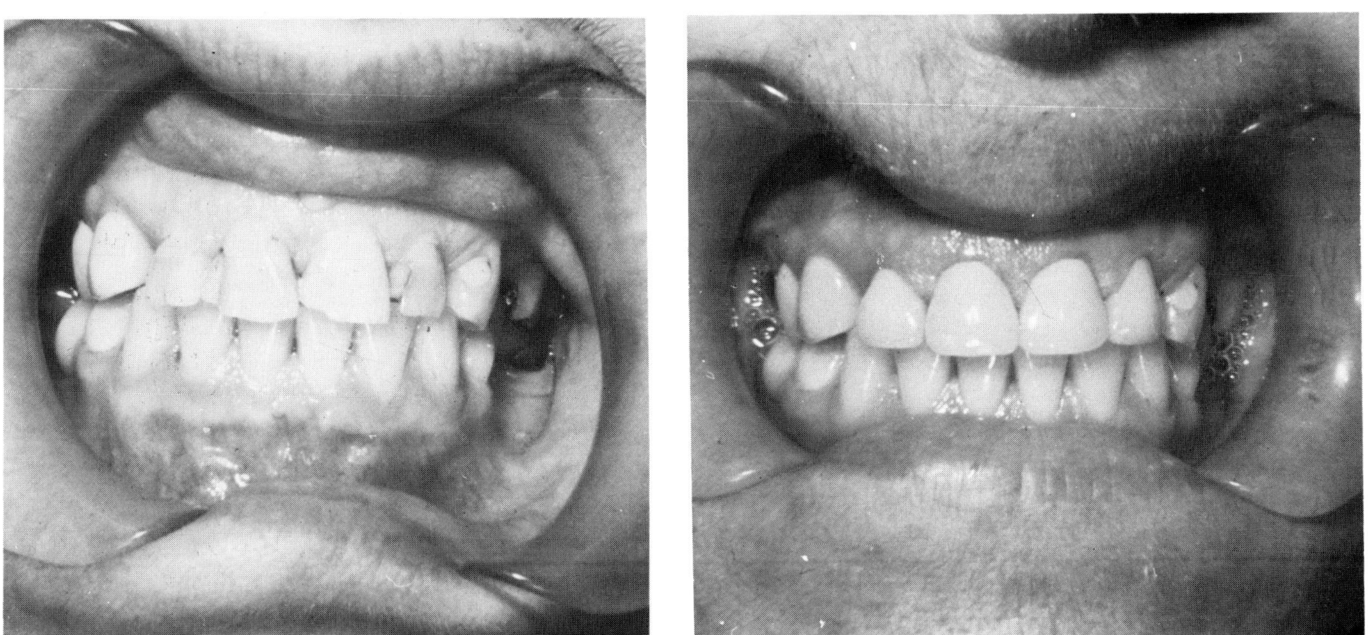

C

Fig. 6–1 *continued.* *B*, Radiographs of the upper anterior teeth demonstrate an extremely high caries rate. This 38-year-old female secretary had less than optimal oral hygiene and a high frequency of sugar intake in the diet. *C*, The left clinical picture shows the same teeth 2 years after environmental control was begun. No restorations have been placed, but the patient has been conscientiously brushing and flossing daily and has curtailed the sugar intake markedly (losing 15 pounds in the bargain). Daily fluoride rinses were also employed. The clinical picture on the right depicts the definitive restorations 2 years after placement. Note the continued good gingival form and surface texture. There have been no new caries in 5 years. The oral environment now should ensure maximum restorative longevity.

intact coronally (other than for the access opening for the endodontic treatment) does not have an urgent need for definitive restoration and may be left as is indefinitely, provided the patient is aware of the somewhat greater potential for breakage. Even heavily restored anterior teeth following endodontic therapy, while definitely needing crown restorations, have less risk of incurring disastrous fracture than molars. This is because anterior fractures are more often incisal angle fractures or horizontal coronal fractures, and less often vertical radicular fractures. Summarized, this example suggests that relative risk should be assessed when determining the sequence of restorative steps and that potential crises should be anticipated and dealt with in order of their likelihood of occurrence.

Another example of urgency-based sequence is the definitive restoration of periodontally treated teeth whose existing form or restoration predisposes them to further periodontal problems. Rough restorations, irregular anatomy, or overhanging margins, if not corrected prior to periodontal surgery, ought to be corrected as soon after as is practical. The patient's ability to achieve and maintain the healthy oral environment must be enhanced early in the restorative stage.

Patient's felt needs must also be considered in the sequencing of restorative treatment. An esthetic improvement may have a low priority in the dentist's restorative picture, but be of prime importance to the patient, and after all, treatment is done for the benefit of the patient.

After urgent restorative needs are addressed, efficiency dictates the sequence of restorative treatment. A good example of this concept involves clinical situations requiring definitive (crown or fixed prosthetic) procedures in both anterior and posterior areas of the mouth. The proper sequence depends on the situation. When loss of posterior support has compromised vertical dimension and created excessive wear or shifting of anterior teeth, it may be critically important in the restorative stage to reestablish good bilateral posterior occlusion so as to allow anterior restoration and ensure its viability. Conversely, a similar situation may call for definitive restoration of the anterior segment so as to establish effective guidance factors in excursive movements, which then allow posterior restorations of normal occlusal anatomy.

When there is no clear-cut indication, patient preference may be taken into account. Here, too, situations vary. In many cases, patients may opt for definitive anterior restorations because of esthetic concerns. A fear often expressed in dental-school clinics is that once the anterior is restored and looks good, the patient may never return for the necessary posterior restoration. This may be less of a problem in a private practice, particularly when the patient has been involved in diagnosis and treatment planning and is fully aware of the restorative needs. Indeed, a great many patients, when given the choice, opt for posterior definitive restoration first (if anterior esthetics are not lacking) because of their desire for comfort, function, and security in mastication.

In certain situations, simultaneous anterior/posterior restorations are indicated. This would be true when altering (regaining) vertical dimension, when the establishment of tooth-guidance factors involves both anterior and posterior teeth, or when the required restorative treatment (long-span bridge or removable partial denture) is an anteroposterior restoration. There are also situations in which it makes no difference to anyone what segment is treated first; in that case, the dentist may choose randomly where to begin.

The important concept to be grasped in this discussion of the anterior/posterior restorative case is that a sequence of treatment must be based on good clinical reasoning. There is seldom a "right" way to sequence treatment, a hard-and-fast rule that can be applied. In sequencing any restorative treatment, alternatives should be considered and reasons proposed for the eventual decision.

Other treatment sequences, such as the sequence involving crowns or fixed prosthesis combined in an arch with removable prosthesis, are routine. Unless one enjoys the challenge of fabricating crowns underneath an existing partial denture, the sequence is self-evident and needs little justification.

Another alternative in sequencing restorative treatment is the anticipatory restoration. The prime example of this would be placement of an upper posterior bridge in a quadrant with no opposing lower posterior teeth. Such a prosthesis is often made in anticipation of the lower restoration (fixed prosthetics generally preceding removable). In that light, the anatomy and curve of occlusion should be designed so as to *anticipate* the later opposing restoration. In such situations, it is often useful to wax the fixed prosthesis against a trial setup of denture teeth representing the future prosthesis. Using those same teeth when the prosthesis is made simplifies the setup and ensures an occlusion of maximum harmony and efficiency.

The same principle applies if upper and lower crowns are to be placed opposing one another and time or financial limitations require the restorations to be done one arch or quadrant at a time. If the lower arch is restored first, the anatomy may be established not to match the existing upper teeth (which may be flat, rough, uneven), but to anticipate future work on the upper arch. It may be necessary or useful to grossly recontour the upper teeth to allow a good anatomic form and curve of occlusion to be established. Lower restorations must harmonize with the as yet untreated upper teeth (that is, make light occlusal contact and be free of interferences in excursions) even though they do not occlude as such. It is often useful to reduce the occlusals of the postponed opposing teeth on the laboratory model and place wax cones for a wax-to-wax build-up of the occlusion. When those postponed teeth are later restored, the anatomy of the previously treated arch will serve to recapture that original cusp-fossa relationship as waxed. Another example of anticipatory restoration is the patient whose upper arch is edentulous and who has periodontal and restorative problems in the lower arch. If an upper full denture is urgently needed because of poor fit or mechanical breakdown, while the lower arch demands a much longer course of treatment prior to restoration of the occlusion, the upper full denture might be made in anticipation of the lower restoration, which will follow periodontal therapy and extractions. Once again, the upper prosthesis can harmonize with existing lower occlusal patterns without actually matching them, so that restoration of the lower arch at a later time can be done to match a good anatomy and curve of occlusion.

The importance of careful and thorough treatment planning was never so obvious as in anticipatory restoration. With careful planning, a long sequence of steps will fall into place at the end. Without this planning, the end result can be very disappointing.

The end point in the restorative stage is an oral cavity possessing a dentition (natural or prosthetic) that provides good form, function, and esthetics. Assuming the first stage was effectively carried out, the clinical picture can be described as a healthy, well-restored mouth. This is a goal that every dentist can appreciate, understand, and strive for, and that, if approached carefully, competently, and in a logical sequence, is attainable. Unfortunately, even the finest clinicians who are flushed with the success of having rehabilitated a mouth may neglect the next stage in goal-oriented treatment—namely, the maintenance of the healthy oral environment and the restorations placed therein.

Maintenance of the Oral Environment and Its Restorations

An effective maintenance program, more than any other step, must be tailored to each patient. No single recall interval, no routine set of procedures will be universally appropriate or effective. Furthermore, the long-term success of a maintenance program depends primarily on patient involvement and commitment, which must be established from the very start of the dentist-patient relationship in order to be carried effectively into a maintenance program. Basic oral-health theory and practice must be operating throughout the entire treatment sequence, not started at its conclusion. Finally, the maintenance stage of the treatment sequence must address both environmental and mechanical maintenance.

Environmental Maintenance. It is fairly obvious that the kinds of strategies employed in the establishment of a healthy oral environment must be used in its maintenance. Most critical is the review, refinement, and reinforcement of the patient's daily preventive regimen. Human nature is such that enthusiasm wanes and skills deteriorate over time. Periodic recall/maintenance sessions must provide a review of motor skills and positive reinforcement of whatever success (no matter how limited) the patient has had, along with sincere encouragement toward improvement when necessary. A hearty pat on the back, coupled with a gentle kick in the pants can be an effective combination. The frequency of the review/reinforcement sessions is critical. Some highly self-motivated patients, having thoroughly mastered oral-health maintenance skills, show little loss of enthusiasm or effectiveness when seen on annual recall. Other patients (perhaps most patients) need review and reinforcement more frequently; visits at intervals of 3 to 4 months are not unrealistic in many cases. The patient should be involved in establishing an appropriate interval between visits that is based on a personal assessment of skills, motivation, and need for review.

Periodic maintenance programs must also be tailored to individual problems. Patients who presented with a high caries rate or extreme periodontal breakdown at an early age should be maintained much more carefully and seen more frequently than those whose dental problems were minimal. Indeed, the greater the adjustment the patient needed to make in lifestyle (diet patterns, oral hygiene, or acceptance of prosthetic appliances), the greater the need for close, careful maintenance and reinforcement of the changes. Many patients, despite their best efforts (and ours as well), are unable to achieve a consistent level of oral-health maintenance and may require more dentist-oriented service. The handicapped, the retarded, the emotionally disturbed may not be able to master the basic, necessary skills. Many normal, healthy people are not endowed with the manual dexterity and fine motor skills necessary for total plaque control. While the dentist cannot accept total responsibility for his patient's oral-health maintenance, monthly or even biweekly maintenance visits might be helpful. The specific elements of maintenance sessions are also highly individualized. Review and reinforcement of the patient's daily oral-health regimen are practically universal, but the amount of time and emphasis placed upon them depends entirely on the patient's needs. Mechanical removal of hard deposits (calculus) and stains is generally assumed to be a maintenance procedure, but may not be necessary in every case. Indeed, the most common maintenance procedure, the so-called "pumice prophy," is primarily psychologic in its effect and not at all lasting in its benefit; unless there are disfiguring stains that cannot be removed with brush and floss, the procedure is often unnecessary. Therefore, flexibility and good judgment must be exercised when establishing the frequency and specific components of maintenance sessions.

Finally, in terms of maintenance of the oral environment, we must consider where and to what extent our treatment has altered that environment and help the patient adjust the regimen originally established to deal with those changes. The most striking example of this is the postperiodontal-surgery situation, in which the entire topography of the mouth may have been altered. Gingival position may be different; certainly, more surface areas are exposed for plaque removal in most cases. Relearning plaque-removal methods and the operation of additional devices may be necessary. Even a very localized procedure, such as a sliding flap or frenectomy and vestibular extension, will alter the topography sufficiently to require the patient's retraining.

Similar changes occur with extensive restorations, extractions, and any kind of prosthetic appliance. Each represents change in the oral environment and each requires individual strategies for health maintenance in, under, and around them. The most typical example is a soldered joint, whether in a fixed partial denture or in a splint. Threading techniques to pass floss beneath the joint in order to clean the proximal sulcus and/or pontic area must be taught carefully and reinforced regularly. Any type of removable partial denture presents special maintenance challenges, both in the anatomic irregularities created for rests, clasps, and the like, and in the greater tendency for plaque accumulation under and around the removable appliance. Once again, the techniques required to maintain oral health and to clean the appliance are not likely to materialize suddenly; they must be taught, corrected, and reinforced positively.

In many cases, completion of the restorative phase does not complicate the oral-health regimen, but it may simplify it. Replacement of removable partial dentures with fixed appliances often eliminates many plaque-accumulation areas. Replacement of rough, overhanging, and poorly contoured fillings with restorations compatible with oral-health maintenance makes environmental control possible in cases in which it would otherwise be an exercise in frustration. Even when maintenance of oral health has been made easier in the course of dental treatment, it is necessary to assist the patient in discovering that fact and in adjusting his oral-health regimen to the new situation.

Mechanical Maintenance. Dentists are often victims of their own terminology. How often, for example, do you hear the term "permanent" filling or "permanent" bridge as opposed to the term "temporary" restoration? To most people, the connotation is clear: the restoration will last forever without any maintenance. No wonder dentists are often frustrated. Fabricating a miniature mechanical device expected to perform comfortably and efficiently 24 hours a day, year in and year out, in a hostile, biomechanical environment is difficult enough. That the device should also last forever without any upkeep is expecting a bit much; yet, we create just that expectation if we fail to establish the need for regular mechanical-maintenance treatment and an understanding on the part of the patient that mechanical devices do deteriorate and break just as natural teeth do, if not faster. If a less durable material (silver amalgam instead of cast-gold alloy) is chosen because of the patient's financial limitations, the patient must understand the need for maintenance and/or replacement. Mechanical maintenance involves advising the patient as to the likelihood of future restorative needs.

The dentition can be likened to any mechanical device. For example, even a new automobile requires maintenance and occasional repairs in normal use, and no matter how costly or well maintained, it is going to wear out some day. A healthy environment is absolutely essential to the survival of mechanical restorations and makes their replacement (if and when the restorations wear out) possible.

TREATMENT SEQUENCES

A sequential approach to treatment that is based first on urgency and then on efficiency in achieving treatment goals has been established in general terms. Priorities within each of those phases have been discussed. Using these general concepts as guides, a model can now be developed that places specific treatment steps into the sequence. It must be remembered, however, that this model is based on the urgency/efficiency concept and should serve as a guideline, not an absolute set of rules. Exceptions and modifications must be made in accordance with the basic principles behind the format.

Systemic

Systemic treatment addresses the general health status of the patient and its relationship to the oral cavity and dental treatment. It may include the elements listed below (not necessarily in sequence):

Treatment of systemic disease (referral/consultation):

1. Dentist detects potential hypertension problem and refers patient for medical evaluation and/or treatment.
2. Dentist suspects or detects possible diabetic condition and refers patient for medical evaluation and/or treatment.

Systemic treatment of oral disease, or coordination of systemic treatment already in progress:

1. Dentist performs a biopsy of an oral lesion. The results of the biopsy, which suggest a malignancy, are referred to physician for further (head-neck) evaluation and treatment.
2. Dentist prescribes penicillin for dental cellulitis, takes patient off medically prescribed tetracycline acne regimen and informs the dermatologist.

Prevention of systemic disease by premedication:

1. A prophylactic antibiotic regimen is prescribed for patients with rheumatic or valvular problems prior to any procedure involving soft tissue.
2. Presurgical antibiotic coverage is given to infection-susceptible patients—that is, brittle diabetics, debilitated individuals, or others with history of poor resistance to infection.

Emergency/Investigative

Emergency/investigative treatment addresses those dental problems that constitute the patient's chief complaint, are producing symptoms, or are potential sources of acute symptoms. The following are examples of this treatment:

1. Relief of dental pain due to pulpal involvement is accomplished through excavation/sedative temporary restoration (reversible pulpal hyperemia), or through opening for drainage, pulpotomy, or pulpectomy (irreversible pulpal pathology).
2. Relief of dental pain due to periodontal involvement is achieved through irrigation, curettage, or incision/drainage.
3. Appropriate analgesic/antibiotic agents are prescribed for the above problems (also a systemic treatment).
4. Definitive or palliative treatment of soft-tissue lesions is accomplished through excision, cautery, or topical medication.
5. Any dental treatment procedure that is exploratory in nature—that is, performed in order to determine the feasibility of further treatment—includes excavations of deep carious lesions, initiation of endodontic procedures to assess likely prognosis, and periodontal flap procedures to assess actual bone levels.
6. Any definitive treatment done to relieve immediate symptoms, i.e., removal of symptomatic, partially impacted third molar. Even a procedure such as cast crown preparation might, in some cases, be appropriate as an "emergency" treatment, but care must be taken in doing such treatment that the entire dental and oral situation is taken into account. Complicated and irreversible procedures should, whenever practical, await a thorough examination and diagnosis before being placed in their proper sequence in the treatment.

Preparatory

Preparatory treatment includes those steps aimed at the establishment of a healthy oral environment. The sequence within this category is flexible, and should be based on goal-oriented efficiency. Examples of this type of treatment follow:

1. Preventive counselling and plaque-control instructions
2. Dietary analysis and counselling
3. Fluoride therapy, systemic and topical
4. Periodontal therapy, including scaling/pumicing (prophylaxis), deep scaling and curettage, definitive surgery for pocket elimination, or repair/enhancement of periodontal apparatus
5. Oral surgery, including removal of teeth, cysts, foreign bodies, exostoses, or modification of the soft tissue to facilitate later treatment; orthognathic surgery in concert with orthodontic correction
6. Endodontic therapy
7. Caries control, either through excavation/temporary or definitive restoration with "interim" materials (such as amalgam or resin). Restoration with castings should generally await completion of all preparatory procedures.
8. Modification of the occlusion, including orthodontic treatment—minor tooth movement, or comprehensive therapy
9. Occlusal adjustment to harmonize occlusal function with TMJ, relieve symptoms, or facilitate later treatment
10. Restoration of lost vertical dimension to alleviate symptoms and/or facilitate later treatment

Corrective

Corrective treatment includes those procedures aimed at the restoration of form, function, and esthetics. The sequence within this category is flexible, but often critical, since in many complex restorative efforts, each step must dovetail properly into the next. For example, a cast post and core on a lower tooth might have to be fabricated not only with the individual tooth in mind, but also with a mind to establish parallelism with another tooth, leaving space for partial denture attachments (intra- or extracoronal), and its relationship with the opposing teeth. The following are examples of corrective treatment:

1. Operative dentistry, including cast restorations and interim materials. This is especially true when further treatment of a prosthetic nature is not indicated.
2. Fixed prosthetics and individual cast crowns
3. Removable prosthetics, including partial denture prostheses and full dentures
4. Maxillofacial prosthetic devices, including obturators and facial reconstructive appliances

Maintenance

Maintenance treatments are aimed at effectively maintaining the healthy environment and the restorations placed within it. In establishing a sequence within this category, timing is all important. The need for maintenance of the healthy environment commences as soon as that environment is created; therefore, maintenance treatment might be commenced in some areas even before corrective treatment is complete, and perhaps even before it is begun. Although a course of dental treatment is often carried out in a very short time, it more often extends over weeks, months, or years. An effective maintenance-treatment schedule, then, must be instituted independent of long-term preparatory and corrective treatment. Finally, although frequency and timing are critical in this phase, the actual content of a maintenance program must be tailored to the individual patient's needs. Examples of this treatment follow:

1. Review of principles and modification of home-care techniques following periodontal, restorative, and prosthetic treatment
2. Periodic review and reinforcement of same
3. Periodic examination and radiographs to monitor status of restorations and prostheses and to detect incipient pathology
4. Periodic scaling/pumicing (where indicated)
5. Fluoride therapy
6. Modification, adjustment, repair, and replacement of restorative and prosthetic hardware

This outline of five treatment stages and examples of the types of treatment likely to be done in each should be viewed only as a guide. The basic principles cited earlier in this chapter must be applied in all cases. A good example of the flexibility necessary is that of bite-plane therapy. A simple occlusal-coverage splint, fabricated over the maxillary teeth and allowing full occlusal contact without lateral interference, is a useful therapeutic dental appliance, yet it cannot be automatically fixed into a treatment sequence.[2] It may be an emergency/investigative device, relieving acute TMJ symptoms and allowing for a truer assessment of centric relation position. It may just as easily be a preparatory treatment that relieves occlusal traumatism within the course of periodontal therapy or aids in re-establishing lost vertical dimension. It may even be used in the maintenance phase, if symptoms develop following corrective treatment or a recurrent bruxism threatens the mechanical integrity of dental restorations.

Flexibility may also be required in altering the normal sequence to accommodate a patient's felt need. The most common example of this is the definitive restoration of an anterior tooth when esthetics is a problem prior to other, more likely, procedures in the preparatory phase. Obviously, such a deviation from standard procedure should be carefully considered in light of the overall treatment plan, and the patient fully informed of any potential risks associated with deviation from normal sequence. In the first case, one would like to avoid extraction, endodontic therapy, or major periodontal alteration of a newly crowned tooth; secondly, if the unusual sequencing jeopardizes the long-term result, the patient must accept the responsibility. With those provisions in mind, occasional deviations from the normal sequence are acceptable and often make for better patient rapport and satisfaction.

Once the list of necessary procedures has been arranged in the proper *sequence*, those general procedures can be analyzed and broken into discrete, *specific procedures*. This is done in order to produce an estimate of the required investment of time and money. It is necessary for both the dentist and patient to know approximately how many visits, over what period of time, and at what cost the treatment will be carried out. At this juncture, it is also possible to consider alternative treatment options as a function of time and money. A beautifully conceived treatment plan requiring 6 to 8 months to carry out can be only of academic interest to the patient who is only available for treatment for 3 to 4 months. Likewise, a treatment plan requiring an investment of thousands of dollars may not be appropriate for the

Appt.		SERVICES NECESSARY		FEES		
	1					
	2					
(5)	3	MOD/alloy, base, anes.	37			
	4	DO/alloy, base	22			
	5					
(4)	6	G/composite, base, anes.	22			
	7	M/composite, base				
?–	8	Cast dowel & core, P/G crn		90 + 290 (elective)		
	9	M/composite (acid etch) base	27			
	10					
	11					
	12					
	13					
(6)	14	MOL/alloy, base, anes.	37			
	15					
2 wks. (8)	16	Surgical removal, tissue	45			
	17	" " impactions	45			
2 wks (9)	18	Full cast gold crown				
(10)	19	Gold pontic	735			
	20	Gold 3/4 crown				
	21					
	22					
	23					
	24					
	25					
	26					
	27					
	28					
	29					
(7)	30	MODB/alloy, base, anes.	47			
	31					
2 wks (1)	32	Surgical removal, partial tissue impaction	45			
1 wk (2) (3)		Preventive visits (2) incl. oral health maintenance instructions, scaling, pumicing, and topical F	40			
		Appointments numbered in probable sequence.				
		Approximate total time: 3 months, allowing for healing of 3rd molar extractions.				

Fig. 6–2. Using a treatment planning form, specific procedures and fees are listed tooth by tooth. Appointments are numbered according to the sequence established, and time intervals estimated when necessary. For example, operative dentistry appointment could be spaced at any interval (4,5,6) but 2 weeks must be allowed between preparation and insertion of the bridge (9,10), and healing time is allotted after surgical removal of a wisdom tooth (1).

patient having difficulty keeping up with costs of food, clothing, and shelter. Possible options in such situations range from the selection of alternative treatment approaches requiring less time and/or money (and providing a lesser service) to phasing the treatment over time, which will be discussed in the next chapter. In any event, it is the responsibility of the dentist to present all the available treatment options to the patient, especially the course of treatment that the dentist feels can provide the best result over the longest time. The decision to accept such a course or to opt for a lesser or delayed approach must rest with the patient. We must not prejudge the patient's willingness to accept good treatment or his ability to pay for it. Even when severe financial limitations have been cited prior to treatment planning, the patient should be informed of the optimal courses of treatment and their cost. Financial situations change, priorities change, and people change. The dentist, while tailoring his services to the individual needs and desires of each patient, must give each and every patient the option of optimal treatment, or at least make the patient aware that such treatment is available. The patient who chooses an alternative approach does so as a result of an informed decision. The dentist need not consider that choice a defeat or a failure in case presentation or personal appeal, but as a decision made by a patient based on good information provided by the dentist. This in itself is a service we can be proud of, and patients appreciate the care that goes into thoughtful treatment planning.

TREATMENT-PLANNING FORMAT

Specific procedures are usually planned and time and money estimated on a tooth-by-tooth basis, with general procedures listed separately. This is generally done out of convenience in correlating information from the examination/diagnosis to the treatment plan, even though the sequence may be different. (We examine and diagnose teeth numerically or by quadrant, even though we may not treat them in that order.) The following examples of treatment sequences broken into specific procedures illustrate the process.

Systemic:

1. Refer for HBsAg determination; positive history of hepatitis 2 years ago

SERVICES NECESSARY	FEES I	FEES II	FEES III
~~1~~			
~~2~~			
3 ENDO, ROOT AMP, FCC / EXT	570	30	30
~~4~~ P/G PONTIC	300		
5 ENDO, POST & CORE, P/G / EXT	515	30	30
6 P/G	300	300	300
~~7~~ P/G PONTIC	300	300	300
8 P/G	300	300	300
9 P/G	300	300	300
~~10~~ P/G PONTIC	300	300	300
11 P/G	300	300	300
~~12~~ P/G PONTIC	300		
~~13~~ P/G PONTIC	300		
~~14~~ GOLD PONTIC	285		
15 FCC / MO/ALLOY	285	285	35
~~16~~ SEMI-PRECISION CAST BASE RPD		950 /	
17 CHROME COBALT & ACRYLIC RPD			650
18	4355	3095	2540
19			
20			
21			
22			
23			
24			
25			
26			
27			
28			
29			
30			
31			
32			

TREATMENT PLAN OPTIONS: MAXILLA

I KEEP ALL MAXILLARY TEETH--IDEAL, BUT HIGHEST COST & RISK
ENDO AND DB ROOT AMPUTATION #3, ENDO AND POST & CORE #5
FIXED BRIDGES: 3--5-6-8 9-11---15
(DESIGN 5-6 & 11 FOR RPD LATER--IF NECESSARY)

II MAXILLARY REMOVABLE PARTIAL--LESS IDEAL, BUT LESS RISK
EXTRACT #3 & 5
FIXED BRIDGE: 6--8-9--11 FULL CAST CROWN #15
MAXILLARY PRECISION OR SEMI-PRECISION CAST METAL
BASE (MUCOSTATIC) RPD

III LEAST COSTLY VIABLE ALTERNATIVE
EXTRACT #3 & 5
FIXED BRIDGES: 6--8 9--11 MO/ALLOY #15
MAXILLARY CHROME COBALT & ACRYLIC RPD (ALTERED CAST)

Fig. 6–3. This detailed list of procedures and fees depicts a complex case (maxilla only) and includes three possible options. Heavy slash marks indicate specific choices of treatment on individual teeth. Such a blueprint is essential to clearly define the cost differential of the various options.

Emergency/investigative:
1. Removal of partially impacted no. 32; chief complaint of recurring pericoronitis

Preparatory:
1. Oral-health maintenance instructions, especially flossing
2. Scaling/pumicing
3. Minor operative dentistry—composite resin on three anterior teeth and amalgam on four posterior teeth.
4. Removal of impacted third molars, nos. 16 and 17—elective timing

Corrective:
1. Fixed bridge replacing missing no. 19
2. Eventual dowel and core and porcelain-fused-to-gold crown for endodontically treated central incisior, no. 8

Maintenance:
1. Periodic recall (6 months), review maintenance, scaling/polishing

This sequential treatment can then be broken into specific procedures, with appointments planned and numbered in sequence (Fig. 6–2). The second example is a more complex case, and demonstrates use of alternative treatment approaches (Fig. 6–3).

In the final analysis, the treatment plan, in its sequential outline and specific breakdown, is a detailed map. It must be accurate and complete to be of value, but just as important, it must be a map that will lead to the destination selected by the patient. Goal-oriented treatment planning is just that—a treatment plan, or map, showing the most effective approach to the goal agreed upon by dentist and patient. Life is seldom so simple, however, and the succeeding chapters will attempt to address some of the complexities inherent in preparing a treatment plan.

REFERENCES

1. Brackett, R.C.: Periodic recall program. *In* Clinical Dentistry. Vol. 2. Edited by J.W. Clark. Hagerstown, Harper and Row, 1979.
2. Butler, J.H., Bush, F.M., Abbott, D.M., and Green, E.: Occlusal guards and bite planes. *In* Clinical Dentistry. Vol. 2. Edited by J.W. Clark. Hagerstown, Harper and Row, 1979.
3. Gier, R.E.: Problem-oriented case analysis. *In* Clinical Dentistry. Vol. 1. Edited by J.W. Clark. Hagerstown, Harper and Row, 1979.
4. Kerr, D.A., Ash, M.M., and Millard, H.D.: Oral Diagnosis. 4th ed. St. Louis, C.V. Mosby, 1974.
5. Mitchell, D.F., Standish, S.M., and Fast, T.B.: Oral Diagnosis: Oral Medicine. 2nd ed. Philadelphia, Lea & Febiger, 1971.
6. Ranly, D.M., et al.: The formocresol pulpotomy: The past, the present, and the future. J. Pedod., *2*:115–127, 1978.

SECTION 3

Principles of Complex Treatment Planning

In the preceding chapters, a systematic approach leading to the synthesis of a treatment plan was established. The resultant treatment plan was problem-oriented, patient-oriented, complete in scope, and rational in sequence. If this approach were applied universally, it would ensure effective dental treatment in the majority of cases. Certain situations, however, call for more sophisticated treatment planning. In the succeeding chapters, general concepts and specific techniques will be presented to address these situations. Creativity and imagination must be applied in many situations in which the mechanical, routine approach does not suffice.

Chapter 7 will deal with phasing of dental treatment, in which the timing of the treatment is significant. Chapter 8 will offer a number of concepts aimed at simplification of treatment on the theory that, if fewer treatment steps are employed, it is harder to fail. If complex treatment situations can be converted into simple situations, the likelihood of success increases. Chapter 9 deals with the likelihood of success and failure and addresses the prognosis of dental treatment. No two patients are alike, and the same treatment regimen carried out on two different patients may succeed in one and fail in the other. In most cases, we must make at least an educated guess as to the probable outcome of treatment and discuss it openly and honestly with the patient before proceeding with treatment.

CHAPTER 7

Phasing Dental Treatment

My daughter's getting married, and I need it done by Saturday!

NEW PATIENT, THURSDAY AFTERNOON

The traditional method of selecting a treatment plan from a range of approaches has been to base the decision on the relative quality of treatment as reflected by its price. That is, the ideal, or optimal, treatment approach carrying the highest price tag is at one end of the spectrum, and minimal, or "patchwork," treatment with a more modest fee is at the other. Between the two extremes may be one or more "middle" options, but the basic assumption is that treatment will be done now, and the plan chosen will vary in quality based on its price. This model fixes time as a constant and quality as the variable and derives directly from the common, dental-school treatment model; that is, the typical dental student, given a patient to complete (or having requirements for graduation reflected in a patient's treatment needs), must treat that patient immediately. Periodontal therapy, extractions, or other treatment must be done quickly to allow time (usually a minimal amount) for healing prior to operative procedures, crowns, and the partial denture that will allow the student to graduate.

This urgency to proceed with complete and comprehensive treatment in as little time as possible does not always serve the needs of the patient, and if carried into a dental practice, results in the time-constant/quality-variable model just described (Fig. 7–1). The late Dr. Robert Barkley addressed this problem in his writings and offered some possible solutions in the design of patient treatment in dental schools.[1] I can agree that one option in the phasing of dental treatment is to alter the equation so that quality remains the constant, and time the variable (Fig. 7–2).

TRADITIONAL MODEL

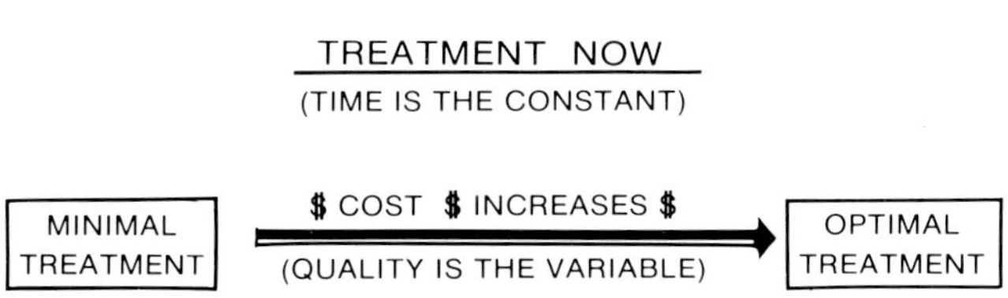

Fig. 7–1. Traditional model of dental treatment.

TIME VARIABLE MODEL

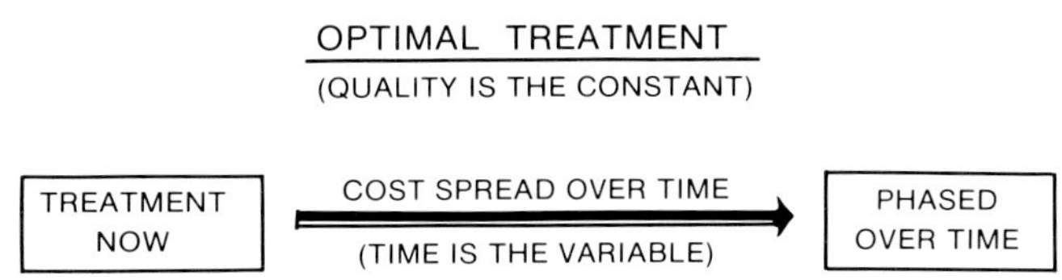

Fig. 7–2. Time variable model of dental treatment.

OPTIMAL TREATMENT MODEL

Most patients who have been involved in their diagnosis and treatment planning can appreciate the intrinsic value of optimal dental treatment. Most patients would prefer the highest available level of treatment for themselves and their families. However, real or perceived financial limitations may deter them from committing to such a treatment approach. The solution in a phased treatment plan is to do the minimal necessary treatment, the urgency-based treatment, as the first phase of an extended course of treatment. These procedures, then, rather than being substandard, final treatments, are simply the beginning steps in optimal treatment. There is more than a semantic difference between these treatments, but the semantic difference itself is not inconsequential. To the patient, it means proceeding with dental treatment toward an optimal goal at an acceptable economic pace. Financial commitments may be made one step at a time; furthermore, the patient has the opportunity to "try out" some dental treatment on a limited basis before committing to extensive and costly plans. To the dentist, it can mean that nearly every patient in the practice has accepted and is involved in an optimal course of treatment. Some are receiving that treatment immediately, some over an agreed period of time, and some over an indefinite period of time. The satisfaction derived from performing preliminary procedures is greater than that derived from doing patchwork dentistry. Lastly, we do not need to label patients as "minimal-treatment," or "low-dental-I.Q." individuals merely because they cannot afford maximum treatment immediately.

This approach to the phasing of dental treatment, while having many advantages, has several possible drawbacks as well. The most serious of these is an overall oral condition that is so debilitated that treatment in segments or over time is technically impossible. The most obvious example might be a loss of vertical dimension, for if it is to be regained, treatment generally must be done throughout the mouth at one time. It is certainly impractical to place one crown restoration at a new vertical dimension and wait a year to place another. On the other hand, removable bite planes are often used in such cases to establish the new dimension, and it might be possible to restore anterior segments to the new dimension using interim, removable appliances in the posterior.

Another potential problem with time phasing is that caries control may require some fairly sound interim restorations (such as large alloys) to be followed by cast crowns in the not too distant future. Thus, some areas might be treated twice in a period of months or years. In many cases, this is not a serious drawback, because excavation of caries and old restorations often precede placement of cast restorations. Examples of hypothetical treatment plans (and approximate fees) applying a phased approach would better serve to illustrate this point.

The following treatment plan presents an optimal approach to dental treatment, and could, if the patient is willing and able to do so, be carried out almost immediately.

Optimal Treatment Plan.

1. Premedicate for all tissue-manipulation procedures; history of rheumatic fever
2. Removal of partially erupted lower right third molar, which is currently symptomatic — $50.
3. Scaling/pumicing and plaque-control instructions, especially stressing floss (two sessions) — $50.
4. Endodontic therapy for upper left central incisor; no. 9 tooth nonvital and darkened subsequent to trauma 3 to 4 years ago; periapical lesion visible on radiograph — $125.
5. Operative dentistry: composite resins on teeth nos. 7 and 8, and silver amalgams on teeth nos. 3, 4, 14, and 29 — $125.
6. Cast crown restoration on tooth no. 30 — $225.
   Fixed bridge replacing missing tooth no. 19; abutments—full crown for no. 18 and 3/4 crown for no. 20 — $675.
   Cast dowel and core for no. 9 — $100.
   Porcelain-fused-to-gold crown restoration for no. 9 — $275.
7. Recall/maintenance session following completion of treatment — $25.

Approximate time: 4 to 6 mos.

Total fee: $1650.

This plan could also be carried out through time phasing over a 3-year period. The treatment plan would then look like this:

Phase 1. Establishing a healthy environment.

1. Premedicate PRN
2. Removal of no. 32 — $50.
3. Scaling/pumicing and plaque control (two sessions) — $50.
4. Endodontic therapy for no. 9 — $125.
5. Operative dentistry as before, including an amalgam core restoration for no 30, and temporary restoration for no. 18 — $175.

Approximate time: 2 to 3 mos.

Total fee: $400.

Phase 2 (second year). Replacing a missing tooth.

1. Fixed bridge for nos. 18 to 20 — $675.
2. Recall/maintenance (two sessions) — $50.

Approximate time: 3 to 4 wks.

Total fee: $725.

Phase 3 (third year). Definitive restorations on nos. 9 and 30.

1. Cast dowel and core for no. 9 — $100.
   Porcelain-fused-to-gold for crown no. 9 — $275.
   Cast crown restorations for no. 30 — $225.
2. Recall/maintenance (two sessions) — $50.

Approximate time: 6 to 8 wks.

Total fee: $650.

With this phased treatment plan, the optimal treatment is carried out at a more comfortable financial pace. Regular payments of less than $50 a month would allow the entire course of treatment to be paid for as it was completed. Fees could be held at the estimated level provided the phases were carried out as planned, or they could be adjusted yearly to reflect necessary fee increases, and the patient advised accordingly. Finally, this same plan could be phased over an indefinite period of time (should circumstances require it), in which case it would look like this:

Phase 1. Establishing a healthy environment.

1. Premedicate PRN
2. Removal of no. 32 — $50.
3. Scaling/pumicing and plaque control (two sessions) — $50.
4. Operative dentistry as before, including an amalgam core for no. 32 and an amalgam restoration for no. 18 — $185.

Approximate time: 2 to 3 mos.

Total fee: $285.

Phase 2. Postponed indefinitely, but patient is monitored regularly.

1. Recall/maintenance sessions twice yearly to scale/pumice/review and reinforce plaque control; monitor clinically and radiographically tooth no. 9, which will need endodontic therapy at some point; monitor space area no. 19 (missing) which will need a fixed bridge and may require a space maintainer should space loss be detected — $50./yr.

It is important to differentiate between such a time-phased approach and the concept of minimal treatment. Although the actual procedures are the same, time phasing provides a goal of eventual, optimal treatment for both patient and dentist and does not label that patient as poor or unreceptive.

PHASING BY QUADRANT

Another application of time phasing is the restoration by quadrants, using interim and temporary materials and methods on the unrestored quadrants, while performing optimal dental procedures one quadrant at a time. This can then be spaced over a period of months or even years.

A striking example of time phasing is the following case history. The patient was a mason contractor with an end-to-end occlusal relationship who had $^{3}/_{4}$ crowns placed on four lower incisors because of severe wear. The crowns, which were placed in 1966, were the first of many optimal restorations placed over a 14-year period. At no time did the patient feel he could afford to restore all the teeth at once, but in the reconstruction carried out over 14 years, over twenty units of crown and fixed-bridge restorations were placed. With the bite relationship and the continual cement dust exposure, the original crowns are now nearly worn through and must soon be replaced. Because of the long-term, goal-oriented treatment, the patient understands and accepts this and realizes that the posterior restorations placed and his excellent oral-health maintenance make another set of crown restorations possible. It is gratifying to see restorations wear out from many years of good and trouble-free service in a healthy environment. If our mechanical miniatures do not last forever (and few will), we should hope that they wear out from daily use, rather than from premature fracture or leakage, or the ravages of uncontrolled dental disease.

PHASING BY LEVEL OF ORAL HEALTH

The subject of uncontrolled dental disease leads directly to another approach in the phasing of dental treatment—namely, phasing by level of oral health. We have previously discussed the chronic nature of most dental diseases and the futility of any dental treatment in the face of uncontrolled disease. All too often, total definitive treatment is carried out without regard to the ability or willingness of the patient to achieve and maintain the healthy oral environment essential to its success. Considerable time, effort, and expense may be wasted in such premature treatment, with the result that the patient, finding himself once again with dental disease and in distress, is emotionally and financially drained and discouraged from further necessary treatment.

In phasing treatment by level of oral health, we do not deny treatment to patients who do not perform up to our standards for oral-health maintenance. To do so would be arbitrary and foolish, since we must always deal with human beings, not automatons. To accept our patients as human beings is to accept both success and failure, enthusiasm and apathy. The patient must be dealt with at his present level of understanding, ability, and motivation. The type of treatment rendered, however, and the timing of that treatment must also reflect that level or be doomed to fail.

PHASING BY CARIES CONTROL

The patient exhibiting a high caries rate must be dealt with through four methods almost simultaneously: plaque control, dietary control, fluoride therapy, and the elimination of carious lesions. Two of those methods require patient initiative, and two are somewhat more passive, but all are essential to effective control of extensive dental caries.

The patient must learn and practice effective daily *plaque control* with a toothbrush and dental floss. The role of the dental team is intructional at the outset and motivational as the techniques are reviewed and reinforced.

The patient must also practice *dietary control* and assess his intake of fermentable carbohydrates, particularly sucrose, as to amount and frequency and effectively eliminate or reduce that intake. The dental team must assist in the dietary assessment and can offer possible dietary alternatives, encouraging this essential step.

These two, primary methods of caries control are almost completely under the control of the patient. In many cases, they require a striking change in lifestyle and daily routine. Such changes do not come easily, and time must be allowed for assimilation, relapse and failure, and hopefully, for renewed efforts leading to some level of success. We must also be prepared to accept less than total plaque and dietary control, given the human factors already discussed. We must consider that the patient who has the personality and self-discipline to exercise total plaque and dietary control is not likely to suffer excessive caries in the first place. The essential concept here is that both the timing and the content of our dental treatment plan must reflect the level of success the patient can attain in caries control and not create a situation in which failure is inevitable.

Fluoride therapy is effective in the control of excessive caries and must be considered in our treatment. The patient should become actively involved in the use of a fluoride dentifrice and home-use gels or rinses as prescribed or recommended. Intensive, therapeutic, topical fluorides can also play an important role in caries control.

The elimination of carious lesions prevents further loss of tooth structure, eliminates plaque formation and retention areas (the lesions themselves), and may serve to alter the oral environment in the direction of health and away from disease. This obvious step is sometimes overlooked in our enthusiasm for patient-oriented treatment, but it remains an essential step in caries control. The critical question that arises concerns not the removal of carious tooth structure, but the methods and materials employed in filling the space created by excavation. Few would advocate placing extensive, porcelain-fused-to-metal crown restorations as an immediate treatment for rampant caries, and we see such treatment fail dismally when it is carried out before good caries control has been established. Resin-reinforced, zinc oxide-eugenol materials, the so-called "intermediate" materials, can be of great value in this area, owing to their economy, ease of placement, caries-inhibitory and sedative nature, and relatively good longevity of 6 months to a year, or more. When greater strength, retention, or longevity is required, silver amalgam, composite resin, or stainless steel crowns can be employed, and in some cases, will serve as the definitive restoration.

If we are basing our timing of further treatment on caries control, we must be able to assess whether that control has been established. We can do this in one of two ways: patient testimony or direct observation.

If the patient reports that he is doing daily, effective plaque removal, has eliminated, substituted, or controlled sucrose and other carbohydrate intake, is carrying out the prescribed fluoride regimen, and we can observe the results of the plaque control directly, we may wish to assume that caries control has been accomplished. This presupposes that carious lesions have been or are about to be eliminated. It also presupposes that the patient is doing what he claims to be doing. While that supposition is reasonable in some cases, it may not be in others.

A more realistic assessment of caries control is obtained by direct observation of the extent and rate of caries activity. Careful re-examination, both clinically and with radiographs, should determine whether or not caries have been controlled. This assessment requires a minimum of 6 months, but 1 to 2 years is a more reasonable estimate. The benefits to be gained are well worth the wait for both patient and dentist. If effective caries control has been established over a 1- to 2- year period, both patient and dentist can proceed with other treatment with confidence in the patient's ability to maintain a healthy oral environment and in the resultant good prognosis for further treatment. On the other hand, should assessment of caries control reveal a continuing problem, that problem can be addressed without the added complication of failed extensive, definitive treatment. We can illustrate this approach with the following hypothetical treatment plans, which are phased by caries control.

The first treatment plan is for a 14-year-old girl who presented with 18 carious lesions on 12 teeth and a Class II malocclusion with bilateral posterior crossbites.

Phase 1. Caries control.

1. Plaque-control counselling
2. Dietary analysis and counselling
3. Topical-fluoride application and home-use prescription
4. Excavation of three deep carious lesions with potential pulpal involvement

5. Removal of all caries; restoration with silver amalgam and composite resin when practical; stainless steel crowns or pin-retained amalgam cores when necessary
6. Recall/maintenance at 3- to 4-month intervals to include review-reinforcement, topical fluoride, and re-examination for caries. This is to continue for 1 to 2 years.

Phase 2. Orthodontic and restorative.

1. Assuming that no new carious lesions are detected and that the patient is able to maintain a healthy oral environment, full orthodontics can be carried out to improve function and esthetics. All caries-control modalities must be continued throughout orthodontic treatment.
2. Porcelain-fused-to-gold crowns to replace interim restorations when indicated following orthodontic treatment.

Unless caries control is effective, phase 2 is not recommended. The advantages of earlier orthodontic intervention are, in this case, more than offset by the risks of applying full-banded appliances in a high-caries environment.

The second treatment plan is for a 45-year-old male who presented with extensive restorations, including crown and fixed-bridge restorations, and had 22 carious lesions (predominately gingival and root caries) on 19 teeth.

Phase 1. Caries control.

1. Plaque control, dietary control, and fluoride therapy
2. Removal of all carious lesions, which will require extensive excavation under and around existing crowns and bridges. Crowns and bridges will be adapted as interim restorations when possible, or removed and replaced with stainless steel or acrylic shell crowns.

Phase 2. Reconstruction.

Assuming that caries control is effective, restoring the teeth to proper form and function will require multiple crowns and fixed-bridge restorations. The investment in time and money is likely to be extensive and should not be undertaken unless the tooth-decay problem is effectively controlled.

Alternative to phase 2.

Should caries not be brought under control, the alternative treatment approach is minimal restoration and patching where possible, leading to eventual extraction of nonrestorable teeth and removable prosthesis.

The alternative to phase 2 constitutes some of the most difficult and least rewarding dental treatment the dentist may perform. It is preferable, however, to helplessly witnessing the collapse and failure of massive reconstruction efforts, and for some patients, it is the most logical, appropriate treatment.

PHASING BY PERIODONTAL MAINTENANCE

Periodontal disease is so closely related to behavior that maintenance must precede almost any dental treatment, including definitive periodontal therapy. If the patient is unwilling or unable to carry out effective daily plaque control, our treatment efforts are doomed to fail. On the other hand, environmental factors may be present at the outset that contribute significantly to the disease (occlusal traumatism) or prevent effective plaque control (rough, overhanging restorations, impassable contacts, or open, food-impaction areas). Severe malocclusion may also inhibit plaque control and presents a special challenge in phasing treatment.

Fortunately, periodontal-maintenance efforts can be evaluated easily by using a number of standardized systems. Disclosants reveal plaque accumulations on teeth, which can be grossly evaluated (slight, moderate, heavy) or quantified through a plaque index (P.I.) and assigned a numerical value. Steady progress in reduction of plaque levels indicates cooperation and some degree of success on the patient's part, whereas no significant reduction in plaque levels bodes ill for the success of long-term treatment. Treatment should not be ruled out if plaque control is not immediately achieved, but the type of treatment rendered and the pace at which it is carried out must relate to observed behavior, which indicates the patient's control of periodontal disease.

In addition to the plaque indices, acute periodontal conditions can be monitored using other indices, such as a gingival-bleeding index, or by periodic observations of the apparent degree of inflammation, tissue puffiness, and bleeding. Even in the presence of deep pockets and bone loss, diligent plaque control by the patient can generally produce observable improvements in gingival tone, color, and architecture.

It is possible, through frequent prophylaxes (scaling, pumicing), to achieve similar improvements without effective plaque control on the part of the patient. While twice weekly or weekly sessions may be desirable in some cases to control inflammation quickly, they may also induce a false sense of security in both patient and dentist, since it is impractical to maintain such a regimen for extended periods of time. At some point, the patient must accept responsibility for his own oral health. While a few wealthy people might wish to present for thrice-weekly deplaquing by a dentist or dental hygienist for the rest of their lives, most people must deal with their own plaque.

While the patient is learning to deal with plaque, the dentist must see to it that environmental factors present in the mouth are not preventing effective periodontal maintenance. Occlusal traumatism must be controlled by minor selective grinding, complete equilibration, protective appliances, or a combination of these approaches. It is critical that plaque control be facilitated when necessary by the removal of overhanging restorations (recontouring or replacement), smoothing of extremely rough restorations or tooth surfaces, and correction of impassable contacts or open contacts. Whenever possible, minimum treatment should be applied to this end, since later evaluation and possible definitive periodontal therapy may dictate removal of some teeth or require specific definitive restorations not foreseen early in the treatment.

Unfortunately, some environmental factors are not readily controlled—severe malocclusion is a good example. Extremely crowded, malposed teeth may make effective periodontal maintenance nearly impossible; yet applying orthodontic appliances and attempting tooth movement in the presence of periodontal inflammation is risky.

In this situation, the dental team may have to carry out plaque control for the patient on a frequent recall basis (at the least, every other week; ideally 2 to 3 times a week). Such a regimen should not supplant the patient's home care, but supplement it until the severe malocclusion has been corrected to a maintainable state.

Nothing in periodontal maintenance is analogous to the intensive fluoride therapy available in caries control, so patient behavior, in terms of effective plaque control, is all the more essential. Fortunately, the usual slow, progressive nature of periodontal disease allows considerable time to assist the patient in gaining control of his disease. Definitive periodontal therapy can be, and often is, postponed for months or years without a striking effect on the long-term prognosis.

A hypothetical treatment plan based on periodontal maintenance illustrates this concept. The patient is a 42-year-old female who presents with moderate to severe periodontitis, generalized pocket depths of 3 to 7 mm, many old, large amalgam restorations, and a heavy plaque and calculus level.

Phase 1. Periodontal control.

1. Plaque-control counselling, including intensive instruction/coaching in sulcular brushing and flossing
2. Calculus removal, including thorough scaling, root planing, and curettage of sulcular epithelium
3. Selective grinding to relieve gross occlusal traumatism, and recontouring of restorations where necessary to facilitate plaque control
4. Periodic re-evaluation of plaque control and tissue condition, along with follow-up scaling/curettage

This regimen should be followed for a period of 3 to 12 months, the goal being effective plaque control throughout the mouth, and the greatest possible tissue health prior to further treatment.

Phase 2. Definitive periodontal therapy.

1. Surgical procedures to eliminate pockets, eliminate and recontour bony defects, and create a physiologic and maintainable periodontium
2. Complete review and modification of plaque control following alteration of gingival position, architecture, and topography
3. Periodic review of same, with thorough scaling/pumicing

This regimen should not be introduced unless phase 1 goal has been attained. The goal of phase 2 is a healthy periodontium, free of pockets and/or inflammation, which is being effectively maintained (relatively plaque free).

Phase 3. Restorative/prosthetic.

1. Operative dentistry and prosthetics where necessary to provide an atraumatic occlusion, comfort, and function
2. Continued re-evaluation of periodontal maintenance to include review of plaque control and scaling/pumicing

This phase should not be carried out if periodontal inflammation persists due to ineffective maintenance, because the prognosis is poor.

PHASING BY THE SUCCESS OR FAILURE OF PRECEDING STEPS

There are often situations in which a treatment that is carried out entails a risk of failure. That failure may become apparent almost immediately, or it may be a latent problem. When subsequent treatment is carried out based on the anticipation of success of earlier treatment, the risk is magnified. For that reason, it is often prudent to allow a reasonable period of time to elapse after initial treatment to establish some degree of confidence in the result. Examples of several observed situations may illustrate the concept.

1. *Deep excavations of carious lesions.* Placement of sedative bases or liners, or even an entire sedative restoration, is aimed at maintaining pulpal health and stimulating formation of secondary dentin. Failure of such treatment is inevitable if the caries have

already invaded the pulp or if caries removal insults the pulpal tissue beyond its ability for repair. Should irreversible pulpal damage occur prior to excavation or subsequent to it, endodontic therapy may be required to retain the tooth. Treatment should be phased so that definitive restorations (cast crowns, onlays) or prosthetics (use of the tooth as an abutment for a fixed or removable partial denture) are postponed pending evaluation of the pulpal status. Deeply excavated teeth that exhibit no symptoms or signs of pulpal hyperemia or pulpitis over 6 months to 1 year may then be involved in subsequent treatments, although a risk is still present that must be discussed with the patient and anticipated in treatment. On the other hand, deeply excavated teeth that remain sensitive to temperature and/or pressure or that exhibit clinical or radiographic signs of pulpal involvement, however slight, are not good candidates for use in further treatment unless endodontic therapy is performed. It should be stressed that teeth not involved in extensive, further treatment may be watched almost indefinitely, even though slight symptoms persist, while teeth that are involved in further treatment (terminal abutments of long-span bridges, for example) demand endodontic therapy prior to that involvement if doubt about their pulpal status persists.

Allowing a reasonable period of time to elapse between excavation and prosthesis constitutes phasing that is based on the success or failure of the preceding step and enhances the prognosis of subsequent treatment (Fig. 7–3).

2. *Endodontic therapy.* Removal of pulpal tissue and obliteration of the canals is a fairly dependable dental procedure. However, some risk of failure exists in the most carefully performed endodontics, due to conditions beyond the control of the dentist. Failure of endodontic therapy most often results in loss of the tooth unless surgical intervention is practical, and treatment should be phased following endodontic therapy to allow some assessment of the result prior to involving the treated tooth in further treatment. Certainly an asymptomatic tooth is essential; radiographic evidence of bone healing is a very positive finding. A waiting period of 6 to 12 months is advisable in cases in which large, periapical lesions were present, mobility had resulted, or the endodontic procedure itself was complicated by root morphology, canal size, or other unusual conditions (Fig. 7–4).

3. *Periodontal surgery.* Many teeth with severe pockets, osseous defects of various types, or mucogingival defects are treated surgically in hopes of eliminating the problems and establishing a viable periodontal attachment apparatus. When such procedures are attempted, however, further treatment must be phased based on the success or failure of the attempt. A successfully treated second molar, for example, may then serve as a bridge abutment, whereas failure of the periodontal effort would render the tooth unacceptable as an abutment and possibly dictate its removal prior to placement of a distal extension partial denture. When periodontal disease has

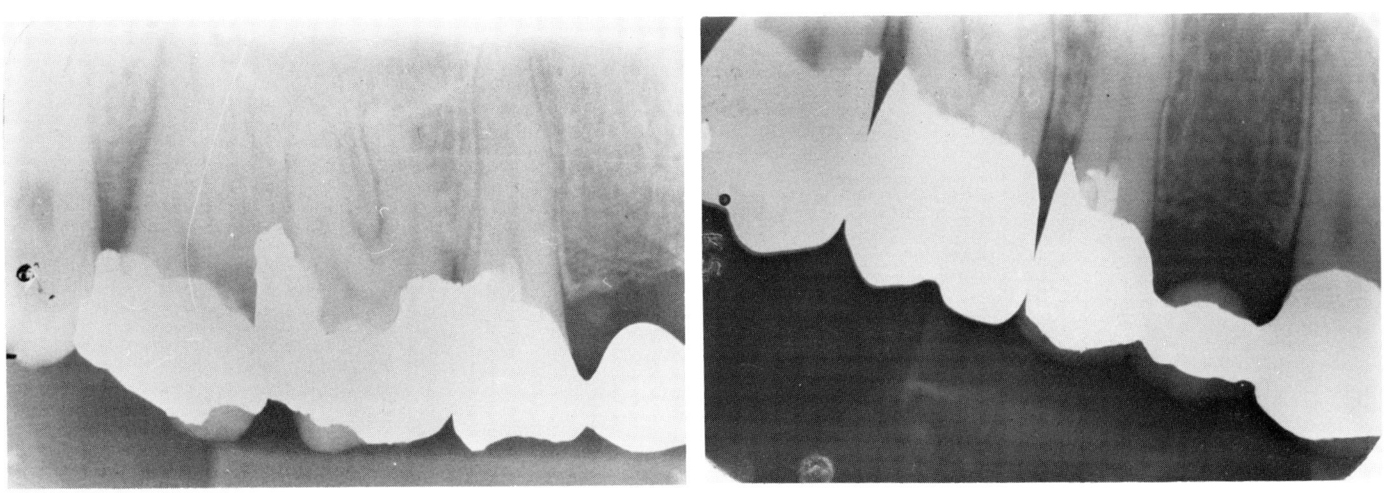

A B

Fig. 7–3. Deep carious lesions on upper first and second molars. *A*, Upon initial examination, caries were removed, and sedative intermediate restoration placed (IRM). This was left in the teeth for 14 months, during which time other restorative treatment was carried out. *B*, Because the teeth remained asymptomatic, cast restorations were placed. This radiograph was taken 5 years after initial excavation of the teeth.

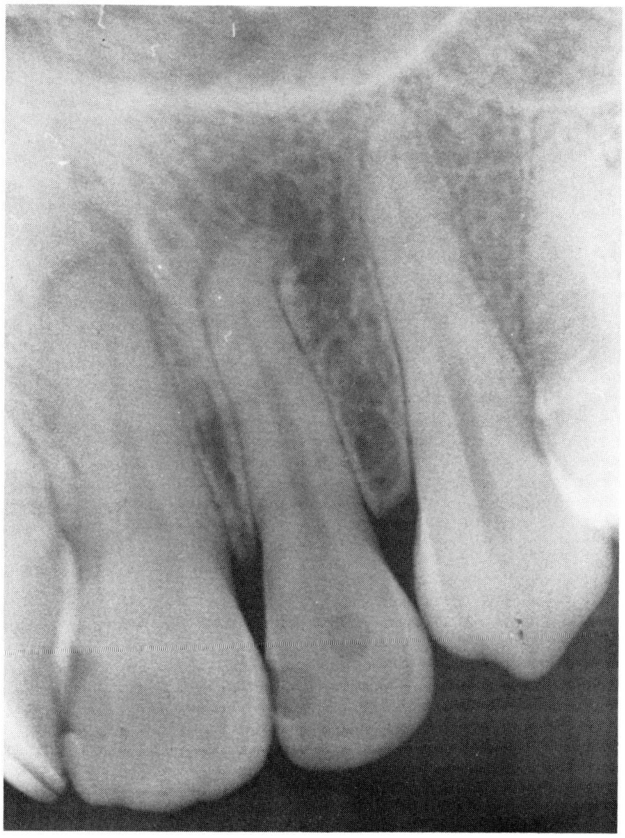

A

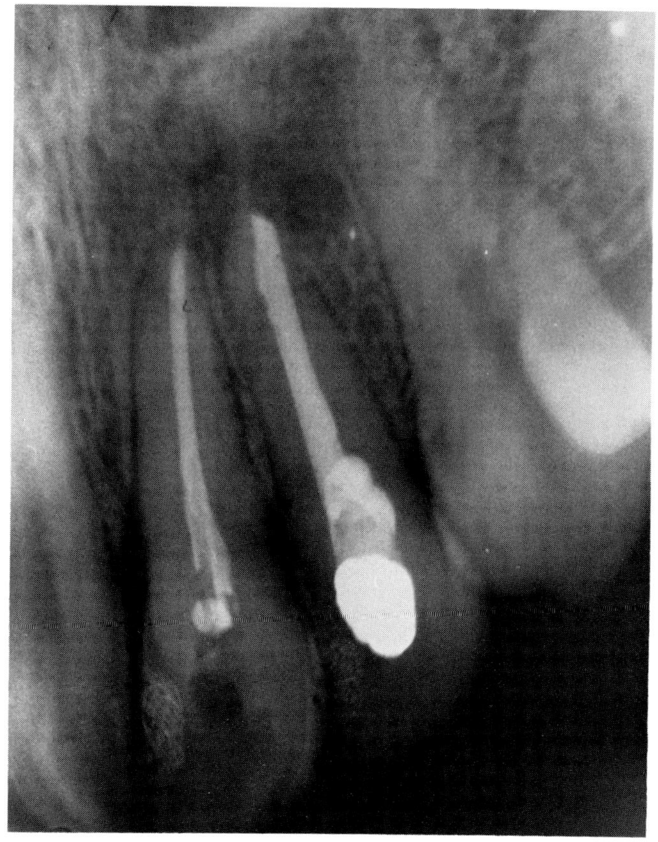

B

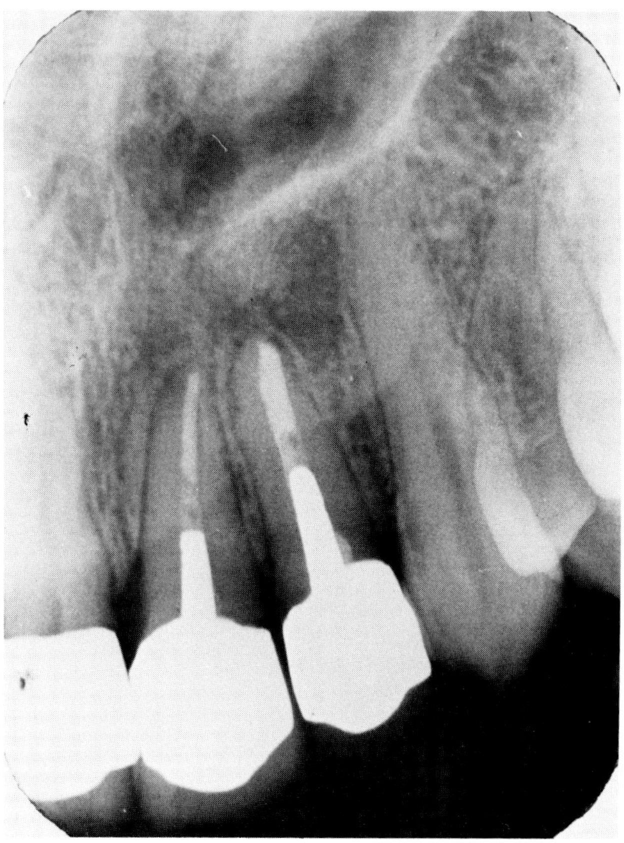

C

Fig. 7–4 Complicated endodontic procedures, treatment pending resolution of lesions.

A, Mobility and large periapical lesions on central and lateral incisors, with severe apical root curvature on lateral incisor.

B, Conservative endodontic therapy carried out on central incisor, apicoectomy on lateral incisor.

C, Definitive restoration with dowel and cores, and porcelain fused to gold crowns. This treatment was not carried out for 2 years after endodontic treatment. By that time, the lesions had resolved completely and no mobility was detectable.

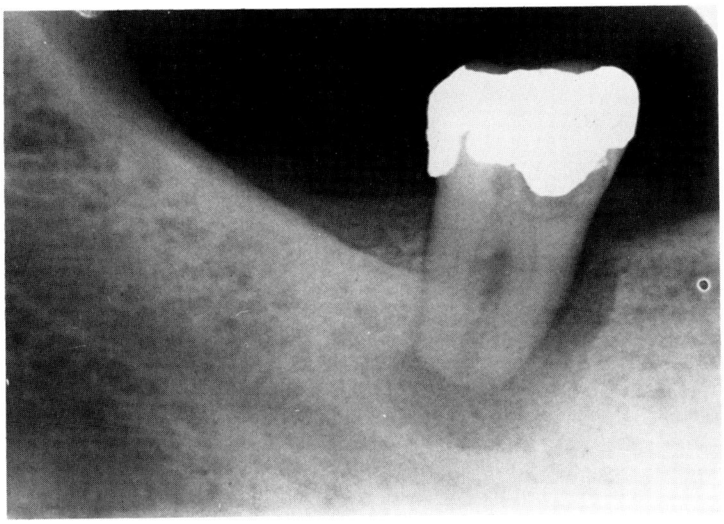

D

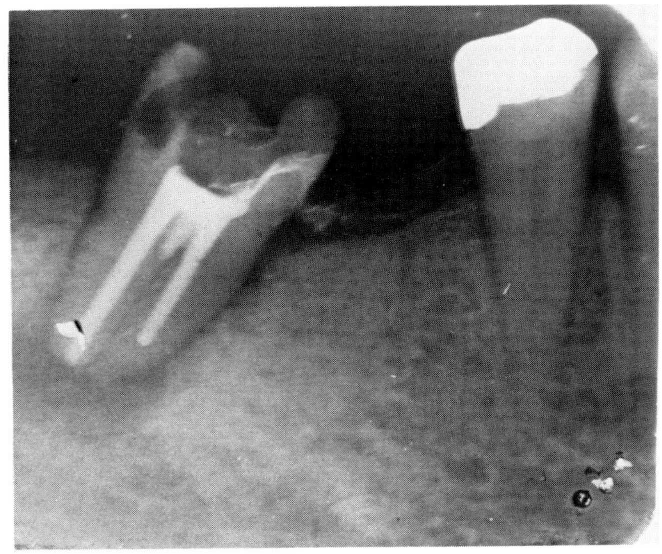

E

Fig. 7–4 *continued.* *D*, Extreme mobility, tenderness, and bone loss required the author to manually stabilize the tooth during endodontic treatment.

E, Endodontic treatment, complicated by calcification of the canals, required fairly heavy "machining" of the canals to permit obturation. Marked decrease in mobility and resolution of the bone lesion is apparent after 6 months.

F, Five years after endodontic treatment, tooth is about to be used as abutment for fixed bridge.

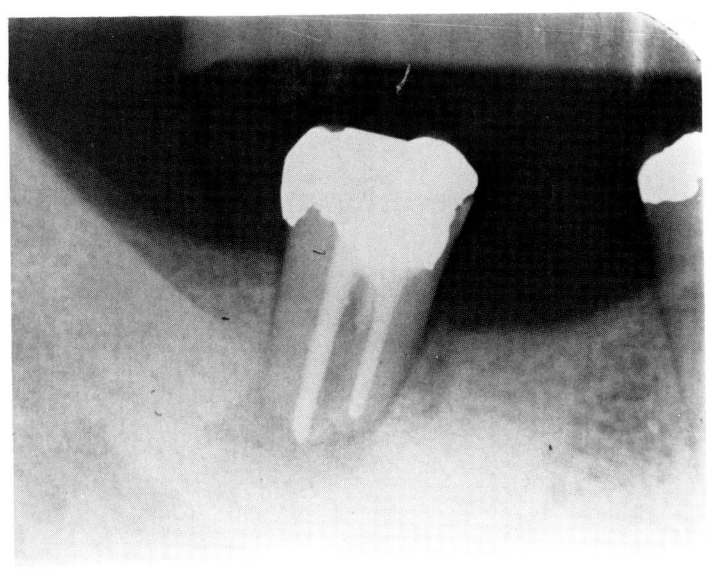

F

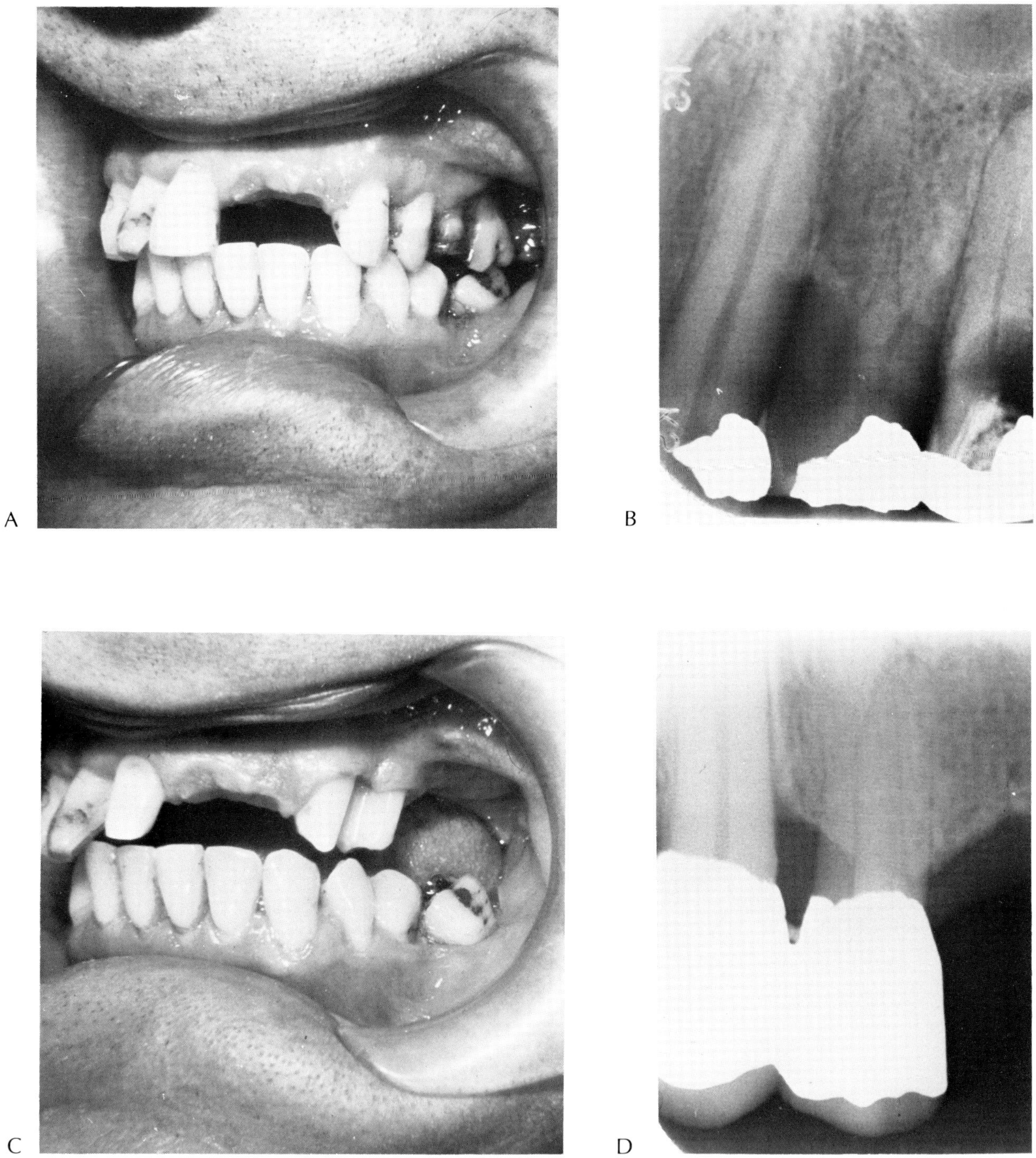

Fig. 7–5. Phasing by periodontal result.

A, 40-year-old man with generalized periodontitis. Consider tooth no. 12, with 6-mm pocket mesial interproximal, mesial root concavity leading to furcation. This tooth is potentially an abutment for both anterior bridge and posterior removable partial.

B, Radiograph of no. 12.

C, Periodontal surgery was performed and an interim acrylic bridge placed pending healing. Here bridge has been removed after 10 weeks to assess status of no. 12. Note the concavity of the mesial aspect of the preparation of no. 12 following the root configuration.

D, Radiograph of no. 12 following cementation of final fixed bridge 16 weeks after surgery. Note the good density of interproximal bone and the contouring that was done during surgery.

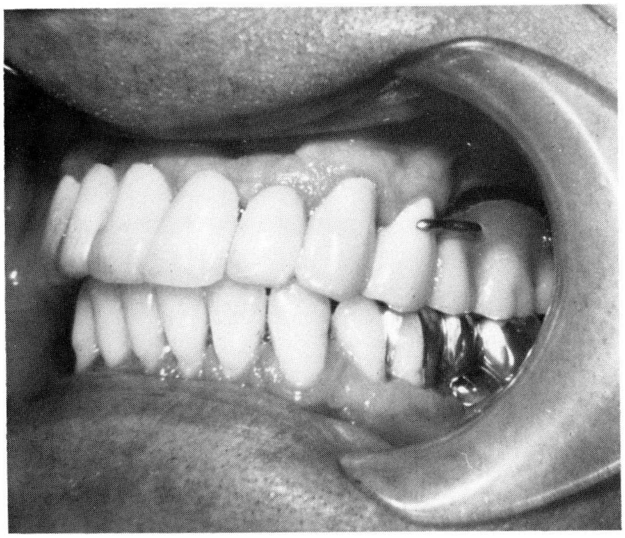

E

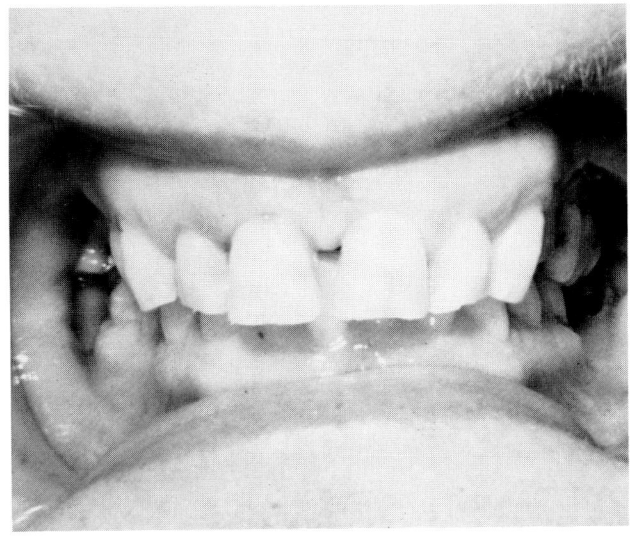

F

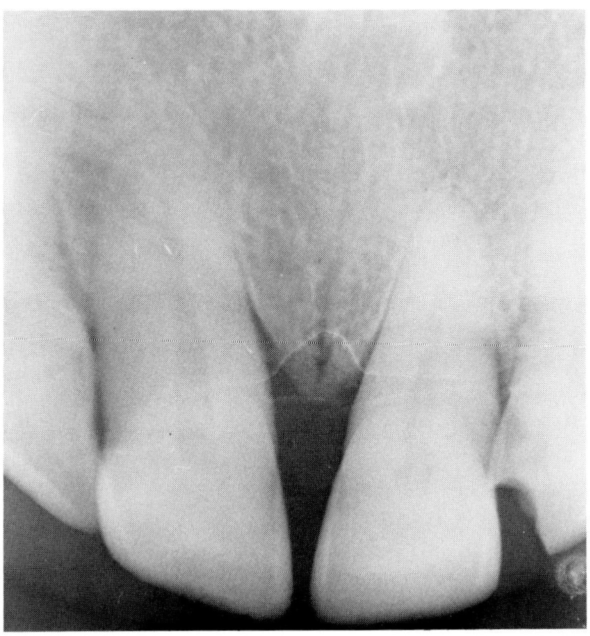

G

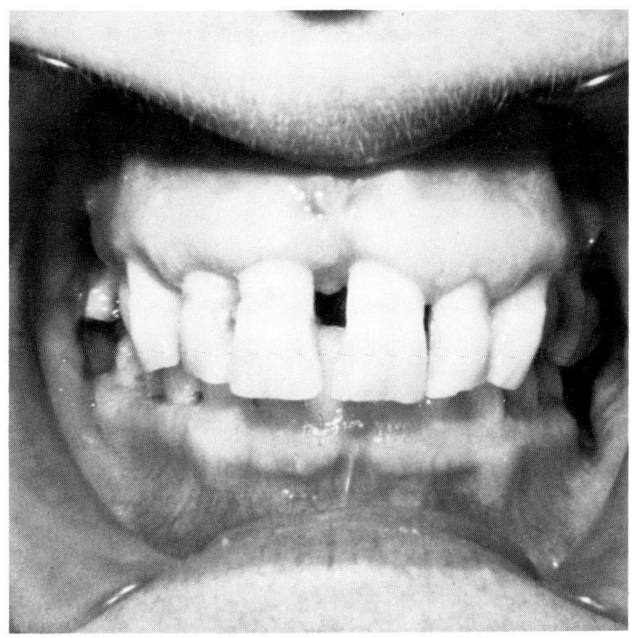

H

Fig. 7–5 *continued.* *E*, Having been established, the periodontal integrity remains excellent in this 5-year follow-up.

F, 48-year-old woman with generalized periodontitis. Consider the maxillary anterior segment. Mobility and pocket depths of 6 to 8 mm were present on all four incisors.

G, Radiograph of central incisors. Note funneling of the alveolar bone. Infrabony pockets were present, especially on lingual.

H, Following surgery, teeth were prepared to shorten the crowns and interim acrylic splints placed for a period of 6 months.

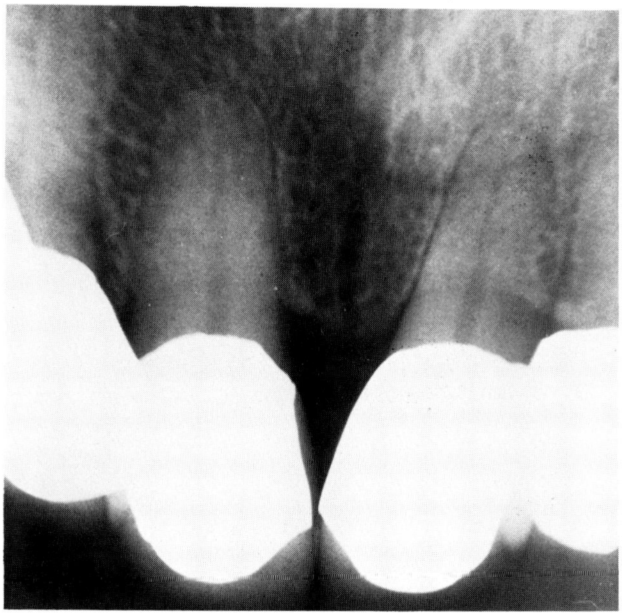

I

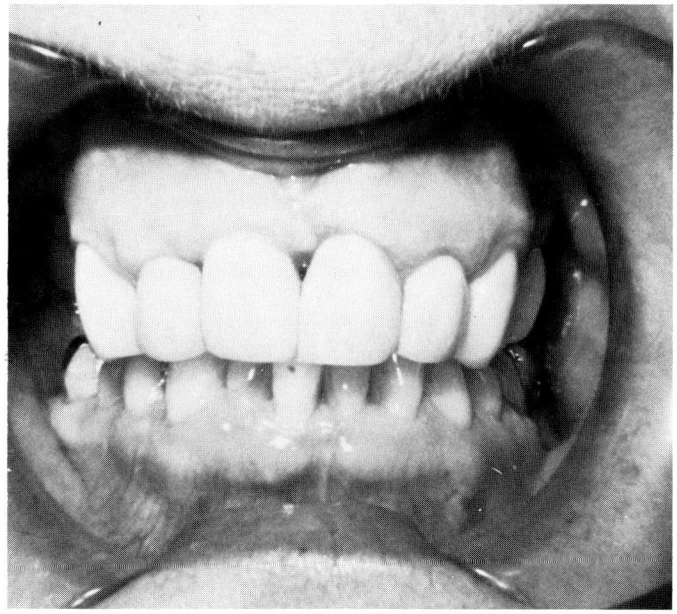

J

Fig. 7–5 *continued.* *I*, Final restorations were made after periodontal result had been determined. Note good density of the bone and improved crown/root ratio despite bone loss.
J, This 5-year follow-up reveals maturation of the tissue and continued periodontal stability.

affected the entire mouth, it is sometimes impossible to intelligently plan definitive treatment until the outcome of periodontal therapy is certain. Let me qualify this point by stating that hopelessly involved teeth can often be identified prior to surgery, and in many cases, should be removed or slated for removal at that time. This avoids the difficult situation of the general or restorative dentist having to tell the patient who has gone through periodontal surgery and has had pockets eliminated that many teeth must be extracted anyway because they are unrestorable or unusable due to inadequate bone support. Thus, phasing by the success or failure of periodontal surgery should involve only those teeth that are potential "keepers" if the periodontal integrity can be reestablished (Fig. 7–5).

Certain treatment planning approaches allow the utilization of questionable teeth in definitive restorations; these approaches will be discussed in Chapter 9.

4. *Orthodontic treatment.* Whether it is minor tooth movement, full-mouth orthodontics, or orthognathic surgery, definitive treatment must be phased according to the relative success or failure of the orthodontic treatment. Furthermore, a period of retention is generally required following tooth movement, and relapse during or after active retention is always a possibility (Fig. 7–6).

The essential concept in phasing by the success or failure of preceding steps is the recognition that, for any number of reasons, failures can and do occur. Unfortunately, such failures are not always immediately apparent and may not become apparent for months or even years. The more treatment steps predicated on a given treatment, the greater the need for caution and careful phasing. Consider two hypothetical situations that illustrate this point.

In the first situation, periodontal surgery has been performed on a second molar tooth in hopes of retaining it despite a distal bone defect and furcation involvement. The subsequent treatment is a Class II amalgam restoration. The restoration can be done almost immediately following the peridontal procedure, since so little time and money is invested. The second situation involves an endodontically treated first molar tooth that is to be reinforced with cast dowel and core and crowned as an abutment for a three-unit bridge. The three-unit bridge will be used as an abutment for a removable partial denture that will replace missing posterior teeth on the opposite side. The need for a phased approach that first assesses the apparent success of the endodontic treatment is obvious. The *number* and *complexity* of succeeding steps dictates the degree of caution required in phasing those steps. Failure of the preceding treatment becomes costly and painful for both patient and

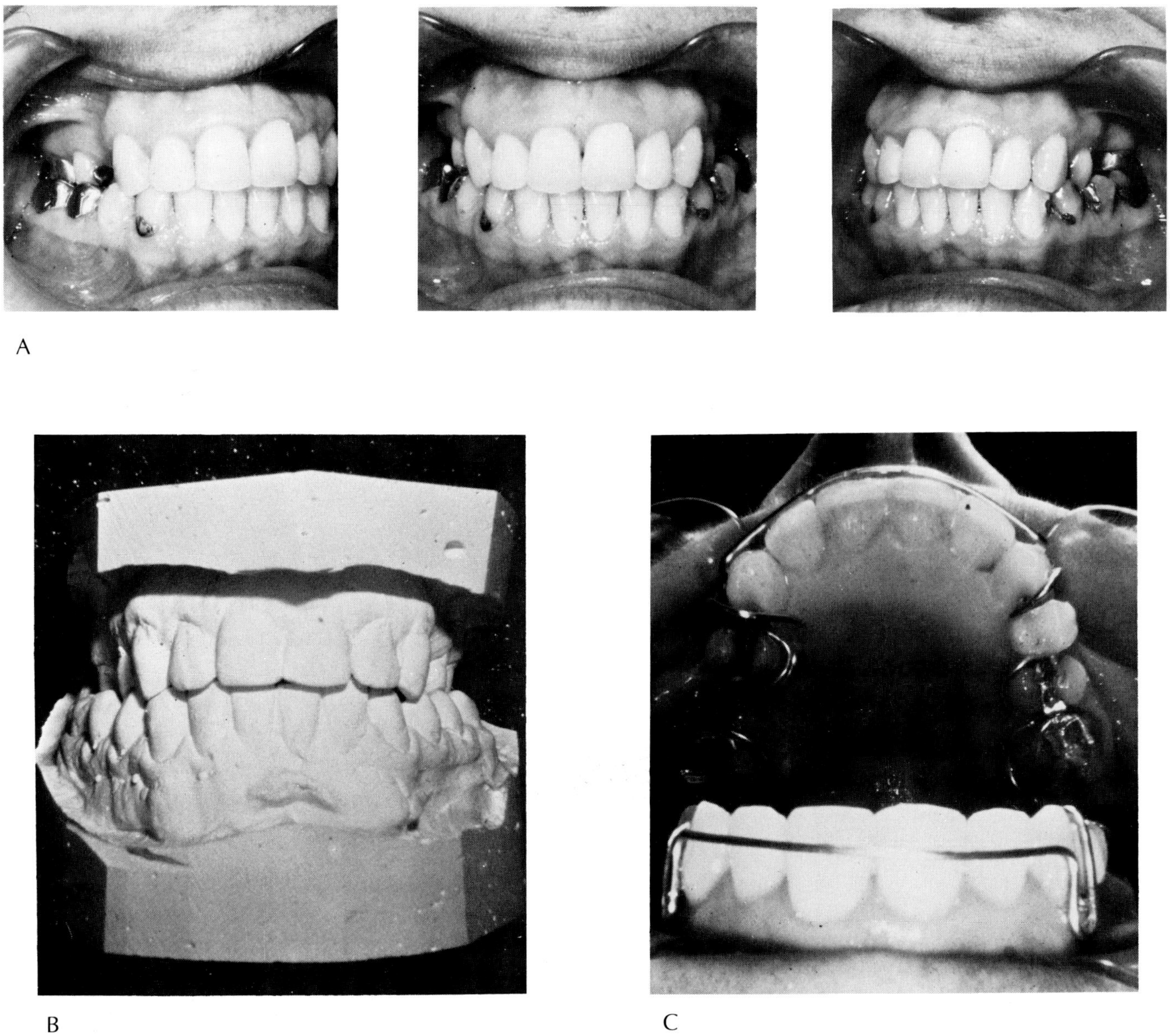

Fig. 7–6. Treatment pending orthodontic result.
A, 38-year-old woman with bilateral posterior crossbite and severe temporomandibular joint pain/dysfunction.
B, Diagnostic casts demonstrating constriction of upper posteriors.
C, Simple Hawley-type orthodontic appliance to expand maxillary posterior arch.

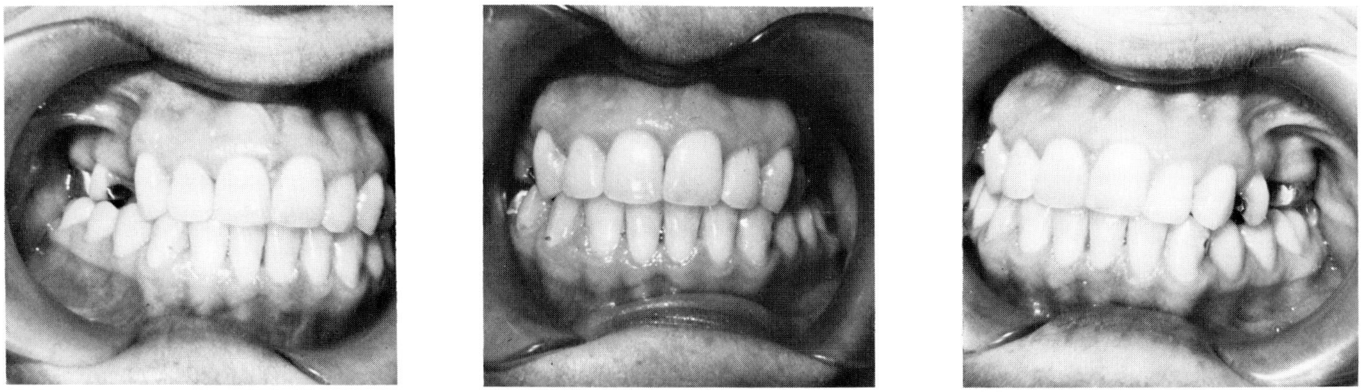

D

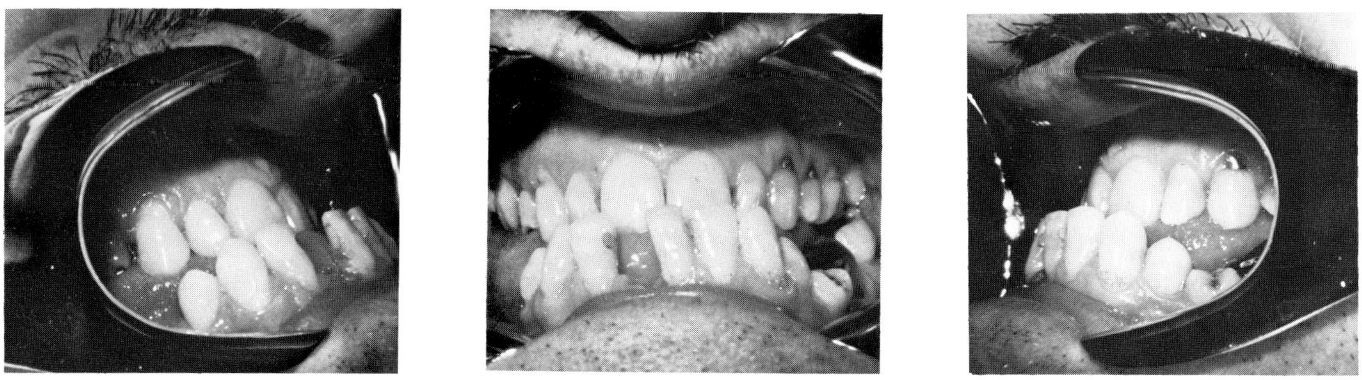

E

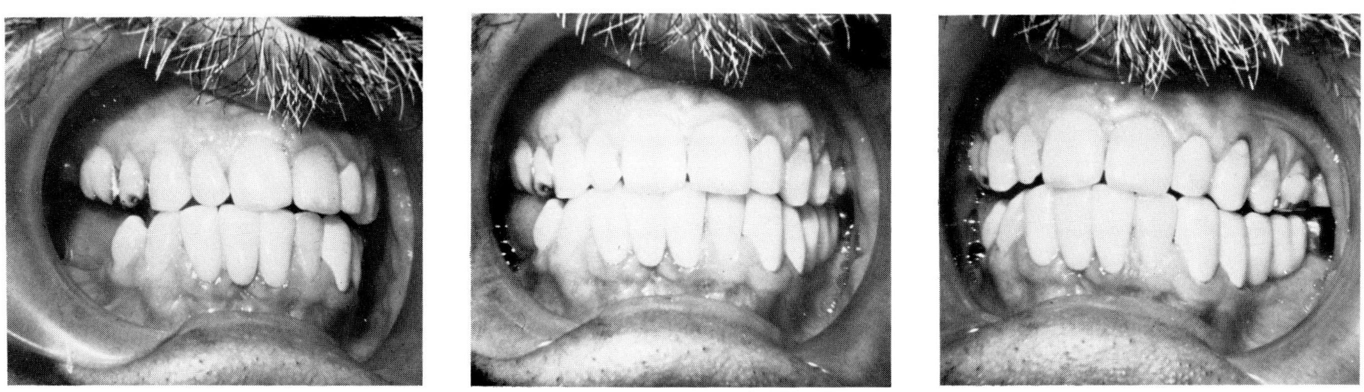

F

Fig. 7–6 *continued.* *D*, Appliance was used as retainer for 3 months, and lower crown restorations were placed in anticipation of upper bridges. Upper arch was observed closely for 3 more months without retention, and when no relapse was noted, fixed bridgework was begun.

E, 43-year-old man with severe Class III occlusion that produced functional disability due to lack of anterior and most posterior occlusion.

F, Orthognathic surgery repositioned the mandible, and intermaxillary fixation was utilized for 6 weeks. Crowns and fixed bridge restorations were placed with temporary cement, so that refinements could be made if needed. Final cementation was carried out after 6 months without detectable change in jaw relations.

dentist. Prudence in phasing further treatment enhances the overall prognosis and the confidence and peace of mind with which the dentist and his patient proceed through treatment.

There are situations in which it is impractical to wait months or years to assess the success or failure of preliminary treatment, and further definitive treatment must be carried out. In Chapter 9, a number of strategies will be discussed that permit such treatment to be carried out with contingency plans.

PHASING IN THIRD-PARTY RELATIONSHIPS

The advent of third-party involvement in dental care has had a tremendous impact on treatment and treatment planning. On the positive side, many patients, who either could not or did not do so prior to the third-party involvement, have availed themselves of dental treatment to the mutual benefit of patient and dentist. At the same time, this third-party involvement tends to complicate the dentist-patient relationship, because restrictions, limitations, and required paperwork take the place of what previously was a simple contract between dentist and patient. These complications can be dealt with in most third-party situations, and a sound and rational plan of treatment can be developed, but it may require more complex planning. Phasing of treatment as it relates to third-party involvement will be discussed in three general situations. In the first, the third party limits the type of treatment and the level of payments and prohibits the dentist from performing more comprehensive services and charging the patient for the difference. Welfare programs such as Title XIX and Veterans Administration programs are in this category. In these situations, treatment planning is difficult if the program will not allow or cover the course of treatment that is best for the patient. Phasing may mean carrying out preliminary procedures only, pending the patient's ability to proceed without the third-party assistance. It should be stressed that, in many cases, these types of programs can and do allow optimal courses of treatment and are highly beneficial to patient and dentist. However, if the financial limitations of a program dictate extremely limited treatment that constitutes irrational or poor dental care, the dentist is faced with a dilemma: to render the optimal treatment free of charge is impossible in most cases, yet to perform the "approved" treatment would constitute substandard care. While there is no solution to the problem, it should be discussed frankly with the patient. Together the dentist and patient must decide on a course of treatment that represents the best available option under the circumstances. In some cases, the dentist may decide not to accept the patient for treatment under the third-party restrictions, and this is his prerogative. Often, however, at least minimal disease control can be carried out within the restrictions of the third-party program, and it represents a first step in a phased treatment plan.

In a second situation, the third party, while limiting certain types of treatment and levels of payment, in no way prohibits more comprehensive approaches, with the patient paying the difference. Most dental insurance plans or prepayment plans operate on this basis. Benefits are provided according to the terms of the individual contract, but no restrictions are placed on the actual treatment chosen by the patient. Phasing in this type of third-party situation can be based on annual benefit limitations or on various waiting periods.

Annual benefit limitations are a common provision of many dental insurance plans. When a proposed course of treatment will significantly exceed the limitation, it may be feasible to perform the same treatment in phases, just as in the quality/time model. This allows the patient to gain maximal financial leverage from the plan (for which he is paying) while receiving optimal treatment. Indeed, it is sometimes possible to perform such treatment in multiyear segments over 3, 4, or even 5 years. If this is to be done effectively, two factors must be considered.

First of all, can the treatment be spread over time safely, without jeopardizing the result? Obviously, active disease cannot be ignored. Interim restorations may have to be placed in areas in which definitive treatment is being postponed. Anterior fixed bridgework prior to posterior removable prostheses may be subject to excessive stress and even breakage if posterior support is not established in a reasonable amount of time. Some form of treatment partial appliance might be employed in this situation, but it is often difficult. In our desire to assist the patient financially through maximal insurance benefits, we must take care not to compromise the results of the treatment.

A possible solution in some cases is to carry the treatment out in a time frame that encompasses the end of one policy year and the beginning of the next. Thus, within a 2-month course of treatment, 2 years of insurance benefits may be available. It is essential that dates of services rendered and fees charged be recorded and reported accurately and truthfully; to do otherwise can be construed as fraud and can place the dentist in a legally untenable position. Careful appointment scheduling is essential and requires equally careful treatment planning. The main drawback to this approach is that many plans are based on a calendar year, and combining 2 years' benefits means that a course of treatment will be carried out in December and January, which can be a very busy time of year because of holidays and vacations. If a large number of patients are involved with this strategy, it can become impractical.

Finally, some situations preclude this strategy altogether. A long-span fixed bridge, for example, may significantly exceed an annual allowance. The temptation to charge and submit a claim for the service as two separate procedures should be avoided, because it would be a fraudulent act. In rare cases, such a prosthesis could legitimately be made as two separate bridges, inserted with temporary cement in separate procedures before and after the benefit date of the policy, and splinted together if indicated at a later time. Such machinations can lead to many complications and should be avoided if possible. We must be sure to treat patients and their dental conditions, not their insurance contracts.

Secondly, is there sufficient stability in the dentist/patient/third-party arrangement to permit long-term planning? Complex insurance-related phasing presupposes that the present insurance plan will remain in effect, that the patient will remain employed so as to be eligible under the plan, and that the patient will not be transferred or elect to move during the course of treatment. If there is a good chance of any of these occurrences, long-term phasing may be contraindicated. At the very least, phasing treatment to accommodate third-party involvement and ensure maximal benefit must adhere to all general principles of rational treatment planning so that, should the extended course be disrupted, the patient will be stable and under good control. As long as this is the case, the balance of treatment can be performed at a later time or in another place with minor modifications.

Waiting periods associated with third-party plans can take various forms. The most common situation involves a patient in need of dental care who is not under a dental plan, but who will be coming under a plan at some future date. It is certainly reasonable to initiate disease-control procedures and postpone definitive treatment until the patient is covered. Likewise, most dental plans limit coverage on replacement of existing prostheses until they have been in the mouth for some period of time (often 5 years). Phasing treatment so as to postpone needed replacement until coverage is available is possible if the existing defective prosthesis can be patched, or otherwise made to serve in the meantime. While this is often possible, there are situations in which it is not—when the defect is too striking or the time too long to safely postpone replacement, for example. Finally, a number of dental plans are designed to provide increasing benefits over the period of years that the policy is in effect. If sound principles are followed, comprehensive treatment can often be postponed or phased over time to allow the patient to take advantage of the higher benefit. While treatment planning under these circumstances is often complex, challenging, and a bit frustrating, it can be beneficial to both patient and dentist. The principle of quality as a constant and time as the variable also applies when a third party is involved, and it can help produce excellent results in dental treatment.

When discussing treatment planning with third-party involvement, we must consider the alternative treatment approaches dictated by the third party. Many such contracts call for coverage of the "minimum acceptable" treatment approach in any given case. For example, in a treatment plan calling for two fixed bridges replacing missing teeth on either side of an arch, insurance coverage might be limited to allowance for a removable partial denture, since that is a less costly, "acceptable" alternative.

Similar conditions arise when a large amalgam-restoration fee might be allowed rather than a fee for a cast crown. Such alternate-treatment provisions create difficulties in two regards. First, it is difficult for the dentist to understand how a third-party administrator, even a dentist/consultant, can determine the feasibility of an alternate treatment approach without ever having seen the patient. Secondly, even though the third-party insists that they are not dictating what treatment course the dentist and patient must pursue, the differential in level of benefit between an optimal course of treatment and the alternate plan proposed by the third party can dissuade or prevent the patient from pursuing the former, even when the latter is not a reasonable approach in his situation.

A possible solution to the problem lies in the dentist/patient relationship and communication with the third party. If the dentist and patient have developed a reasonable treatment approach based on established goals, then the level of third-party benefits should be less critical. Indeed, if the only reason for pursuing treatment is that third-party coverage is available, and if the type and extent of treatment is to be based solely on the limits of that coverage, we are then treating an insurance plan, not a patient. There are times when extensive and costly treatment is not indicated, even though generous benefits are available through a third-party arrangement. Here again, the dentist must avoid the temptation to treat the insurance plan, and instead, concentrate on what is best for the patient.

Many difficulties with third-party involvement in treatment planning can be overcome simply by good communication. Many, if not most, third-party plans require predetermination of benefit level prior to extensive treatment, and such predetermination is valuable whether it is required or not. In submitting a course of treatment and estimated fees for determination of benefit, the dentist should include some of his reasons for selecting that course and indicate significant clinical findings that require, for example, a cast restoration instead of an amalgam. Given this information, it is often possible for the third-party administrator or dental consultant to allow maximal benefits under the contract. Seen as a cooperative venture, third-party involvement in dental treatment planning can be fairly painless and benefit all concerned. If the third party is viewed as an adversary and treated as one, frustration may be the ultimate result.

The third situation involves capitation or HMO, in which the provider, in effect, determines the benefit. Ethically and legally, this type of third-party involvement demands much of the dentist. Needless to say, the immediate performance of all maximal, definitive treatment for every patient within the plan is uncalled for. Not only would such an approach be economically difficult for the provider, it would be impractical from a standpoint of good patient care as it is discussed throughout this text. However, postponing definitive procedures indefinitely or simply not discussing the available options with the patient may constitute professional negligence on the part of the dentist.

In such arrangements, it is extremely beneficial to develop with the patient a written phased treatment plan that is based on any or all of the approaches discussed previously or on any other good rationale. This written plan and the criteria upon which it is based become part of the patient record. It serves to protect the dentist, in justifying what treatment had been done and at what pace, and the patient, in ensuring that his treatment will be based on sound dental principles and serve his specific needs. It also facilitates the peer-review process necessary in this type of third-party system, since both the projected course of treatment and the criteria for its progress through the various phases are immediately apparent.

PLANNING PHASED TREATMENT

Phasing dental treatment can be an effective approach to optimal patient care, but it requires more of the patient and dentist than an immediate-treatment approach. I will discuss some of the requirements that must be considered when phasing dental treatment.

First of all, complex treatment plans that are phased over long periods of time are not easily developed and demand greater *care, skill, and judgment* than simple, immediate plans. Care must be taken to ensure that postponement of a given treatment will not create greater problems. Judgment is required in making some predictive diagnoses—that is, in foreseeing possible developments in the clinical picture and preparing alternative treatment approaches to meet those developments.

Phased treatment planning definitely requires a greater commitment of *time and effort* on the part of the dentist and is often financially unrewarding and not fully appreciated by the patient. The intellectual challenge can be stimulating, however, and the opportunity to seek out other ideas from dentists in complex situations is always educational.

A phased approach to dental treatment (whatever the criteria) also requires patient involvement in treatment planning and *patient commitment* to the plan and his dental-health goals. Phasing is often ineffective without this commitment, because the patient may lose interest and not return, or lapse in his personal, oral-health efforts, which will compromise the overall treatment.

Because the human body and the mouth are dynamic environments, *continual reassessment* is necessary in a phased approach. Factors to be considered include the following:

1. Changes (for better or worse) in the oral clinical picture, in the patient's general systemic condition, or in the patient's lifestyle, job, marriage, outlook on life, or attitude toward dental health.
2. Changes in costs of rendering care and, subsequently, changes in treatment fees; introduction of third-party involvement subsequent to the original treatment plan and phasing.
3. Advances in available techniques and/or materials that might allow or dictate different approaches from an original long-term plan. Examples of such advances include wider use of orthognathic surgery, bonded-resin techniques of various kinds, and application of implants and/or transplants.

Alterations made in the phased treatment plan should be recorded and if necessary, the plan redrawn to address the conditions observed in the periodic reassessment of the patient.

REFERENCES

1. Barkley, R.F.: Must third party dentistry be mediocre? J. South. Cal. Dent. Assoc., *41*:307–310, 1973.
2. Clark, J.W., et al.: Clinical Dentistry. Hagerstown, Harper and Row, 1979.

CHAPTER **8**

Management of Complex Cases

When you're up to your armpits in alligators, it is often difficult to remember that your original intention . . . was to drain the swamp.

ANONYMOUS

Dental treatment situations can be loosely grouped in one of two categories—simple or complex. A simple treatment situation is one in which the sequence and content are fairly obvious, and in which steps in the treatment can be carried out one at a time, if necessary. Such a situation might be one in which a teenager presents with a generally normal, healthy mouth but needs minimal operative dentistry, evaluation, and possible removal of third molars. The course of treatment suggests itself, and it is neither complex nor extensive. Treatment situations can be extensive, however, while remaining simple. An otherwise normal, healthy young adult who presents with missing first permanent molars in three quadrants resulting from severe caries early in life, with little or no tipping of second molars and good CO-CR relationship, can require extensive treatment (9 to 10 units of fixed bridgework involving much of the posterior occlusion), but the procedures themselves are uncomplicated and can be carried out one at a time if desired (Fig. 8–1).

Complex treatment situations, on the other hand, involve multiple problems that require more complicated treatment, which must often be performed either concurrently or in some strict sequence. Patients presenting with moderate-to-severe periodontal disease, multiple missing teeth, misaligned teeth, large CO-CR discrepancies, lost vertical dimension, similar problems, or combinations of these problems require careful handling. Treatment planning becomes complicated, and the treatment regimen itself requires skill, finesse, and careful timing. In general, complex situations do not allow the treatment steps to be carried out separately and independently. Thus, the greater number of problems seen in diagnosis and their dependence on one another in treatment greatly increase the chances of failure in complex situations.

We can illustrate using examples similar to those cited above. If our teenager presents with minor caries and third molars, as well as TMJ symptoms, facial pain, heavy balancing-side contacts in lateral excursions due to an anterior open bite, and resultant lack of guidance on the working side, the situation becomes more complex. If we add to the picture an enamel dysplasia affecting the cusps of the first permanent molars requiring castings for occlusal coverage, we muddy the waters still further. Using the example of the young adult missing three first permanent molars, we could envision a resultant collapse of the dental arches, with severe tipping of second molars, flaring of anteriors, and apparent loss of vertical dimension. The situation is no longer simple; the required treatment involves multiple steps, some quite challenging technically, demanding precise sequencing and timely execution. Two examples serve to illustrate this difference.

In the first example (Fig. 8–2 A), we can foresee the fabrication of a simple, three-unit posterior bridge that will replace the missing first permanent molar—a simple treatment situation. In the second example (Fig. 8–2 B), the second molar is supererupted, tipped, has had extensive caries, and has incipient buccal furcation involvement. Utilizing the tooth in its present state presents a challenge in bridge design and fabrication to obtain parallelism and a good curve of occlusion, in pulpal management owing to previous deep restoration, in periodontal maintenance due to furcal involvement and the likely placement of the crown margin into it. On the other hand, alleviation of these problems might well require a number of

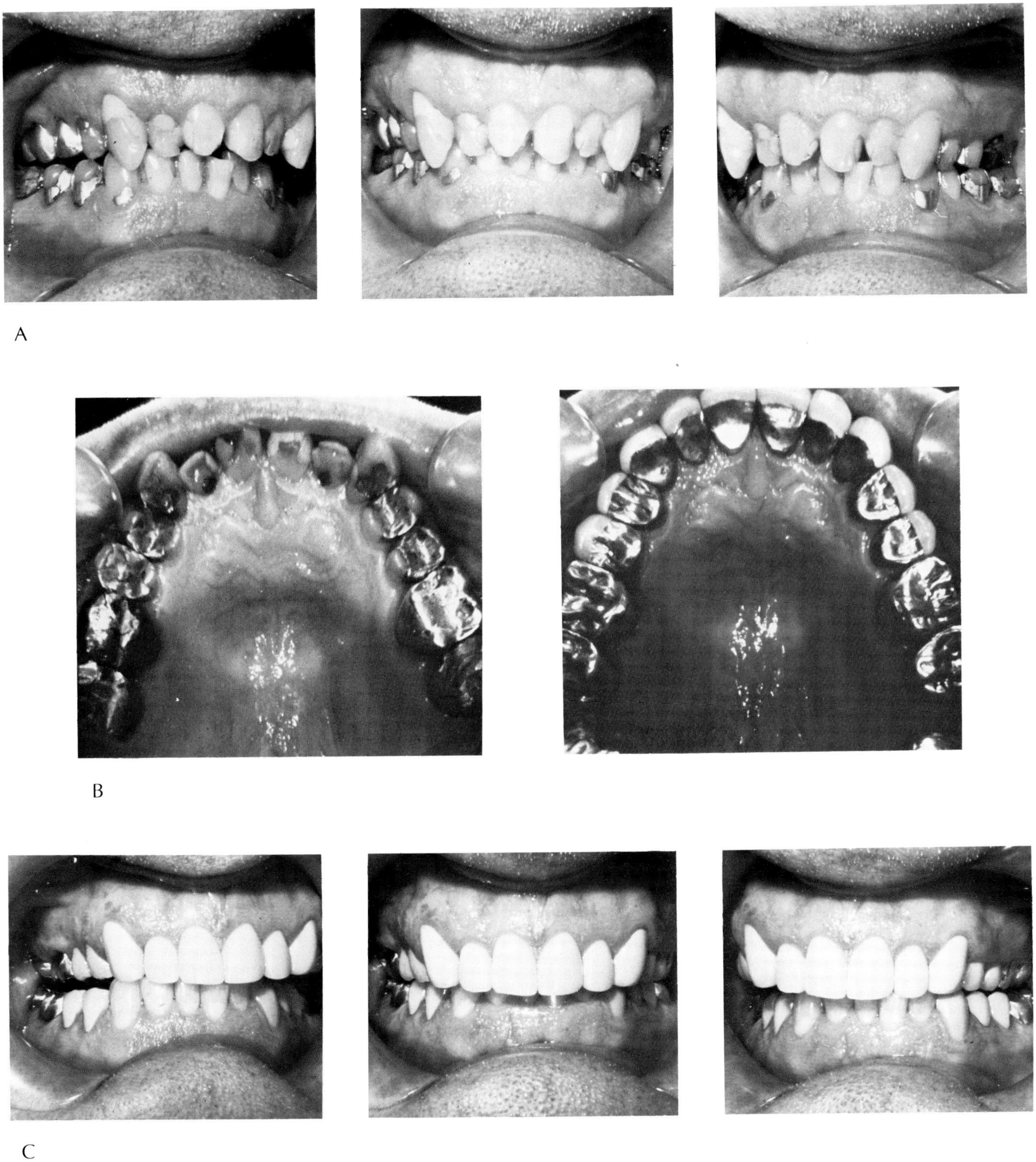

Fig. 8–1. This 66-year-old attorney had experienced gradual dental deterioration for 30 years and, except for one poorly-made cast crown, had been "patched" rather than restored. *A*, Despite the mechanical breakdown, the periodontium was sound, centric occlusion coincided well with centric relation, and anterior disocclusion was available. *B*, Left photo depicts maxillary arch (mirror view) prior to treatment. Right photo shows the rebuilt occlusion. *C*, The crown reconstruction involved 23 units, the other five teeth being restored with acid-etch bonded composite resins. Although extensive, the treatment was simple. It was carried out in three segments, but it could also have been done by quadrant, or even one tooth at a time.

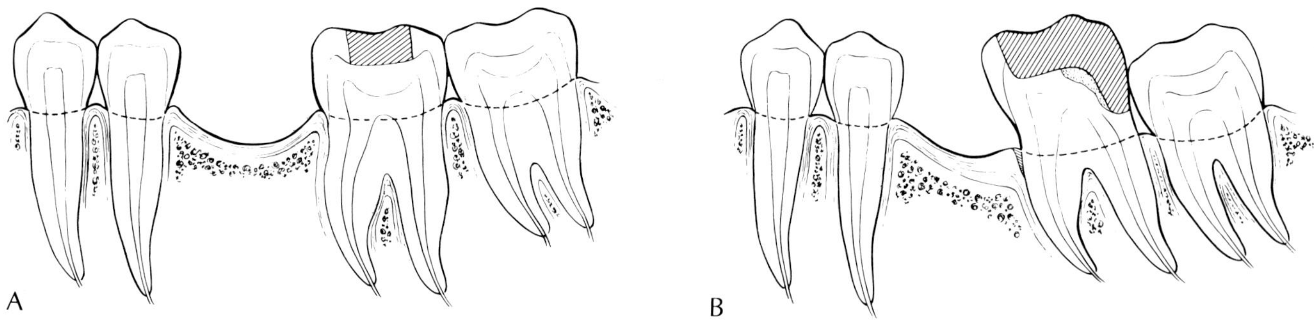

Fig. 8–2 *A*, Simple fixed bridge situation. *B*, Same teeth involved, but situation more complex.

treatment steps, such as endodontic therapy, periodontal correction, and fabrication of a dowel and core. While this approach would assist in bridge fabrication (in terms of parallelism and curve of occlusion), obviate the pulpal question, and allow effective periodontal maintenance, we now have a number of interdependent steps, each with some difficulty, each with some potential for failure that would result in failure of the entire effort. Furthermore, the cost in time and money is significantly greater and adds a further risk factor.

These two examples illustrate clearly the difference between simple and complex treatment situations. The balance of this chapter will consider approaches to complex situations and offer strategies for the simplification of such situations.

APPROACHES TO COMPLEX CASE PLANNING

We must assume that the dentist, in approaching the complex case, recognizes it as such. While many patients present with clinical pictures that are rather awe inspiring in their severity and complexity, others may have problems that are just as complex, but more subtle in appearance (Fig. 8–3). Thorough examination and careful diagnosis are essential, especially when dealing with complex situations.

Key-Tooth Concept

In the midst of complex dental problems, it is helpful, and in many cases, essential to identify those teeth that might be utilized effectively in a course of treatment. We term these "key" teeth, and a key tooth must possess, or be capable of attaining, two attributes: stability and favorable arch position. Such teeth can be depended upon to stand by themselves and provide good function over time, to serve, if necessary, as abutment teeth for fixed or removable prostheses, or to strengthen or reinforce other teeth in splinting procedures. The "model" key teeth are normal healthy canines and first molars, which most often fulfill the criteria of stability and arch position. Indeed, it is sometimes possible to restore and rebuild an entire dental arch using four key teeth—the canines and first molars.

Identifying Key Teeth

In a normal, healthy full complement of teeth, many other teeth might be considered key teeth, but it must be remembered that while some teeth function well by themselves, they may not be dependable for extended purposes. Consider a lower first premolar, canine, and lateral incisor grouping, for example. Should the canine be lost through trauma, the premolar and lateral incisor, while perfectly sound by themselves, may not be well suited as abutments to replace the lost canine, and hence, may not be key teeth. In severely diseased or debilitated mouths, the identification of potential key teeth helps to simplify the clinical picture and provides the clinician with direction as to possible treatment strategies.

We can postulate that the more key teeth present in the mouth, the better the outlook for successful treatment. If the key teeth are well distributed, the treatment possibilities are limitless. In the event of loss or debilitation of the usual key teeth, we can identify others based on stability and favorable arch position.

Stability. A key tooth must have sufficient root surface in healthy bone to act as an abutment tooth, or at the least, to ensure its own retention over time. Factors influencing this include root morphology and the level of the alveolar bone in relation to the tooth length.

Root morphology includes length, diameter, and configuration of the root—that is, the shape and number of roots. Root length obviously influences the total surface in bone and is especially critical when

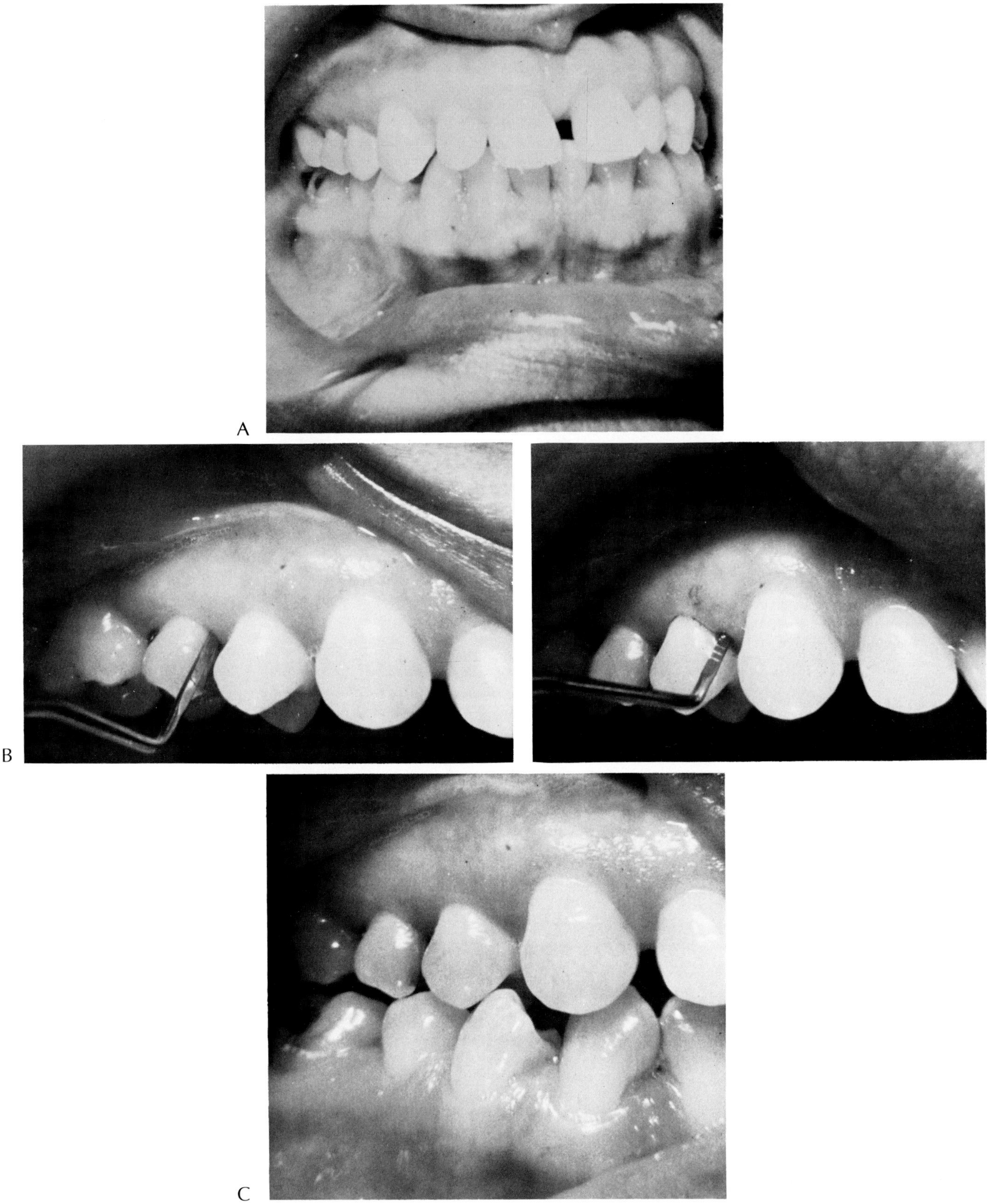

Fig. 8–3. Complex treatment situation, subtle in appearance.

A, This 39–year-old woman complained of pain in the right premolar region. There were no findings of dental origin (caries, periapical involvement), and the general periodontal picture was excellent. Note, however, the space apparent between upper and lower right canine teeth and keep it in mind.

B, A closer look at the radiographs suggested a periodontal source of the pain, and probing of first and second premolars left no question about the diagnosis. Probing the rest of the mouth, however, revealed no pocket depths over 3 mm, and further investigation of this severe localized problem is essential.

C, In lateral excursion, contacts were solely on first and second premolars; canine teeth did not contact in the functional range, despite normal alignment and good vertical overlap. The lack of canine function was contributing directly to the problem on the premolars.

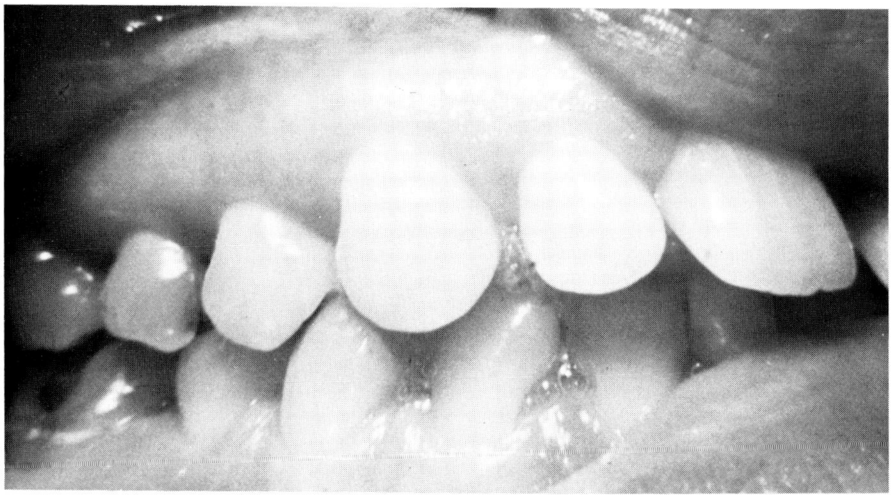

D

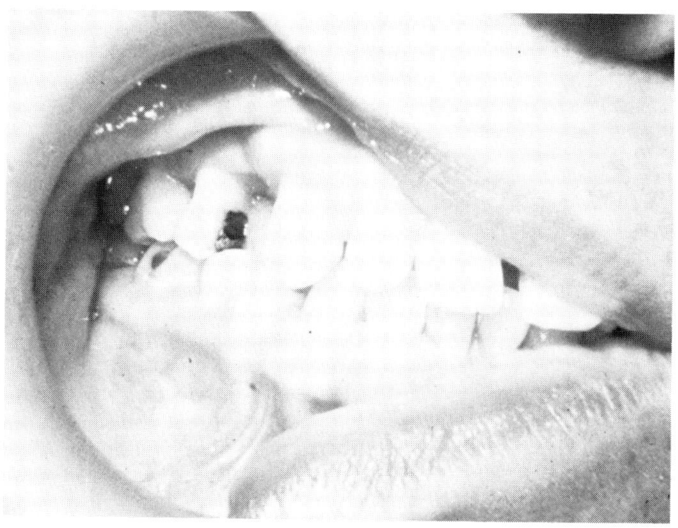

E

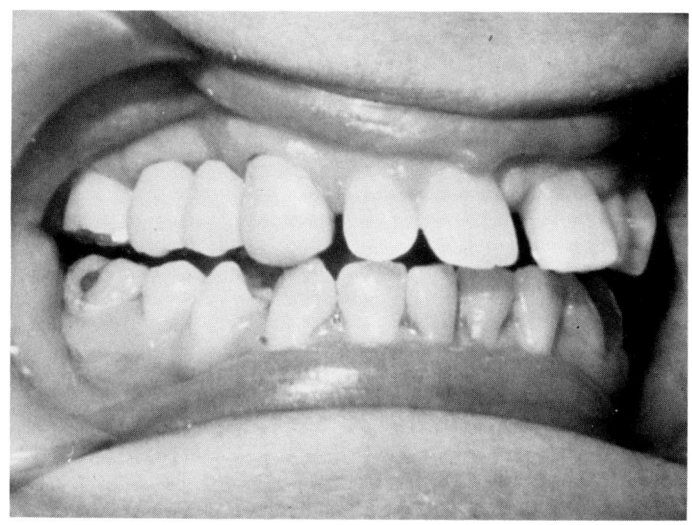

F

Fig. 8–3 *continued.* *D*, Carrying the investigation further, we observe the tongue during a swallow. Consistently interposing between upper and lower anterior teeth, the canines are maintained in open bite, unable to erupt into normal contact.

E, Extraction of first premolar after exploratory periodontal surgery (in which apically repositioned flap and osseous recontouring was performed on the second premolar) eliminated the immediate problem.

F, The restoration, however, was designed with the other etiologic factors in mind and included building the canine into centric contact and lateral function, and double abutting the weakened second premolar with the first molar. Careful observation of the completed bridge over time was done to determine whether tongue pressure might move the entire prosthesis, in which case myofunctional therapy would be required. This photograph was taken 3 years post treatment, and the situation was stable at that time.

lateral forces are likely to be encountered, usually in the anterior region. General bulk (diameter) of the root is often more important than length in assessing key teeth, because the surface area in bone is greatly increased. In terms of configuration, cylindrical roots are preferable to conical roots from a mechanical standpoint; indeed, dilacerated and clubbed roots may greatly enhance stability, provided that endodontic therapy is not likely. Multiple roots are obviously more stable than single roots as long as furcations are well below the bone crest.

Bone level is determined by two factors: loss due to periodontal disease and/or supereruption of the tooth. The ratio of tooth length out of bone to root length in bone has been referred to as crown/root ratio, which should be as small as possible and no greater than 1:1.

Given these general factors, we assess the stability of potential key teeth in relation to certain teeth that are generally considered keystones of the dental arches—the canine teeth and the first permanent molars. Indeed, provided that the crown/root ratio is favorable, these teeth can generally be considered key teeth in any treatment plan. In their absence, however, other teeth may be utilized provided that their root morphology and crown/root ratio compare favorably. This comparison is best made within the mouth in question, because tooth size varies from individual to individual. In addition, a key tooth must have a healthy pulp or be amenable to endodontic therapy if it is to be considered a stable tooth.

Favorable Arch Position. The location and orientation of the tooth are important, since stability alone does not allow effective utilization. The most stable tooth we have seen was a full bony impacted upper canine, with a large root, infinite crown/root ratio, and healthy pulp, but it was of no clinical use whatsoever. Stable teeth that are located outside the range of functional occlusion or that are severely tipped or supererupted are not key teeth. Generally, key teeth should be located somewhere along the normal dental arch from second molar to second molar and be aligned relatively parallel to the forces of occlusion.

Distribution—the number of key teeth present and their relationship to each other—is also an important factor. For example, in a lower arch with only two retained key teeth, the restorative options depend entirely on locations. If the teeth are a lower right second premolar and a first molar, their value is severely limited by lack of anterior and contralateral support. If the two teeth are a lower right second premolar and a lower left first premolar, there is at least bilateral support, and an overdenture is a possibility. If the two teeth are lower right and left canines, the range of options widens greatly, and one may consider overdenture, overdenture built on a bar splint, crowns and a bar splint with partial denture, or anterior bridge canine-canine with partial denture.

Creating Key Teeth

In defining key teeth, it was stipulated that such teeth must possess, or be capable of attaining, two attributes: stability and favorable arch position. It is helpful, and often critical to the treatment plan, to convert questionable teeth into key teeth; this can be accomplished in a number of ways.

Attaining Stability. Methods of restoring or increasing stability include the following:

1. *Endodontic implants.* Metal dowels that obturate the root canal and that are driven well beyond the apex into bone may enhance stability, especially toward lateral stresses.
2. *Periodontal therapy.* Procedures that regain bone support, such as the successful fill of osseous defects or autogenous bone grafts of various types, may greatly enhance the stability of otherwise questionable teeth.
3. *Shortening the crown.* While often necessitating endodontic therapy, reducing the tooth length out of bone improves (reduces) crown/root ratio and thereby enhances stability. The most extreme application of this principle is the overdenture tooth, which is reduced nearly flush with the gingiva or in some techniques, buried entirely beneath the ridge tissues. Shortening is often employed after periodontal therapy, when it can provide esthetic improvement as well as greater stability.
4. *Splinting.* Splinting of two adjacent teeth with crowns cast or soldered together creates, in effect, a multirooted tooth, which may be far more stable than either of the individual teeth. A good example of this method is the use of weakened lower first and second premolars as distal extension partial denture abutments. Neither tooth would serve by itself, but splinted together they create the effect of a molar root system with markedly enhanced stability.

Attaining Favorable Arch Position. Arch-position problems can often be resolved through minor orthodontic procedures. Indeed, if drastic repositioning is required, root length and periodontal stability may be jeopardized. The role of tooth movement in complex cases will be discussed at greater length later in this chapter.

It is technically possible to improve distribution of key teeth by autogenous transplantation—that is, by surgically removing and reimplanting teeth in new locations. Following these procedures, however, such teeth must be considered questionable, due to the possibility of external resorption and other imponderable problems. Therefore, while such procedures may have application in many cases, use of transplanted teeth as key teeth is generally contraindicated.

A similar caution must be applied to the use of implants. While a variety of methods and materials have been used in dental implantology over the last decade, long-term success rates are poor.[20] Bacterial invasion at the "cuff" area, where the implant emerges from the tissue, is the usual cause of loss. If the original tooth loss was periodontally induced, the risk for implants is even higher. When an implant is employed, it cannot be considered a key tooth, and the treatment plan should allow for an alternative approach should the implant fail (see Chap. 9).

The key-tooth concept provides the dentist with a tool in approaching the complex treatment situation in order to identify those teeth that can be effectively utilized in comprehensive treatment. The application of the key-tooth concept requires a systematic approach, which can be referred to as a tooth "inventory."

Tooth Inventory

The tooth inventory is, as the name implies, a counting and evaluation of all teeth present. It is generally carried out in complex cases following the clinical examination and patient interview, with the aid of full-mouth radiographs and in most cases, study models. The dentist must have ascertained that centric relation and centric occlusion coincide, or the study casts should be mounted on a semiadjustable articulator with an arbitrary hinge-axis transfer. More sophisticated fully adjustable instrumentation, hinge-axis location, and excursive records may be helpful in some cases, but are usually not essential.

The primary purpose of the inventory is to locate and identify key teeth; it may also identify teeth that are sound and retainable by themselves, and to identify those teeth that might be eliminated altogether due to their instability, unfavorable arch position, or questionable prognosis in relation to other key teeth. It is useful in the inventory process to assign appropriate symbols to the teeth evaluated, so that upon completion of the inventory, a clear picture emerges. The following symbols will be used in the example cases:

- \+ indicates a key tooth that is stable and in favorable arch position.
- (+) indicates a potential key tooth, which would require some alteration of position or enhancement of stability.
- 0 indicates a sound, retainable tooth, which, while capable of standing by itself, is not necessarily key-tooth material.
- (0) indicates the same type of tooth as above, but one that is in need of some treatment or modification.
- – indicates a tooth that is to be eliminated from the treatment plan.

The factors to be considered in eliminating certain teeth will be discussed in greater detail, but first, examples of the use of the tooth inventory in approaching complex cases will be presented (Fig. 8–4, Cases 1 and 2).

The tooth inventory provides a routine systematic approach to planning complex cases. It enables us to perform, in our mind's eye, multiple dental procedures without actually touching the patient; for example, we can identify key teeth, develop potential key teeth, and eliminate extraneous teeth. The inventory may reveal strikingly simple treatment approaches, or it may confirm the difficulty and complexity of a case. It may also serve as a blueprint for a full diagnostic wax-up, in which teeth are eliminated, moved, and rebuilt in wax on mounted study casts. The diagnostic wax-up itself can reveal much information, but it cannot be done without some definite plan in mind; the inventory serves to suggest that plan.

A number of treatment strategies have been referred to in these case illustrations. These strategies, when applied in the key-tooth concept, result in simplification of the clinical situation, which results in less treatment or simpler treatment in the definitive phase. Some of these strategies are discussed below.

SIMPLIFICATION OF DENTAL TREATMENT

The greater the number, complexity, and interdependence of dental procedures done for a single patient, the greater the chance of failure, and the more catastrophic that failure is likely to be. If we can simplify the clinical situation prior to the definitive restorative phase of treatment, we enhance the prognosis greatly. Three major strategies in the simplification of dental treatment are extraction of teeth, nonreplacement of missing teeth, and movement of teeth, which I will discuss in turn.

Strategic Extraction

Extraction may be to dentistry what amputation is to general medicine. Treatment by gross removal of the affected part is generally not considered advanced. As a result, the conscientious dentist is always thinking about how to save this tooth or that

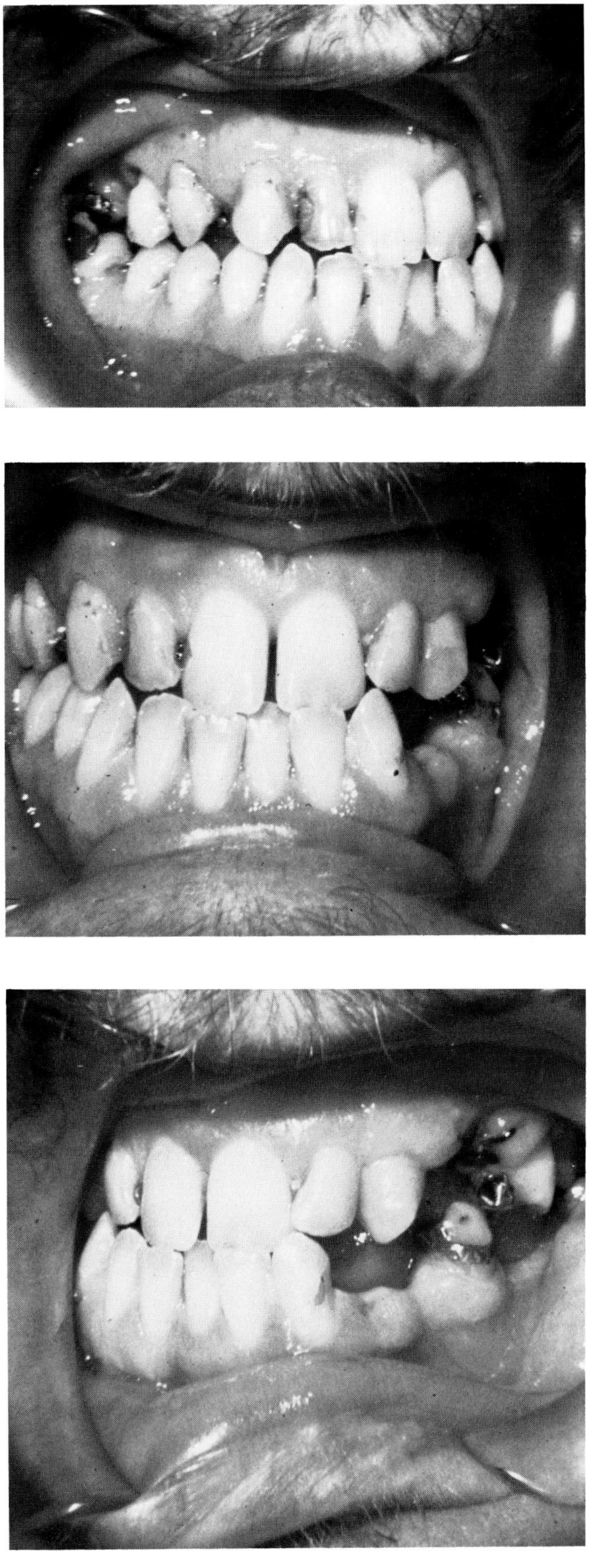

A

Fig. 8–4. Tooth Inventory: Case 1.

A, This 38–year-old male engineer realized that his dentition was in dreadful condition and expressed a desire to keep his teeth and get them into good condition again. Periodontal support was good, although marginal gingivitis was present; tooth no. 12 (already extracted on these photos) had no attached gingiva and nearly half its buccal root was exposed and carious. Centric occlusion (Class III) coincided with centric relation, and anterior teeth were locked in alternating crossbite.

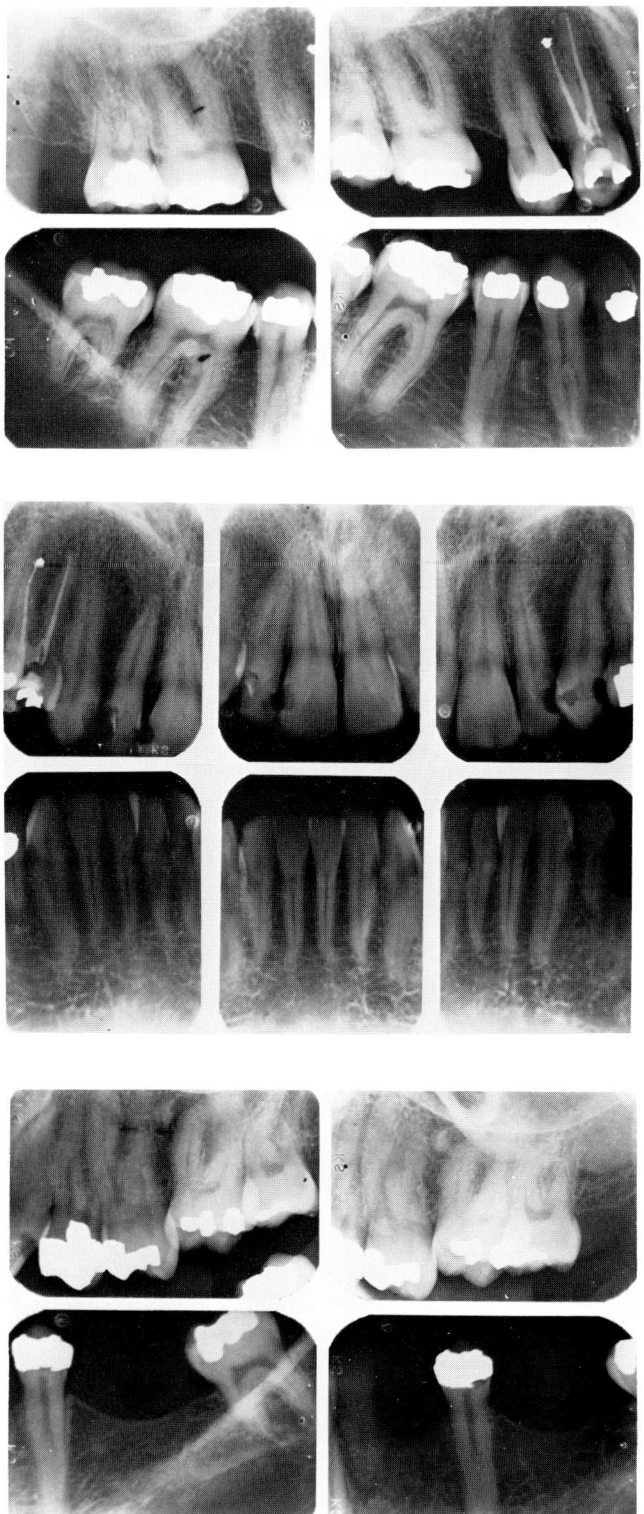

B

Fig. 8–4 *continued.* *B*, Full-mouth radiographs illustrate the good bone support, but note the extensive breakdown, restoration, and loss of teeth that have led to tipping and drifting of posteriors.

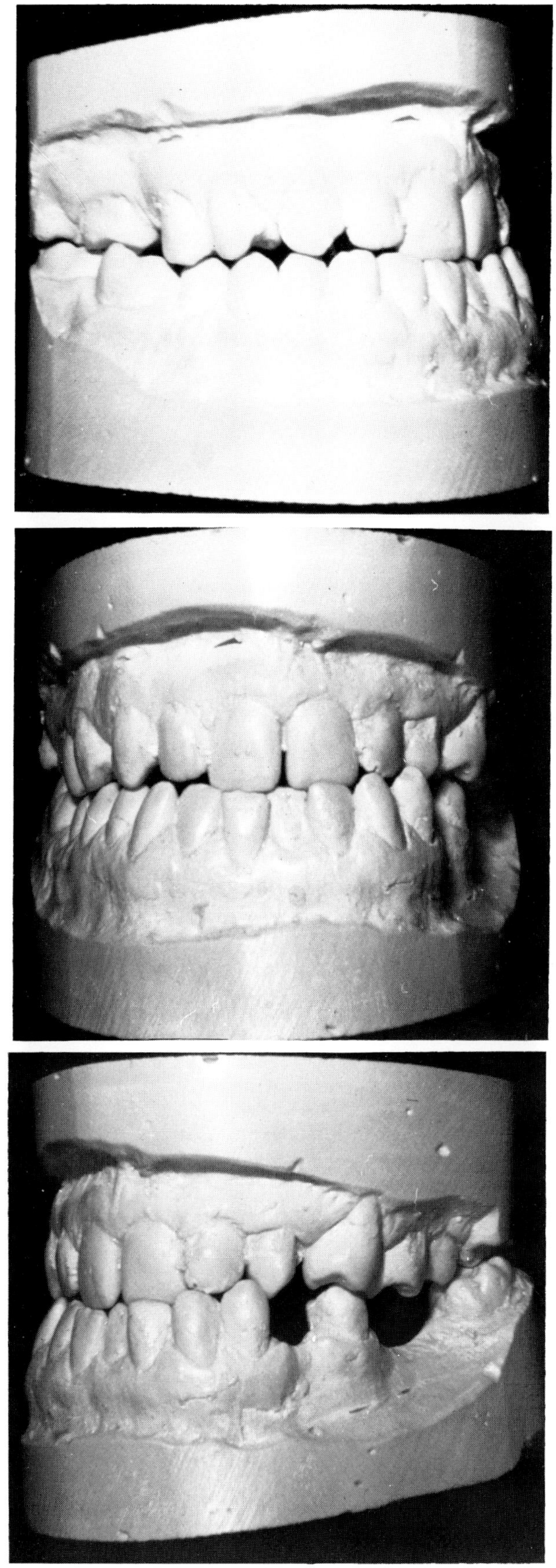

C

Fig. 8–4 *continued.* *C*, Diagnostic casts further illustrate the malposition of posteriors and difficult anterior relationship.

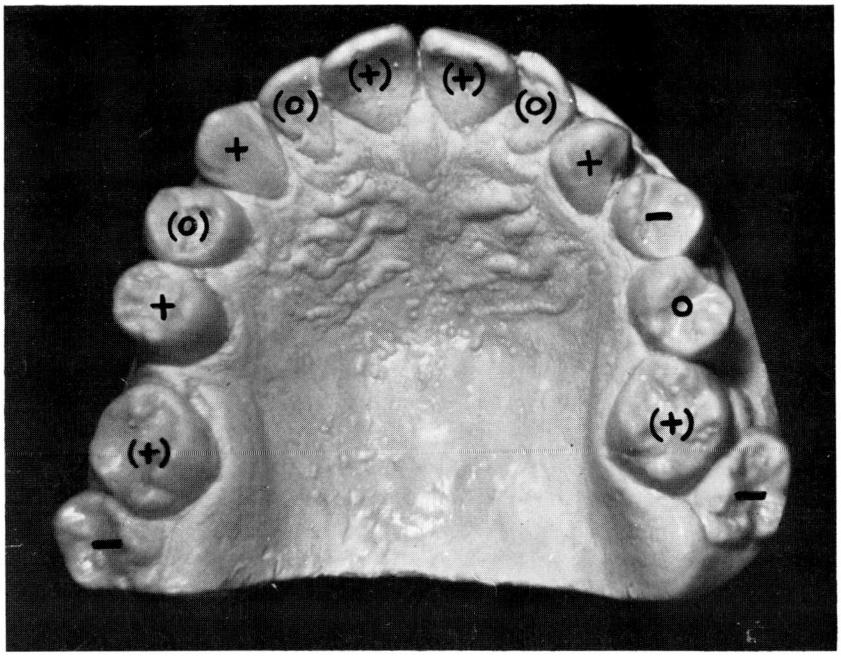

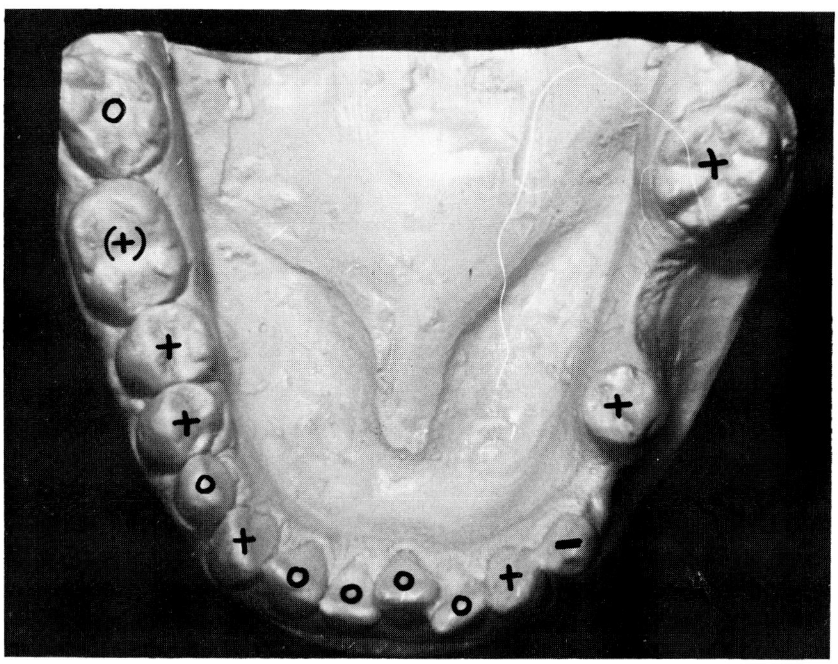

D

Fig. 8–4 *continued.* *D,* A tooth inventory is done from clinical, x-ray, and diagnostic cast information, beginning with tooth no. 1 and proceeding throughout. Teeth are tentatively judged as key teeth, marked "+"; potential key teeth, marked "(+)"; sound teeth, marked "0"; potential sound teeth, marked "(0)"; or candidates for extraction, marked "−." The rationale for judgment in this case is as follows:

No. 1. Third molar, poor root formation, difficult access for plaque removal, and blocking out no. 2; therefore, candidate for extraction—"−"
No. 2. Second molar, excellent root, pulpally sound, but rotated into linguoversion; therefore, a potential key tooth with some orthodontic correction—"(+)"
No. 3. Missing, space partially lost, might be regained
No. 4. Second premolar, excellent root, pulp sound, good position, a key tooth—"+"
No. 5. First premolar, endodontic treatment 18 months previous apparently successful, can be considered at least a sound tooth and possibly a key tooth, but needs definitive restoration—"(0)"
No. 6. Canine, good condition, a key tooth—"+"
No. 7. Lateral incisor, needs extensive restoration, a potential sound tooth—"(0)"
No. 8. Central incisor, good root, but orthodontically deficient, a potential key tooth—"(+)"
No. 9. Same as no. 8—"(+)"
No. 10. Same as no. 7—"(0)"
No. 11. Canine, extensively restored, but pulp has apparently receded successfully, a key tooth—"+"
No 12. First premolar, rotated with root exposure and severe root caries, candidate for extraction—"−"
No. 13. Second premolar, rotated but sound—"0"
No. 14. Missing, space closed
No. 15. Second molar, excellent root, but severely rotated into linguoversion; therefore, a potential key tooth with orthodontic correction—"(+)"
No. 16. Same as no. 1—"−"
No. 17. Third molar, good roots in bone, sound pulp, a key tooth—"+"
No. 18. Missing
No. 19. Missing
No. 20. Second premolar, excellent root in bone, key tooth—"+"
No. 21. Missing
No. ? A deciduous canine, short root, does not contribute to the likely restoration (fixed bridge), but complicates it; therefore, extraction is indicated—"−"
No. 22. Canine, typical key tooth—"+"
No. 23. Lower incisor, sound tooth although slight crowding requires careful maintenance—"0"
No. 24. Same as no. 23—"0"
No. 25. Same as no. 23—"0"
No. 26. Same as no. 23—"0"
No. 27. Canine, typical key tooth—"+"
No. ? The other deciduous canine. Here, however, there is no interference in projected treatment, and the tooth is sound although short of root—"0"
No. 28. First premolar, excellent root in bone, key tooth—"+"
No. 29. Second premolar, same as no. 28—"+"
No. 30. First molar, probably missing since early childhood
No. 31. Second molar, excellent root in bone, but tipping due to loss of no. 30 and rotation of no. 2 requires correction with casting, a potential key tooth—"(+)"
No. 32. Third molar, a fairly sound tooth not interfering with other treatment and accessible for plaque control—"0"

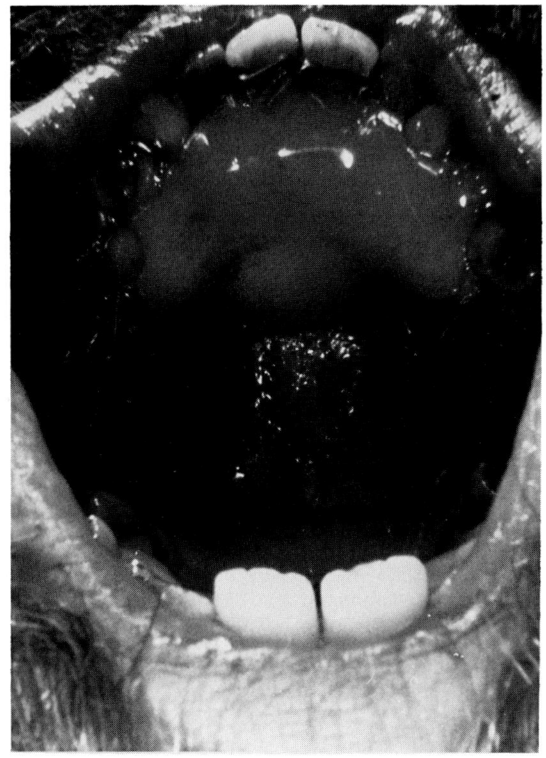

E

Fig. 8–4 ***continued.*** *E*, A simple orthodontic appliance was utilized to develop the potential key teeth. Treatment time was approximately 8 months.

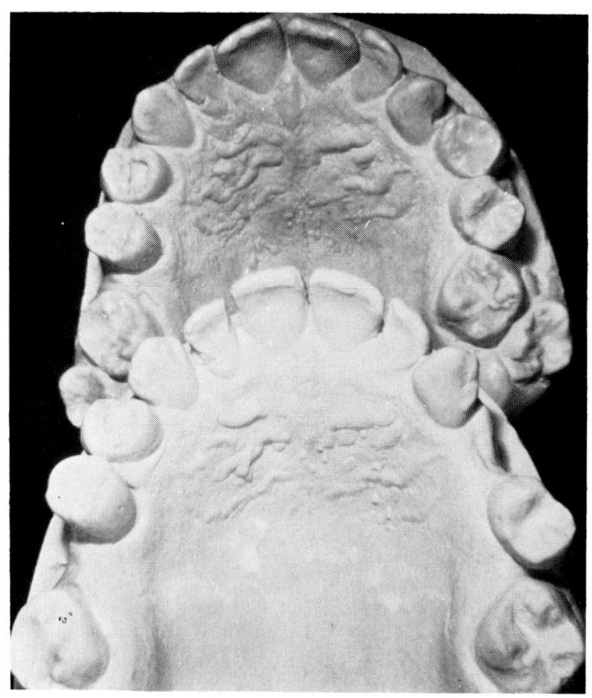

F

Fig. 8–4 ***continued.*** *F*, Comparison of diagnostic casts before (top) and after (bottom) extractions and orthodontic treatment. Note the favorable arch position that has been developed.

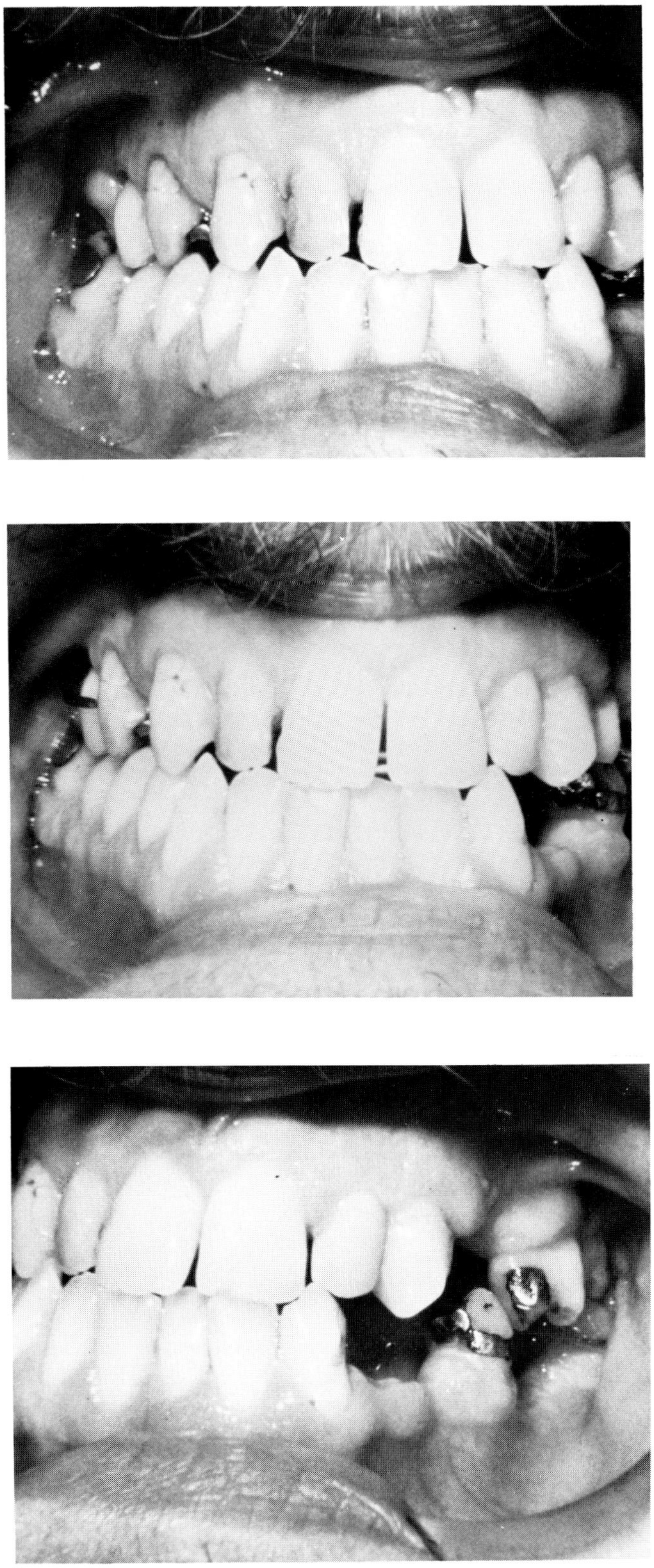

G

Fig. 8–4 *continued.* G, Clinical appearance after 8 months. In addition to orthodontic enhancement, note the tissue health and hygiene that the patient had developed in that time.

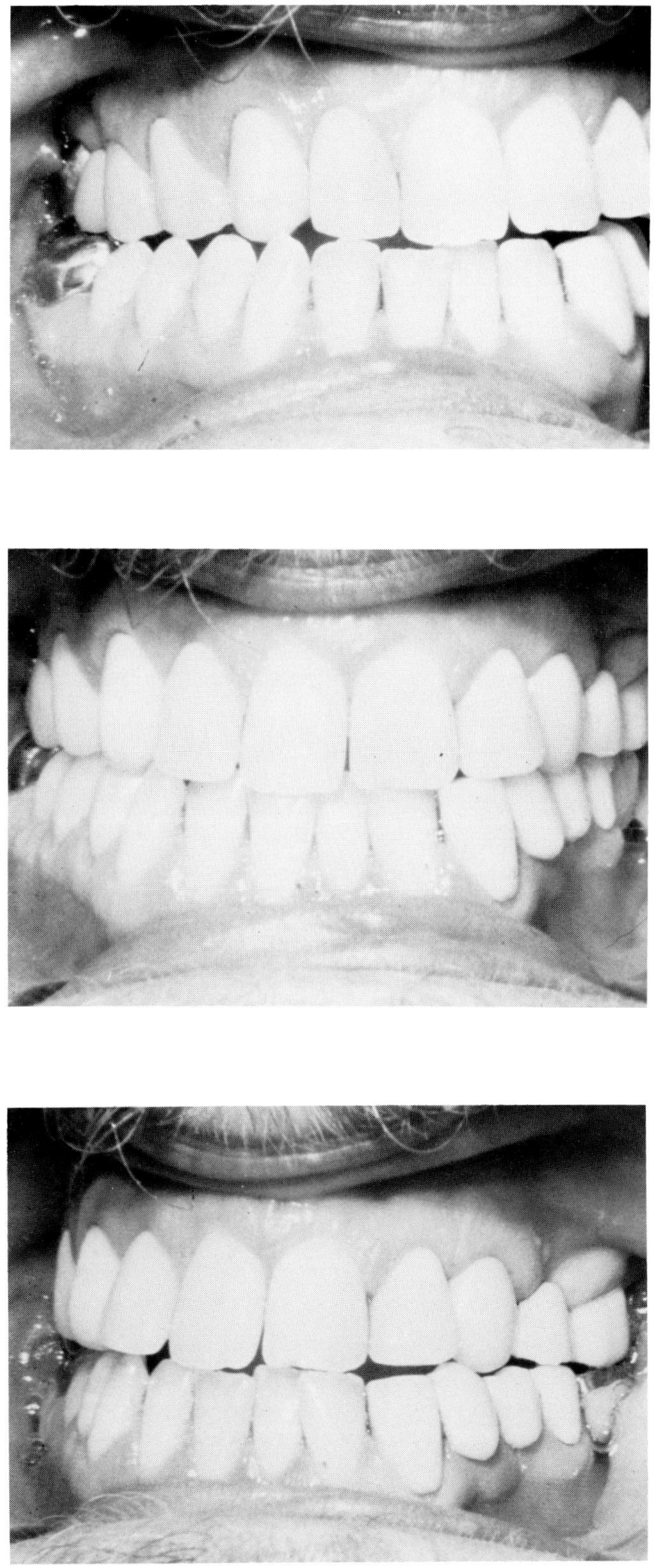

H

Fig. 8–4 *continued.* *H,* Five years after full and final restorative treatment. Note the development of working-side group function in this nearly Class III occlusion. Note also the continued maintenance of a healthy oral environment. As a point of interest, count the lower incisors. The lower left canine was reshaped to mimic an incisor for better esthetics.

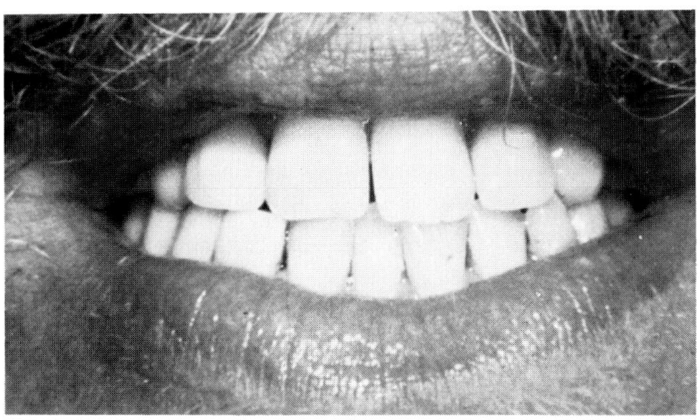

I

Fig. 8–4 *continued.* *I,* A satisfying 5-year result

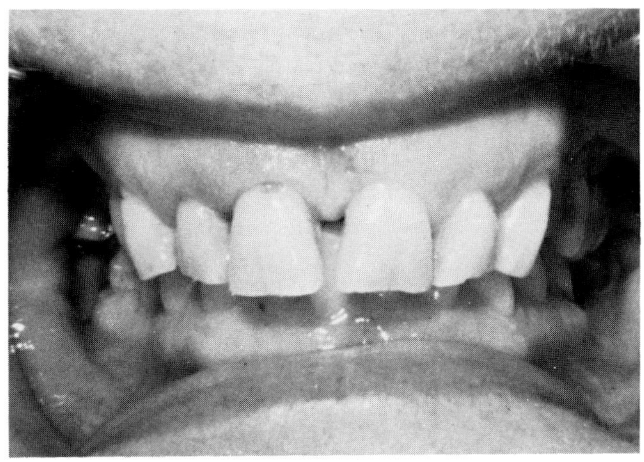

A

Fig. 8–4. Tooth Inventory: Case 2.
A, This 48-year-old woman was aware that something was seriously wrong with her teeth due to the mobility and recurring gum abscesses. She wanted desperately to keep all her teeth; the retention of as many teeth as possible became the primary goal.

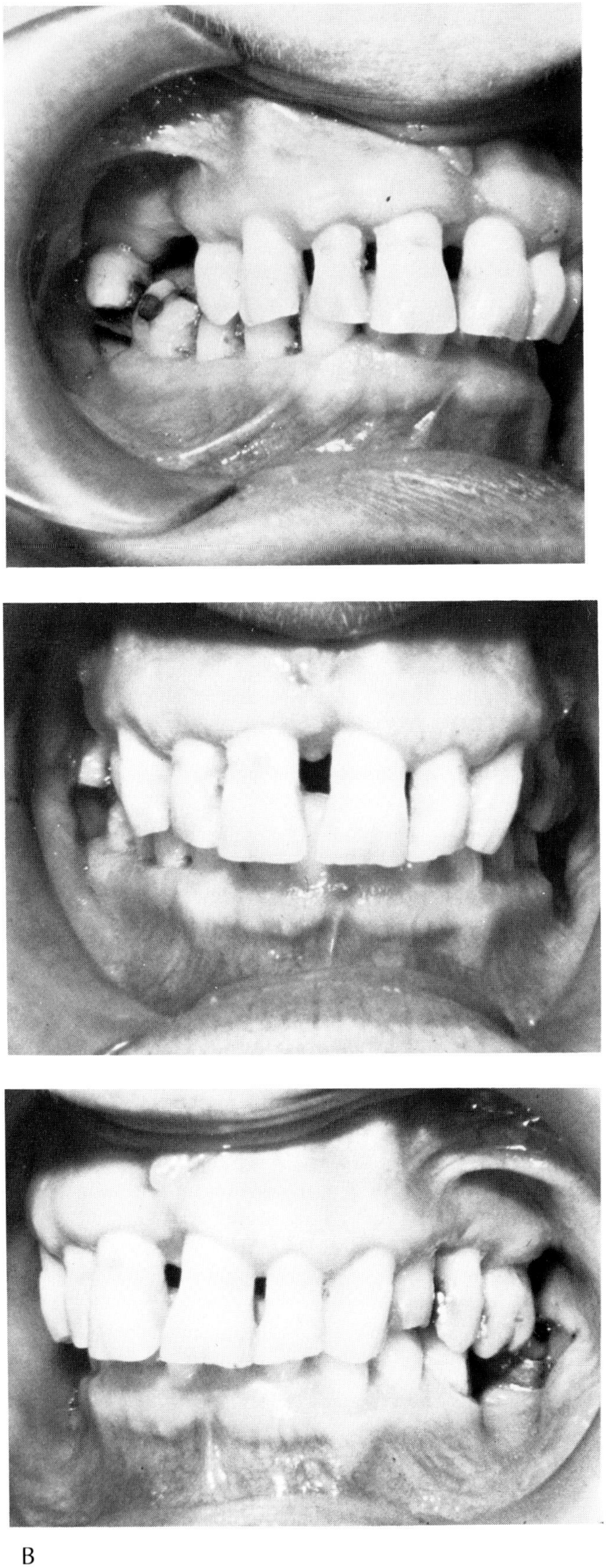

B

Fig. 8–4 *continued.* *B*, The disfigurement resulting from periodontal surgery was anticipated and the patient prepared. Nevertheless, tears were shed when the periodontal pack was removed.

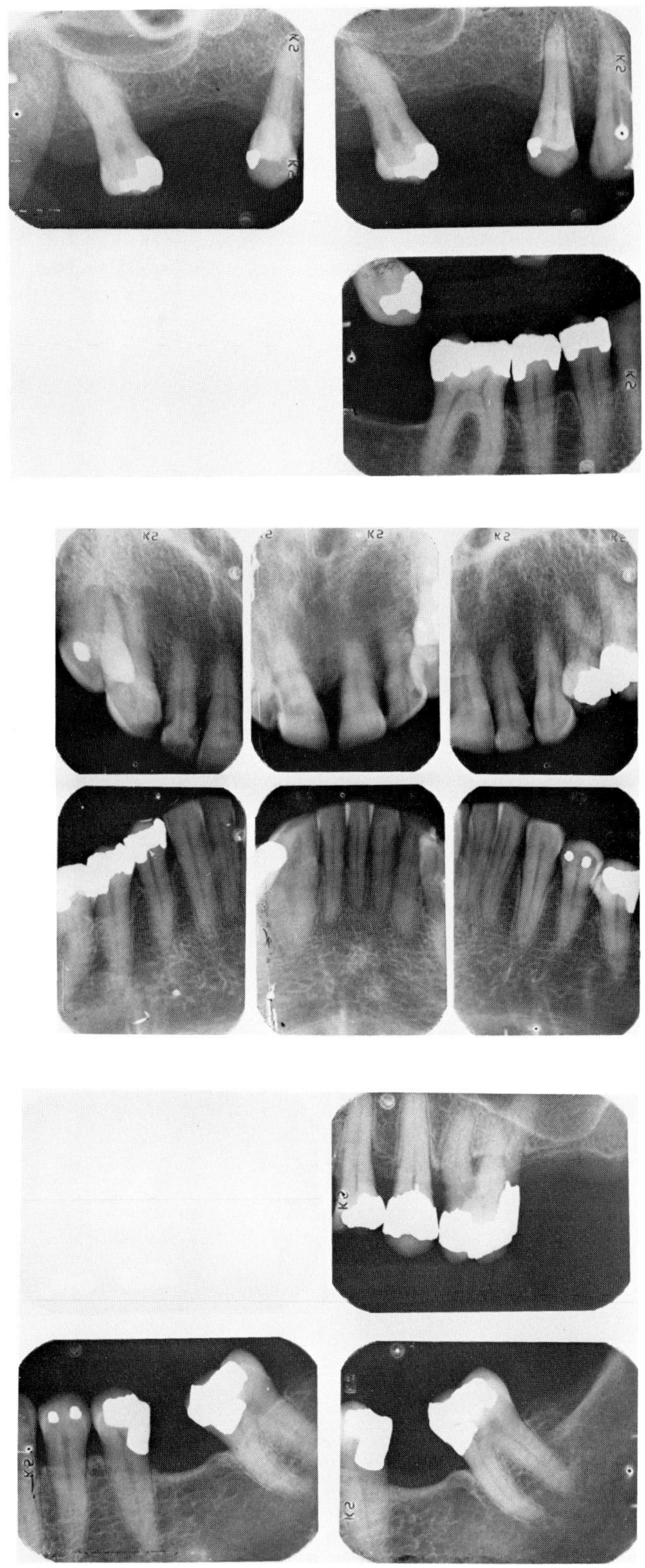

C

Fig. 8–4 *continued.* *C,* Radiographs reveal severe bone loss in maxilla, less advanced in mandible (nos. 28 and 29 had 5 to 6 mm pockets). Generalized pockets in the maxilla were most severe on tooth no. 1 (Class III mobility), tooth no. 5 (Class II mobility—note the hint of the infrabony pocket extending up to the apical third of the root), teeth nos. 7,8,9, and 10 (Class II mobility), tooth no. 12 (Class II mobility), and tooth no. 14 (Class II mobility with suppuration).

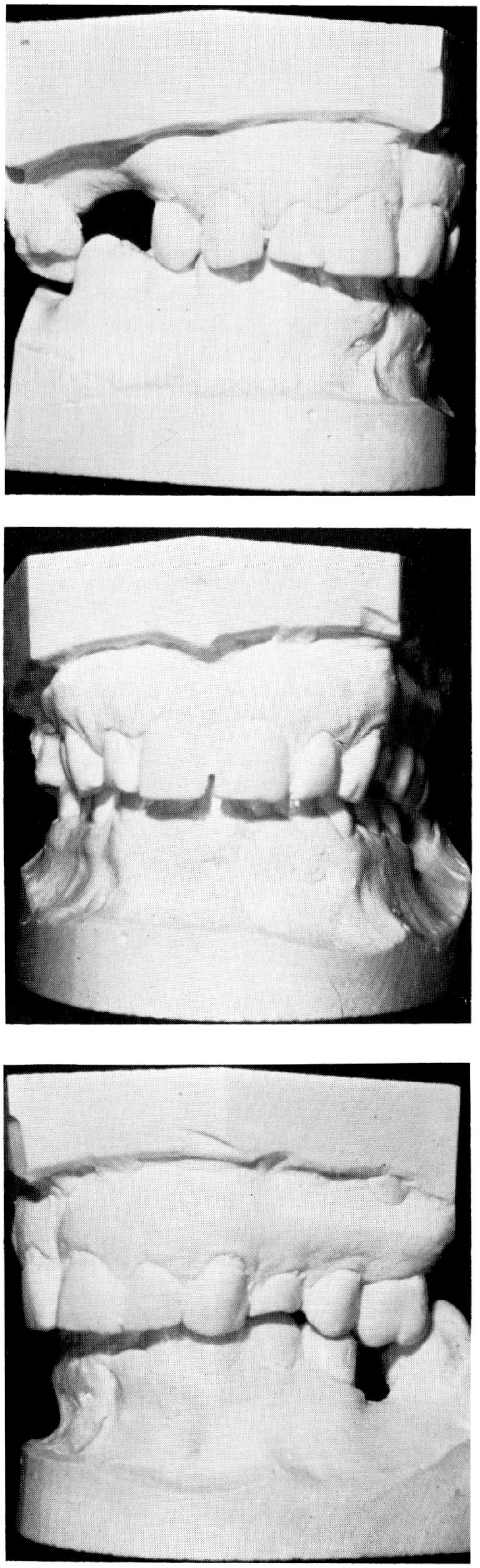

D

Fig. 8–4 ***continued.*** *D,* Diagnostic casts suggest collapse of the bite, which, through wear, migration, and loss of posterior support, may have compromised the vertical dimension. Patient reports that deep overbite seems more pronounced over the past several years than previously.

Fig. 8–4 *continued.* E, A tooth inventory is done as illustrated in Case 1.

- No. 1. Third molar, supererupted, stubby root, and severe periodontal involvement, extract—"–"
- No. 5. First premolar, periodontally condemned—"–"
- No. 6. Canine, although requiring periodontal therapy, a potential key tooth—"(+)"
- No. 7 Lateral incisior, severely involved periodontally, but if treatable may be potentially sound—"(0)"
- No. 8. Same as no. 7—"(0)"
- No. 9. Same as no. 7—"(0)"
- No. 10. Same as no. 7—"(0)"
- No. 11. Canine, requiring periodontal treatment, a potential key tooth—"(+)"
- No. 12. First premolar, requiring periodontal treatment, may be potentially sound—"(0)"
- No. 13. Second premolar, heavily restored, but good root in bone—"0"
- No. 14. First molar, severe periodontal involvement, with caries and supereruption, a hopeless situation—"–"
- No. 18. Second molar, excellent root in bone, slight tipping and large restoration, plus minor periodontal involvement make this a potential key tooth—"(+)"
- No. 20. Second premolar, good root in bone, large restoration and minor periodontal involvement make for potential key tooth—"(+)"
- No. 21. First premolar, even better root in bone; minor periodontal treatment would produce potential key tooth—"(+)"
- No. 22. Canine, typical key tooth—"+"
- No. 23. Lateral incisor, even with slight bone loss a sound tooth—"0"
- No. 24. Same as no. 23—"0"
- No. 25. Same as no 23—"0"
- No. 26. Same as no. 23—"0"
- No. 27. Canine, typical key tooth—"+"
- No. 28. First premolar, Class I mobility with lingual periodontal pockets, sound if treated—"(0)"
- No. 29. Same as no. 28—"(0)"
- No. 30. First molar, good roots in bone, despite some pocketing and bone loss, furcation is unaffected; with treatment, a potential key tooth—"(+)"

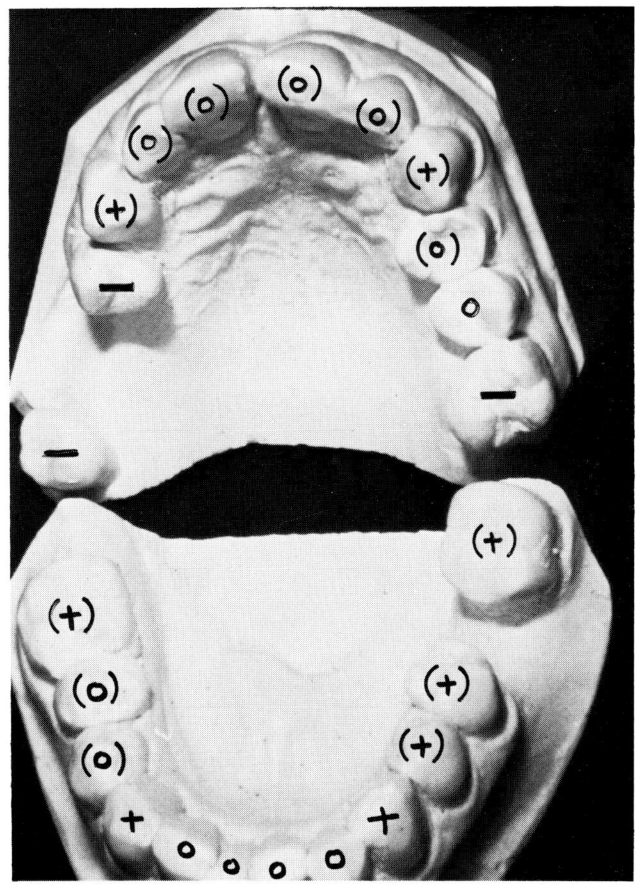

E

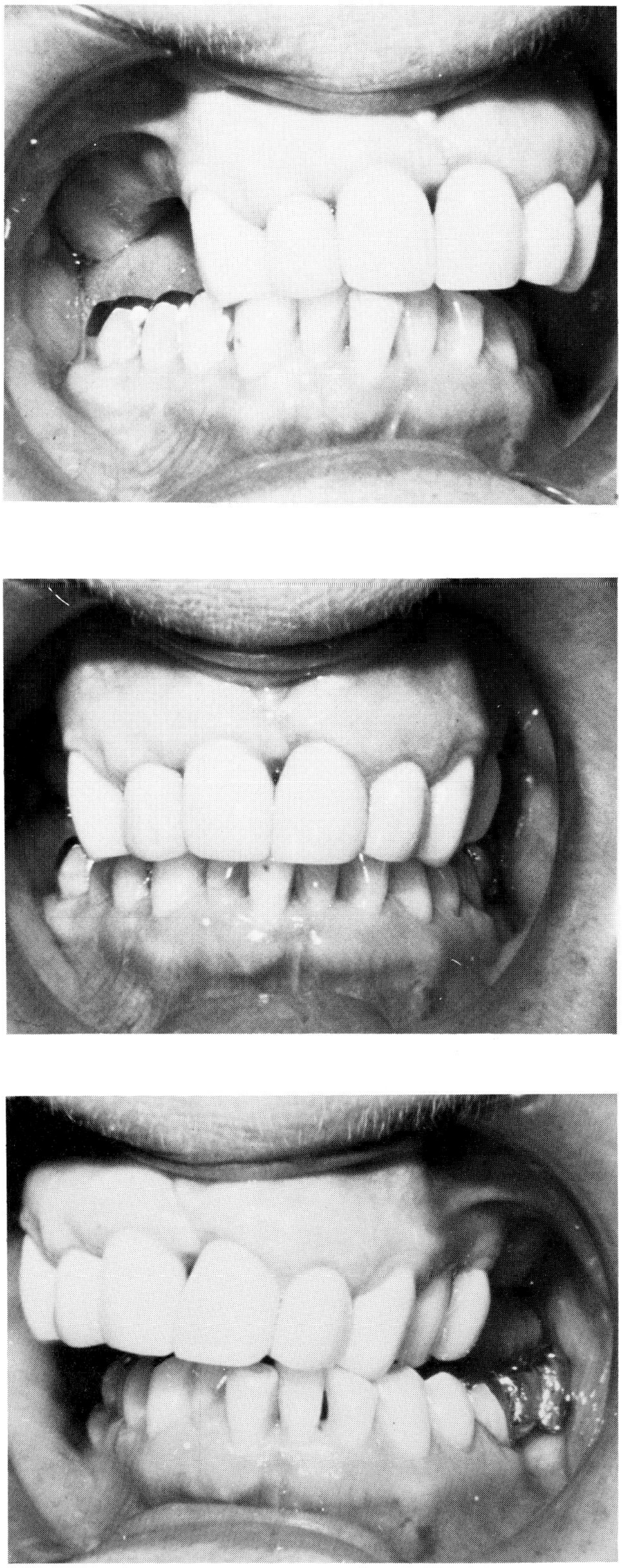

F

Fig. 8–4 *continued.* *F*, Following periodontal therapy, interim splinting, definitive restoration, extraction of the nonviable teeth, all sound or key teeth remain. A number of maxillary teeth were splinted for postperio stability and to enhance the anchorage for a removable partial denture.

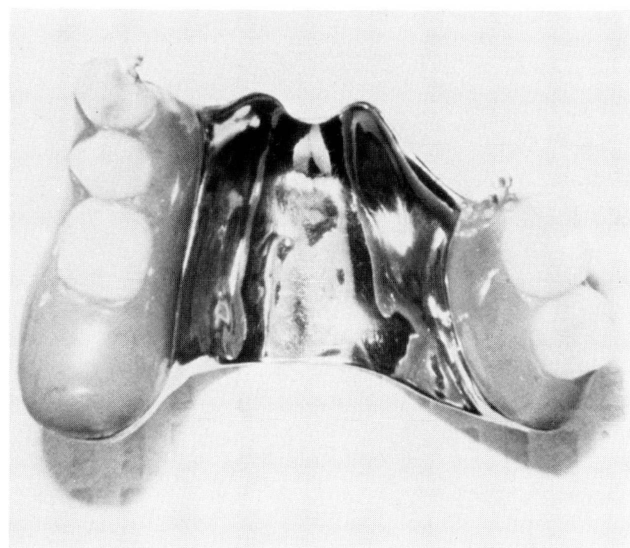

G

Fig. 8–4 *continued.* *G,* Semiprecision attachments keying into splinted abutments provided sufficient retention even without retentive clasps for this cast gold base (mucostatic) removable partial denture.

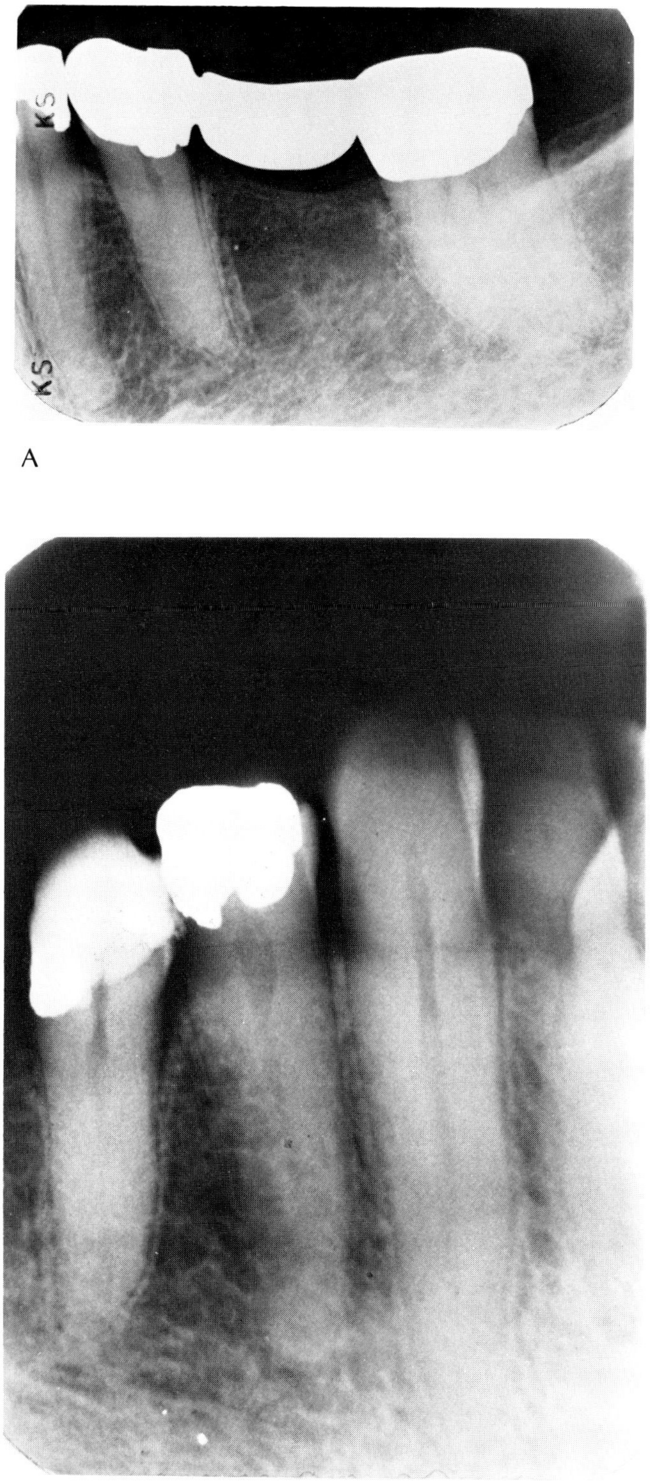

A

B

Fig. 8–5. *A*, Radiograph of lower second premolar bridge abutment that was to have been extracted. *B*, Same tooth (x-ray reversed) 6 months later with sedative restoration in place.

one; indeed, many desperately involved teeth have been saved by the diligence, creativity, and skill of a dentist. It is disheartening and occasionally infuriating to see a patient who has been recently edentulated, whether fully or partially, and to note extraction sites on the radiograph that suggest that ample root was present in the bone to permit retention and utilization of the teeth. When teeth are removed without the patient having been apprised of the potential for their retention, it may constitute professional negligence. If the attending dentist does not or cannot perform the procedures necessary to retain teeth, referral is indicated, if only to allow the patient to make the final decision based on good, ample information. Once the teeth or potential distal abutments have been removed, it is too late. A typical example is illustrated in the radiograph in Figure 8–5A, B. This patient had been referred by her general dentist to an exodontist for the removal of a lower right second premolar due to extensive caries under the three-quarter crown retainer. The patient, preferring not to lose a tooth, sought another opinion. Excavation of the tooth eliminated the caries and did not result in exposure of the pulp (although endodontic therapy was certainly possible had that occurred). After restoration with a sedative temporary material for several months, the tooth was available for use as an abutment once again. Had it been removed, a fixed bridge to replace it would have been longer in span, and considering the relatively poor root structure of the lower first premolar, probably would have required double abutment and anterior extension to the canine, for a total of five units in the prosthesis rather than three.

Because such dubious extractions are a common occurrence, the subject of strategic extractions can be very touchy. It is essential that we remain rational and scientific in our approach to the subject. Some dentists have publicly stated or written that extractions are never justified or necessary, a statement that can be as harmful as the when-in-doubt, take-it-out approach. We must allow some middle ground when considering the removal or retention of teeth. While extraction is not an ideal treatment, dentists are fortunate in that teeth are usually more numerous than other body parts that might be considered for amputation, and the prosthetic possibilities greater. We might liken the situation in treatment planning to the military axiom that one should seek to defend "high ground." If, in desperately trying to save every tooth, we jeopardize the overall result, what is to be gained? In many complex cases, it is advisable to "retreat" to the next "high ground," even though it means cutting losses by strategic extractions. The decision about which teeth to remove and when must be based on sound clinical judgment using good criteria. No one need apologize for extractions proposed or performed on that basis as long as the patient is involved in the decision. I will discuss some criteria for the strategic extraction of teeth, which simplify overall treatment and enhance the prognosis.

First of all, teeth should be extracted if they are so extensively debilitated through periodontal disease, caries, fracture, or pulpal pathology that they cannot be effectively and dependably treated and restored. This depends on the relative severity of any or all the problems involved, with the "bottom line" being the amount and nature of root in bone, as discussed in the key-tooth concept. However, other factors must be considered, three of which I will discuss at this time: ability of the practitioner, availability of specialty practitioners for referral, and availability of other key teeth.

Every practitioner has limits to his ability in given areas. Depth and breadth of training, experience, and individual innate skills will vary. It is no crime, therefore, for a practitioner to admit openly that he does not feel able to perform some complex clinical procedure or group of procedures in a difficult case. It is far better to refer a procedure to another dentist or to select an alternative treatment approach than to perform complicated procedures incompetently. Such alternative treatment approaches often entail the strategic extraction of teeth requiring the complicated procedures. The ethical questions involved in extractions such as these are serious, and there is no justification for wholesale extractions due to a practitioner's inability to perform routine general dental procedures.

Given a severely debilitated tooth that could potentially be retained with periodontal, endodontic, and restorative procedures, one must consider the availability and practicality of multiple referrals if the attending dentist is unable to perform one or more of the necessary steps. If no specialist is available for a given procedure or if the time and distance involved makes referral difficult for the patient to accept (especially if multiple referrals are required for one tooth), extraction may be the logical alternative.

We have previously discussed the concept of referral to other general practitioners for specialty procedures when there are no specialists available and feel that many teeth might be saved through such cooperation. Often, however, the greatest resistance to referral comes from the patient, and his difficulties with time, distance, and dealing with multiple practitioners must be considered.

Perhaps the most important factor in assessing the possible extraction of the badly debilitated tooth is the availability of other teeth for use in an overall treatment plan. Given two relatively similar teeth—for example, lower first permanent molars that are periodontally involved, deeply carious, and possibly in need of endodontic therapy, cast dowel and core, and crown—the decision to extract or to treat and retain can be made on the basis of other available teeth. If a healthy second molar is present and there is the option of a sound, three-unit fixed bridge, extraction might well be the treatment of choice. On the other hand, if a second premolar and a second molar are not present and retention of the first permanent molar is essential to avoid the necessity of a removable prosthesis, more complex procedures might be worth the effort.

After these three factors are considered, the debilitated tooth must be judged for its real value, assuming that the multiple procedures are carried out successfully. Will there be sufficient root in bone to ensure long-term stability? Is the arch position favorable? Can this tooth be utilized effectively in the plan (a key tooth) or will it at least stand on its own indefinitely following the proposed treatments? If there is reasonable doubt that it will, due to the extensive debilitation, extraction might be indicated.

Secondly, teeth should be extracted if they do not contribute to the overall function of the oral cavity or if they tend to complicate the treatment plan.

A typical example of such noncontributory teeth are third molars that are nonfunctional because of their distal location and consequent, habitual cheek biting or because they are unopposed in the opposite arch. Such teeth, while providing no function, stability, or esthetic value, are often the sites of chronic pericoronal infection or, through supereruption, create occlusal interferences.

Retained deciduous teeth or malformed teeth (pegged lateral incisors) that lie in the path of proposed fixed or removable prostheses are typical examples of complicating factors in a treatment plan. If, due to their poor root size or configuration, they do not contribute to the proposed prostheses, extraction and inclusion in the prosthetic plan are often indicated.

Finally, teeth should be extracted if their retention is not cost-effective; that is, when large investments in time and money would be required to obtain little benefit, or when alternative approaches appear to provide equal or better benefit at less cost, extraction may be indicated.

A good example of this is the endodontically involved lower second molar that occludes only partially with the upper molar opposing it. The time and cost of endodontic therapy and possible core and crown restorations must be weighed against the minimal occlusion that will be provided by its retention. Other factors to be considered in such a case are the patient's age, his ability to afford the time and money involved, and the condition of the lower first molar, since the second molar might be needed in the future. Obviously, the patient must be involved in the cost-effectiveness assessment, since it is his time and money being expended, and his benefit being gained or lost.

Another example of the cost-effectiveness criteria is the decision whether to retain a badly broken down and endodontically involved lower first molar when the rest of the lower teeth are present. In one hypothetical situation, the rest of the teeth in the quadrant are virgin teeth or, at least, have not been restored interproximally. Removal of the first molar, while eliminating the time and cost of endodontic procedures and core and crown restorations, would likely necessitate the placement of a three-unit fixed bridge, requiring crown restorations on the previously uninvolved adjacent teeth. Extraction, therefore, may be less cost effective than treatment. If the adjacent teeth are also heavily restored and in need of crown restorations, however, it might be less costly and in the long run, more effective to remove the endodontically involved tooth and fabricate a fixed bridge.

Even if cost is not a significant factor, the time and effort expended must still be considered. We have seen teeth that probably should have been removed in the first place but were subjected to a series of complicated, time consuming, and not altogether pleasant treatments, only to fail within a year or two and require extraction. Therefore, teeth that have been previously treated extensively should be approached with great caution if further problems arise. The conscientious dentist's tendency is to "try, try, again," since large investments have already been made. Too often, however, this is throwing good time and money after bad, and extraction of the failed tooth may be the most rational approach in the long run.

In the cost-effectiveness criteria, we must also consider the patient's ability to afford the treatment necessary to retain a given tooth, or teeth. If funds are limited, the best interests of the patient may dictate extraction of many teeth that could be saved, in order to obtain the best overall clinical result under the circumstances. For example, upper posterior teeth that could be retained with endodontics, root amputation, and fixed bridges might be extracted instead, if, in so doing, the patient could afford a fixed rather than a removable prosthesis in the lower arch. Such decisions are almost always difficult and require patient involvement.

In each criteria, the candidate for extraction is evaluated in light of the overall clinical situation. At all times, we must avoid "tunnel vision," which results in poor judgment. Teeth are components of a system, and *it is the system that we aim to preserve*. Strategic extractions based on sound criteria can often be positive steps in preserving the overall system.

Carried to its extreme, the cost-effectiveness criteria can be applied in selecting a full upper denture as treatment of choice even when restorable teeth are available. When time and/or money are not adequate for full mouth reconstruction, resources can sometimes be concentrated on retaining and restoring the lower arch, while extracting remaining upper teeth and placing a full upper denture. The rationale here is that upper dentures generally are well tolerated and can usually provide good comfort, function, and esthetics, while lower full dentures cannot be counted on to be as well accepted. Thus, if one must choose which arch to preserve, it is usually the mandibular arch that is most critical. Such decisions should not be made lightly, but neither should they be rejected outright.

Cost is not the only factor that might suggest edentulation of the maxilla and a full denture prosthesis. In many cases, a severely debilitated dentition might present such complex challenges in terms of lost vertical dimension, attrition, malocclusion, and esthetics that even full reconstruction of the maxillary arch with crowns and fixed and/or removable partial dentures cannot ensure a good, long-term result. In such situations, a full maxillary denture can greatly simplify the treatment, since vertical dimension and esthetic problems are often managed more easily.

This concept does not apply to the lower arch as well; although edentulation and a full denture prosthesis might cost less than retention or restoration of teeth, the relative difficulty of adapting to and utilizing the full lower prosthesis makes it the least beneficial option we can offer. Most conscientious dentists urge their patients to preserve as much of the mandibular dentition as possible even if the long-term prognosis is poor, due to the great difficulties in both the construction and utilization of the full lower denture.

Recently, an intermediate treatment option has come into use—namely, the overdenture. The concept of preserving viable roots to provide retention, stability, and proprioception, and to maintain the alveolar bone has much to recommend it. A discussion of overdentures and their applications is not within the scope of this text; however, some examples of how an overdenture prosthesis might be applied as an alternative to full edentulation would be in order.

When an upper full denture is chosen as the most cost-effective alternative, retention of at least two key roots under the prosthesis may enhance the prognosis. Retention of multiple roots is also possible, however, since endodontic therapy is nearly always required when the tooth is severed just above the gingival margin and cast dowel/coping restorations are advisable for long-term stability and caries protection, the cost of retaining many roots may approach that of a reconstruction. At the very least, it may significantly reduce the economic advantage of a full prosthesis in some cases. Furthermore, while retention, stability, and proprioception are enhanced utilizing overdenture, the advantage to the maxilla is less, due to the generally good retentive properties already present.

When teeth are available as abutments but they lack sufficient root surface in bone to be dependable, overdenture construction may allow their long-term use. This is especially of value in the lower arch, where sound teeth in unfavorable postions (premolars) or canine teeth having lost significant bone support are not available as partial denture abutments, but can be used under an overdenture. The goal in these applications is to preserve the teeth for as long as possible and to gain the many advantages of their retention.

Overdenture can be applied in many cases as an interim treatment, a means of easing into a full lower denture. When remaining lower teeth are periodontally condemned but relatively asymptomatic, a temporary overdenture can be fabricated Teeth to be retained on a temporary basis can be anesthetized and reduced grossly to a slightly supragingival height, exposing the pulp in the process. A vital pulpotomy can then be performed by removing pulpal tissues another 3 to 5 mm apically and by placing a formocresol preparation, followed by base and amalgam "plug." This can be done even when delivering an immediate denture, by leaving more tooth on the master cast than necessary and by later adding cold-cure acrylic under the denture to provide stops on the amalgam-filled, pulpotomized roots. The goal of this approach is to provide a modicum of additional stability and proprioception in the first months of lower-denture experience, after which the teeth can be extracted prior to the first reline of the immediate denture. The additional cost is modest, representing a nominal fee for vital pulpotomy and amalgam restoration on two teeth.

This approach can be used on teeth that are not condemned when the cost of endodontic therapy and possibly cast dowel/coping restorations discourages the patient from attempting to retain potential overdenture teeth. By allowing the patient to experience the overdenture appliance for 3 to 12 months with minimal investment, we may foster the patient's desire to retain the teeth and allow the financing of the endodontic therapy and definitive restoration to be spread out. The pulpotomy treatment must not be considered a lasting procedure, however, by either patient or dentist; both parties must be prepared for possible symptoms arising at any time that indicate the need for endodontic therapy.

While overdentures provide an intermediate step between full reconstruction and total edentulation, they are not without drawbacks, complications, and expense. The dentist must carefully consider the indications and contraindications in each case before making the option available. Endodontic complications, severe undercuts, and the necessity for stringent periodontal maintenance and caries control are but a few factors that may preclude use of overdentures. While attempting to preserve teeth, we must recognize our own limitations and the inherent limitations in any given treatment modality.

Nonreplacement of Missing Teeth

In listing strategies to simplify dental treatment, we must consider the advantages of nonreplacement of missing teeth. While the concept may seem heretical in the light of traditional dental education, for some patients, it may be the best approach.

A case that comes to mind is that of a gentleman who, being in the dental-supply field and having some knowledge of dental practice, would delight in showing off his edentulous space where the upper right first premolar had been extracted some 40 years previous. Although never bridged, there were no signs of tipping or mesial drift of the second premolar, nor supereruption of the opposing lower tooth. Despite predictions of collapse of the dental arch and recommendations that the tooth be replaced with a fixed bridge, the gentleman, now advanced in years, continues to have a healthy dentition, minus one upper first premolar. Risks are involved in nonreplacement of missing teeth, but risks are also involved in fabrication and placement of a fixed or removable prosthesis, particularly if the potential abutments are virgin or relatively uninvolved teeth. Using again the principle that if more treatment is attempted, there are more opportunities for failure, we must not make prosthetic replacement a reflex act whenever a missing tooth is discovered. Any treatment, especially

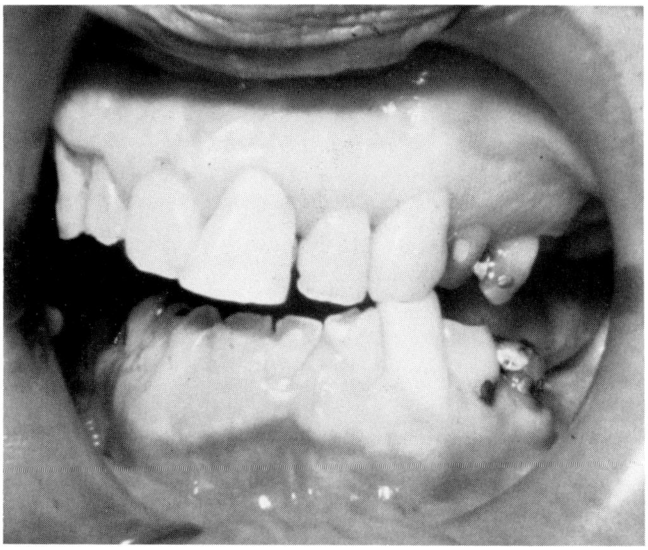

A

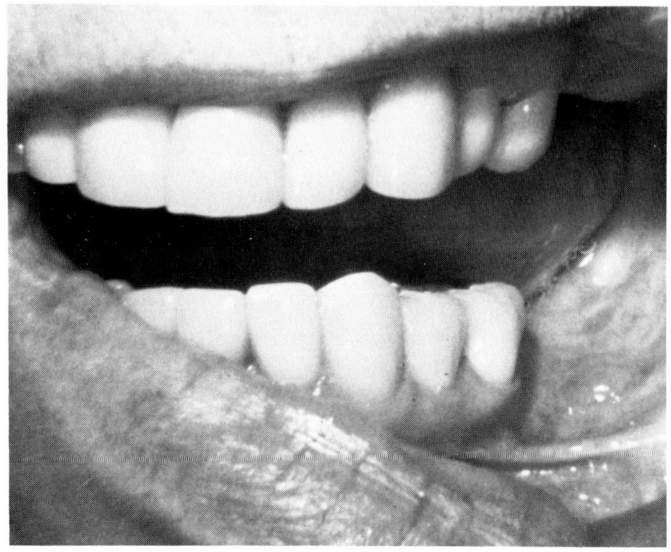

B

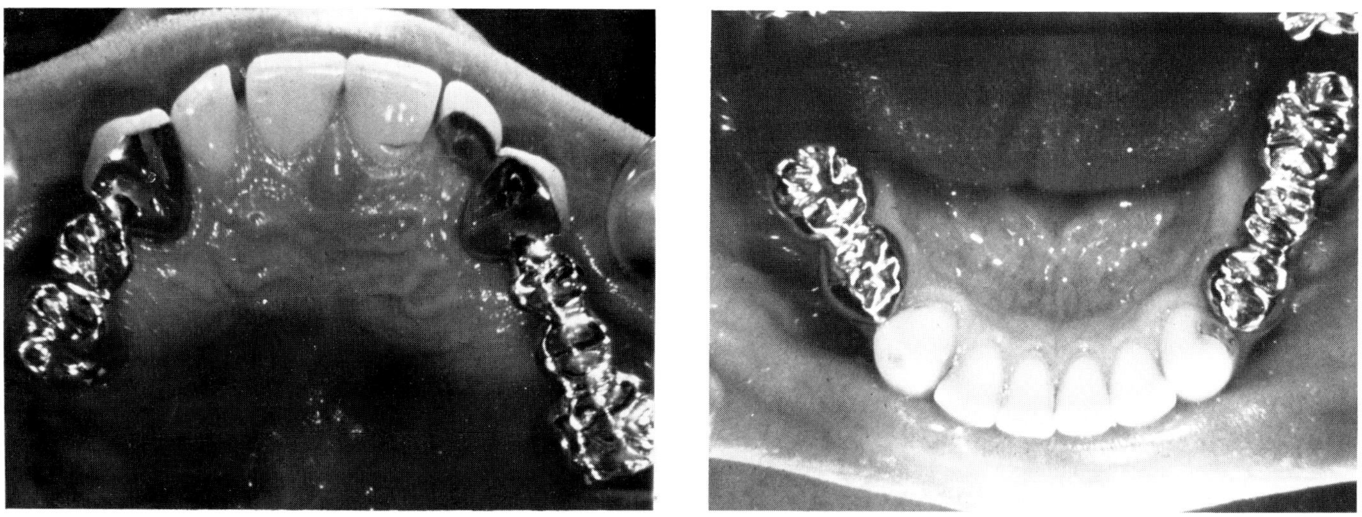

C

Fig. 8–6. Nonreplacement of missing teeth.

A, This 63-year-old woman had gross occlusal wear, and the plan called for full mouth rehabilitation. She had second molar occlusion on the right, but had been missing left molars for over 25 years.

B, Left molar region was left unrestored in reconstruction. Five years later, patient is functional, comfortable, and pleased with the result.

C, This 40-year-old pilot had had two sets of removable partial dentures; neither set was tolerated. Fixed bridges in three quadrants and a two-tooth splint replaced missing teeth and provided full function and comfort. Note the mini-molar occlusal patterns of the second premolars (left side of photos).

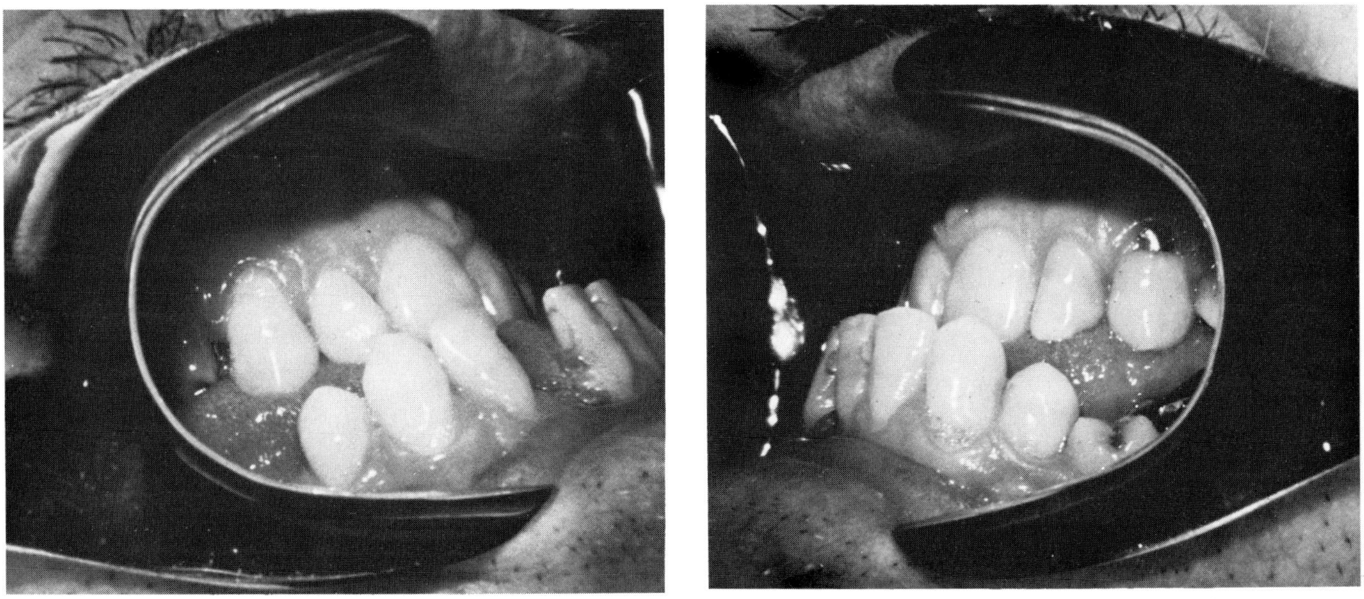

D

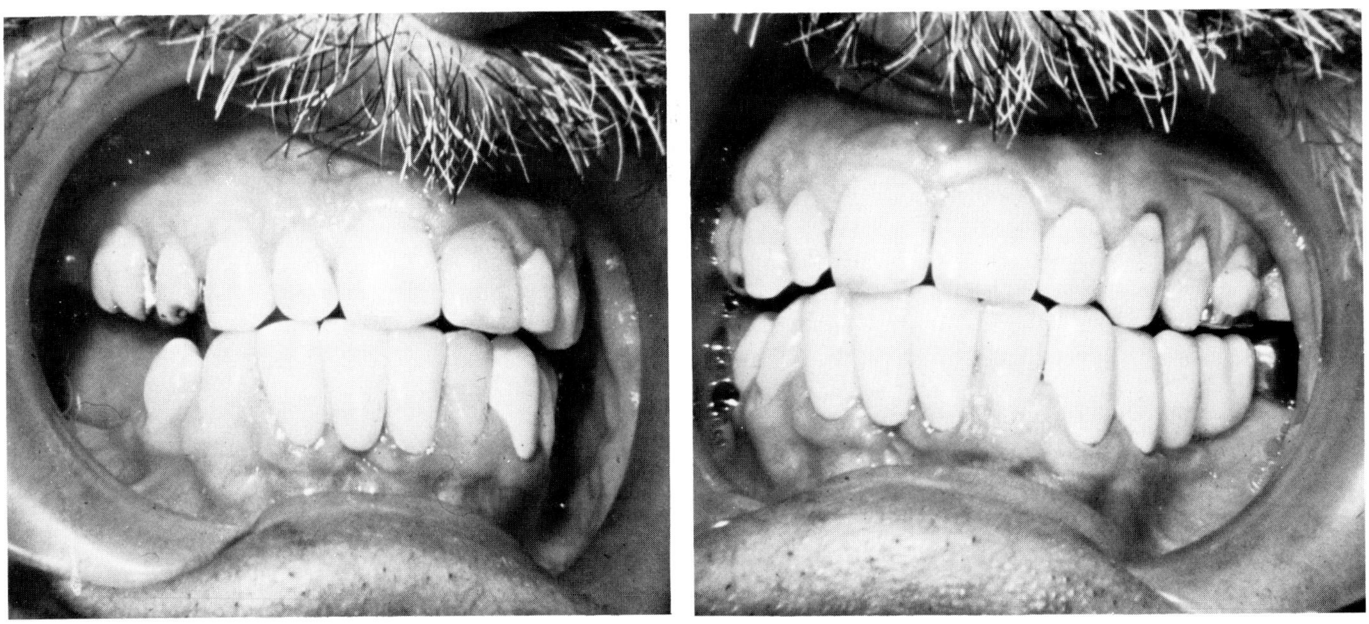

E

Fig. 8–6 *continued.* *D*, For over 40 years this man was without effective anterior or posterior occlusion. Orthognathic surgery was chosen, along with crown and bridge restoration on the left, as the treatment of choice.

E, Following this treatment, the patient was offered the opportunity for removable partial prosthesis on the right side, which he enthusiastically declined.

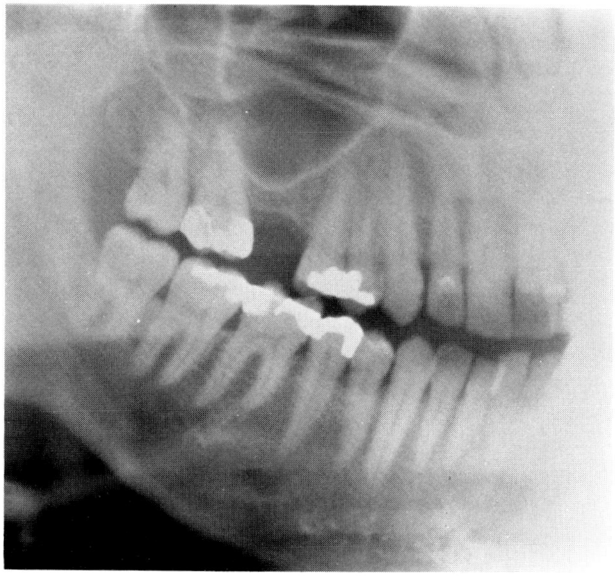

F

Fig. 8–6 *continued.* *F*, Panographic view of edentulous space, upper left molar. The tooth has been missing for 35 years, occlusion is stable, and replacement is contraindicated unless patient perceives a problem.

prosthetic replacement, should be looked at as a solution to a problem. Unless we can identify an actual problem, a solution is neither necessary nor desirable. When considering the edentulous space, we must ask the following questions:

1. Does the patient perceive the edentulous space as an esthetic problem? Is he self-conscious about the space? Does he tend to guard the space in conversation, or when smiling or laughing does he keep his mouth closed or place a hand in front of it? If so, replacement should certainly be considered.

2. Is the patient experiencing any discomfort or perceived loss of function? If the edentulous space bothers the patient, makes chewing difficult, or interferes with speech, replacement is probably indicated.

3. Are there definite signs of pathology as a result of the tooth loss? Periodontal breakdown, excessive mobility, gross wear, and occlusal dysfunction resulting from supereruption are some frank pathologic findings possibly associated with tooth loss. Obviously, replacement should not wait until such conditions are advanced. However, if the edentulous space has been present for some time and frank pathology is *not* present, prosthetic replacement may not be necessary and is certainly not urgent.

4. Are there any signs of tipping, drifting, or supereruption associated with the edentulous space? Is there flaring of anterior teeth with loss of vertical dimension? Are those conditions progressing or arrested? In the absence of frank pathology and subjective symptoms, it is possible to assess over time whether the missing teeth are causing or contributing to deterioration of the dental arch, or whether the arch is stable despite the edentulous area. This can be done if the patient is committed to a preventive recall program at regular intervals. Observations can be made for mobility and/or periodontal breakdown. Actual measurements can be made of edentulous spans intraorally, radiographically, or on study casts.

Such observations and measurements should be made annually (at least) and ideally every 6 months. As long as there is no observable deterioration of the dental arch, prosthetic replacement should be considered an elective procedure. This is true even when some tipping or mesial drift has obviously occurred but is presently stabilized. If deterioration is detected, then replacement should be recommended to prevent frank pathologic changes later. Should the patient's personal or financial situation preclude such treatment, space maintenance in the form of band and loop, bonded resin and wire, or removable temporary appliance ought to be considered as an interim approach.

If, having considered these four questions, nonreplacement of missing teeth appears to be a viable option, we should document that decision and the patient's involvement in it. It should be stressed that the decision not to replace certain missing teeth in no way precludes comprehensive and optimal dental treatment. Indeed, it may be part of an overall treatment approach that involves considerable prosthetic services elsewhere in the mouth. Examples of clinical application of nonreplacement are cited in Figure 8–6. These include examples of missing teeth within the dental arch—that is, with other teeth located both anterior and posterior to the edentulous space, and missing teeth distal to the dental arch, the so-called "free-end" or "distal-extension" situation.

It is clear from some of the examples cited that the question, "How many teeth is enough?" has no firm answer. The dentist, trained on typodont models containing 28 teeth in ideal occlusion and alignment often desires to recreate every dentition in the image of that laboratory model.

A general standard accepted in the dental profession calls for at least first-molar-to-first-molar occlusion in a restored dentition. There is no doubt that, for most individuals, first-molar occlusion can provide good function and support. The point to remember, however, is that each and every patient must be assessed individually to determine the extent of prosthetic replacement that is necessary or desirable.

Many patients we have observed can and have functioned long and well with far fewer than 24 teeth, with no apparent, resultant pathology. Prosthetic appliances are at best rather crude imitations of the real thing. The dentist must realistically assess whether his treatment in the case of missing teeth might be worse than the disease. Indeed, a significant percentage of removable partial dentures are seldom or never worn and end up in a drawer or in a glass.[3] In assessing missing teeth and the prospects for replacement, the dentist must constantly ask himself and the patient, "Is there a problem?" In the absence of pathology, esthetic or functional complaint, or observed deterioration of the system due to the missing teeth, replacement may not be indicated. When replacement of missing teeth is indicated (and it often is), the dentist must always seek the approach that is most likely to be accepted and tolerated by the patient. This will generally prove to be the simplest appliance, whether it is fixed or removable. The less hardware we place in a mouth, the more likely it is that it will be accepted, the easier it will be to clean and maintain, and there should also be less of a potential for breakage and failure. These criteria do not automatically rule out restoration of a 28-tooth, second-molar occlusion. The goal, however, should be to restore the function, comfort, and esthetics of the individual patient; those individuals will vary tremendously in their needs and desires. Once again, it is the *system* that we are attempting to preserve, not our idealized concept of what that system should look like.

Tooth Movement

Tooth movement, whether a simple single-tooth, cross-bite correction or a sophisticated full-mouth treatment involving orthognathic surgery, is one of the most effective strategies the dentist has in the simplification of case planning. Indeed, it is often poor alignment, location, or occlusion that make for a complex treatment situation.

There has been much interest in tooth movement as an adjunct to comprehensive dental treatment, and it is beyond the scope of this text to detail techniques and/or indications for orthodontic treatment. It must be noted, however, that there seems to be a problem of applications similar to that of definitive periodontal therapy—namely, that many, if not most, general practitioner dentists feel incompetent to carry out even relatively simple orthodontic treatments. Few dental curricula include practical application of orthodontic principles that would prepare a graduate dentist to carry out routine, minor tooth movement. Fortunately, texts, articles, and postgraduate lectures and courses dealing with the subject are plentiful, and it behooves the general practitioner to acquire at least a familiarity with available techniques. The application of tooth movement in comprehensive dental treatment, whether it is performed by the general dentist or referred to a specialist, can solve a great many problems for the dentist and his patient. Some of these problems and their possible solutions will be outlined in the balance of this section. All of the clinical examples cited have in common a degree of complexity that is alleviated or removed by tooth movement. Specific techniques employed as well as criteria for assessment may be mentioned, but I will not attempt to advocate any philosophy, technique, or system (Fig. 8–7).

Establishment of Anterior Guidance

The so-called "therapeutic occlusion," which consists of good posterior interdigitation at or near centric relation, with cuspid guidance or anterior group function acting in all excursions to disocclude all posteriors, has much to recommend it. As a means of simplifying the complex case, establishment of anterior guidance can be very effective. Simple equilibration can sometimes result in elimination of posterior, lateral interferences. In some cases, a nonfunctioning canine can be built up on the lingual either with composite resin (interim) or cast lingual—pin ledge or three-quarter crown (definitive). When anterior crowns or a fixed prosthesis is indicated, anterior guidance must be planned and, in most cases, designed into the preparations for best results (Fig. 8–8).

Management of Lost Vertical Dimension

Lost vertical dimension nearly always introduces complexity into a dental treatment situation, and dealing with it presents special challenges to the dentist. Failure to recognize the significance of the problem can be disastrous. In the example shown in Figure 8–9, extensive restorative dentistry had been placed at the patient's present vertical dimension, which was undoubtedly compromised. The result was gross primary-occlusal traumatism, which particularly affected the upper premolar bridge abutment and resulted in pain, tenderness, and a Class III mobility (Fig. 8–9). The upper anterior teeth were crowned and also exhibited mobility with gingival recession. The entire restorative effort was for naught and had to be removed and completely rebuilt with posterior support at the proper vertical dimension.

Regaining lost vertical dimension nearly always involves multiple crown and/or fixed-bridge restorations to achieve and maintain the proper maxil-

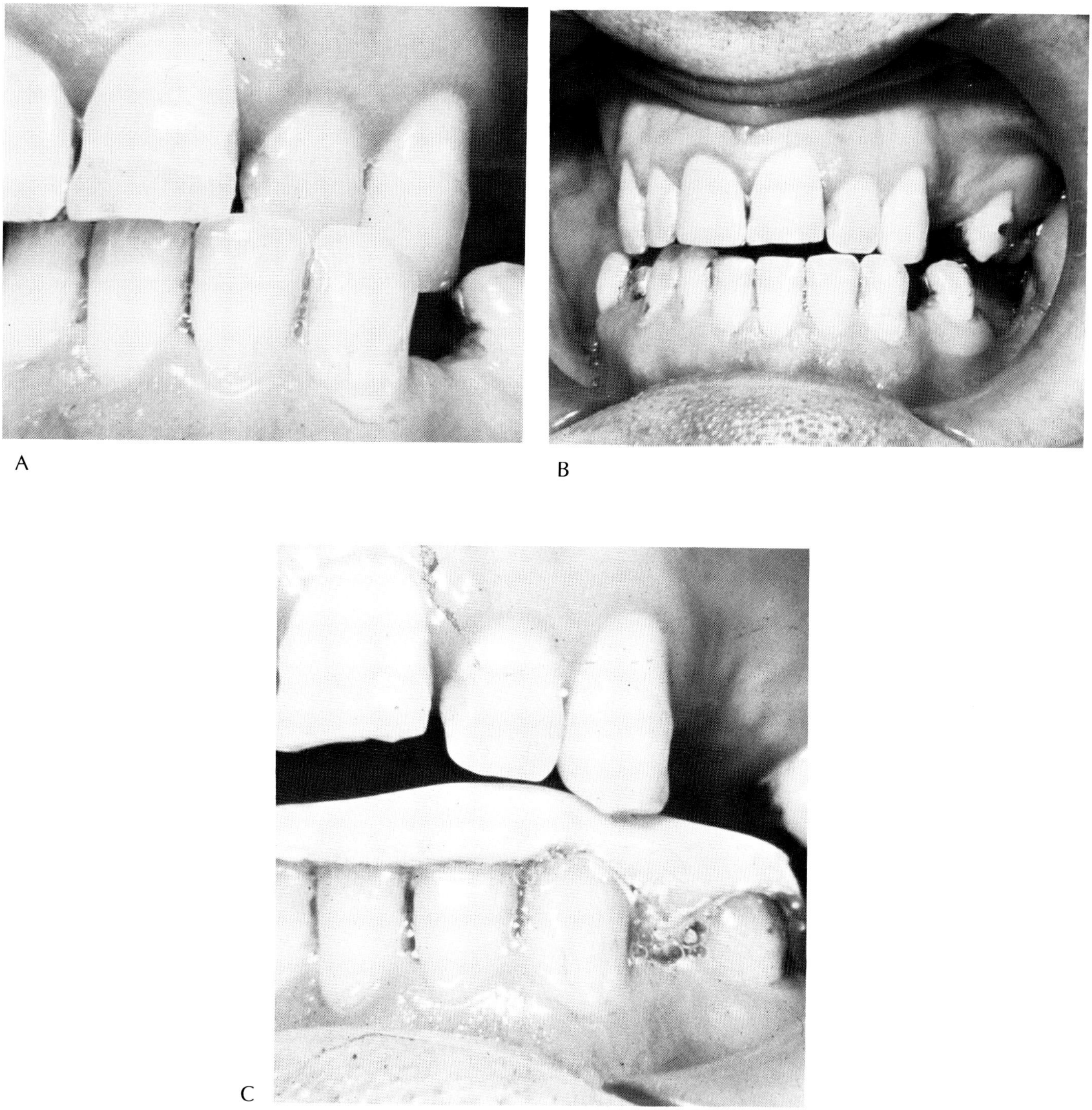

A B C

Fig. 8–7. Movement of teeth.
A, Canine and lateral in crossbite, complicating occlusal scheme in partial denture treatment case.
B, Locating centric relation, we find that crossbite is partially acquired; actual malocclusion is not as severe as first thought.
C, Use of cemented lower-bite ramp to "jump" lingually locked teeth where there are insufficient teeth in maxilla to retain appliance.

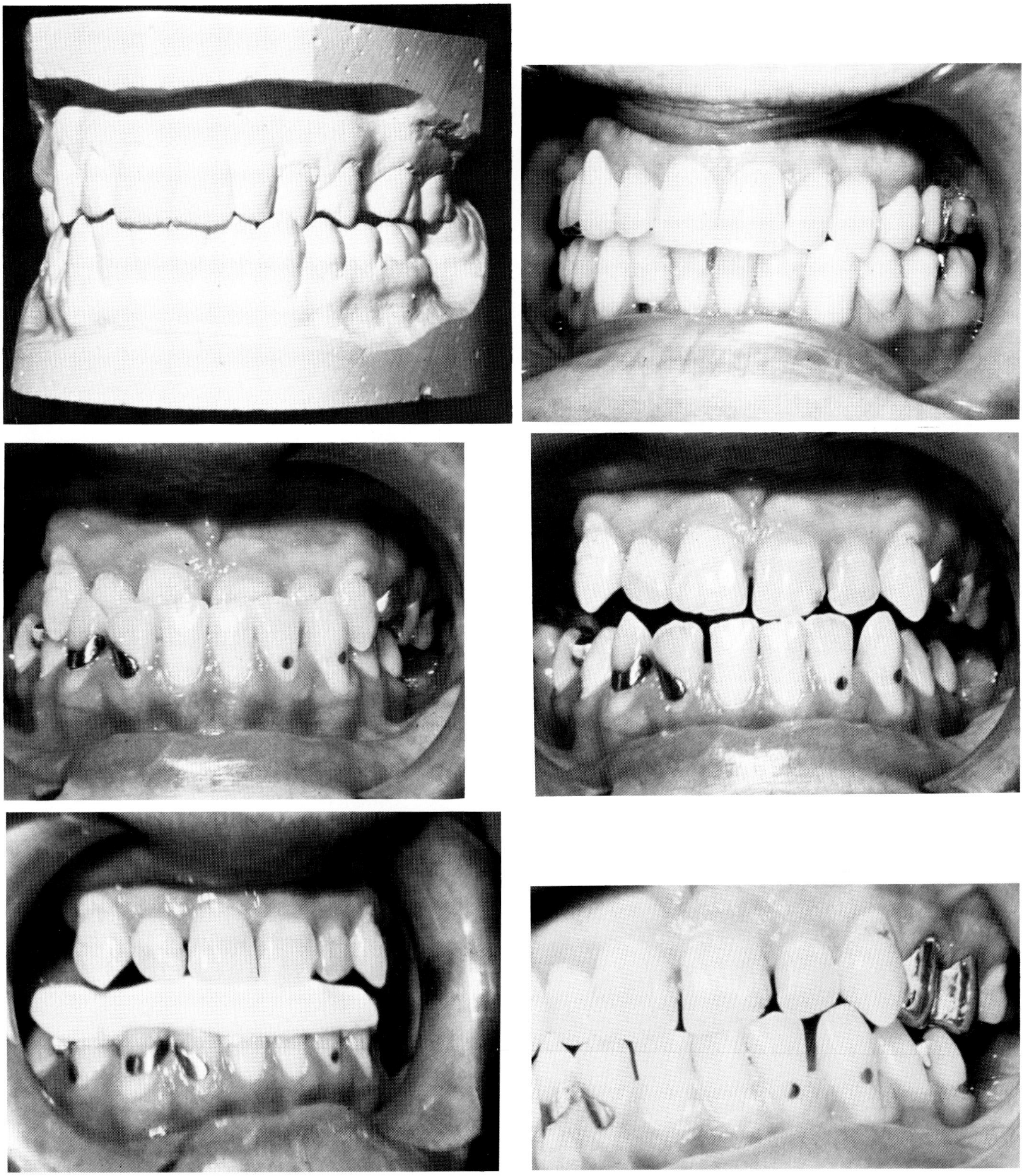

Fig. 8–7 *continued.* *D,* Canine crossbite complicating fixed-bridge treatment case. Simple appliance was used to develop no. 6 into a key tooth.

E, Clinical view 5 years after minor tooth movement and fixed bridgework. Anterior guidance provided by the canine in normal position allows disocclusion of posteriors in lateral excursion.

F, Severe crossbite in apparent Class III occlusion. Posterior support has been lost through extraction.

G, Locating centric relation, we find that crossbite is primarily acquired.

H, Bite ramp employed for 2 weeks.

I, With normal relationship established, stainless steel temporary crowns are placed at the regained vertical dimension. Now greatly simplified, the case can be treated prosthetically.

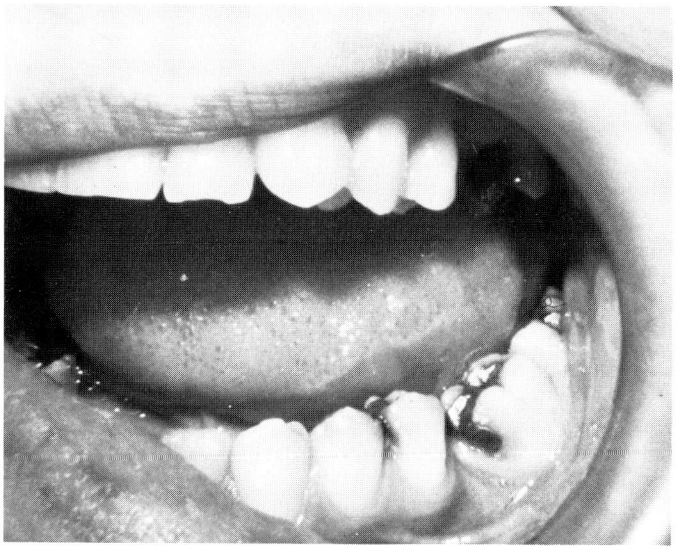

J

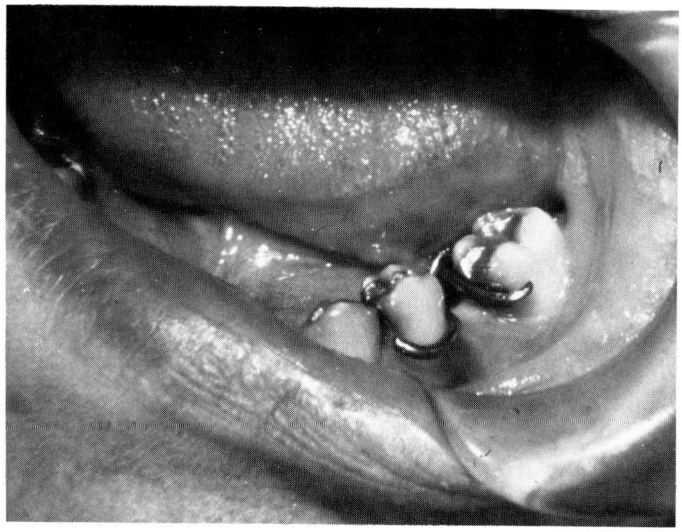

K

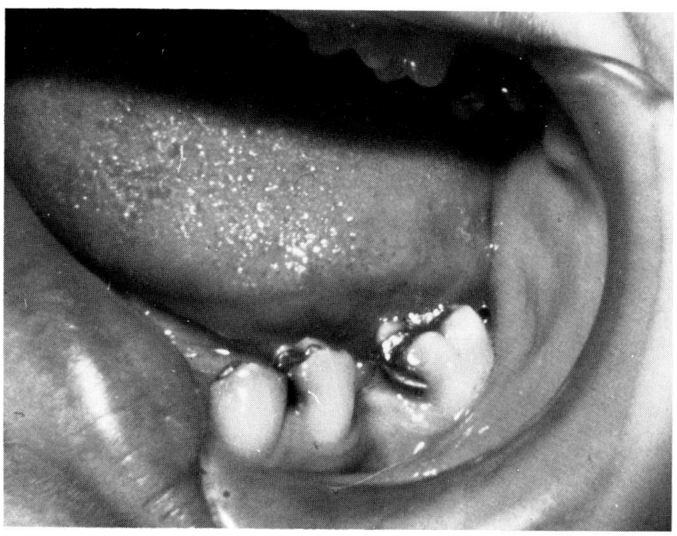

L

Fig. 8–7 *continued.* *J*, Tipped lower molars subsequent to loss of first molar. This common situation complicates fixed prostheses and periodontal maintenance, and creates force distribution problems.

K, Simple removable appliance in place (2 months).

L, Area now prepared for simple fixed bridge with premolar-size pontic (5 months).

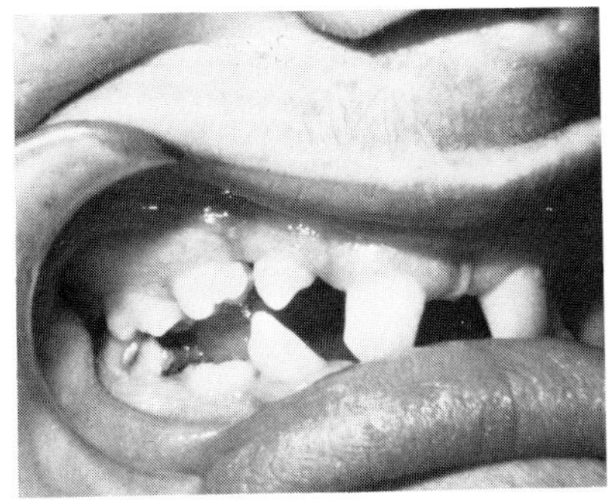

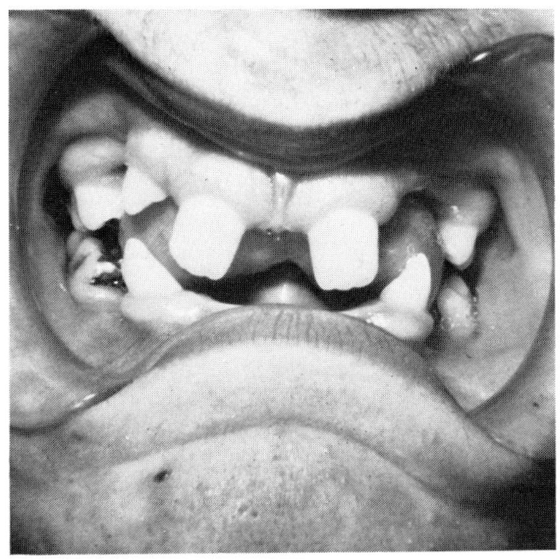

Fig. 8–7 *continued.* *M,* Extremely complex case. This 17-year-old student was missing congenitally all premolars, all lower incisors, upper right lateral incisor, and upper left lateral incisor and canine. Numerous deciduous teeth were retained, but ankylosed, and in some cases, they were buried beneath the tissue. A severe Class II occlusal relationship and malposition of permanent anterior teeth completed the challenge.

M-1. Clinical view as presented.

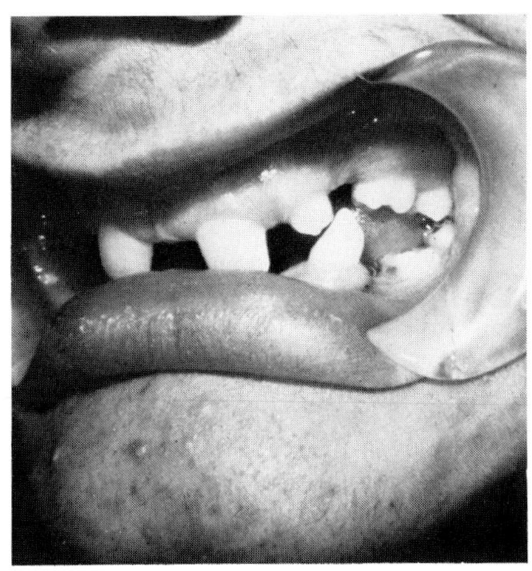

M-1

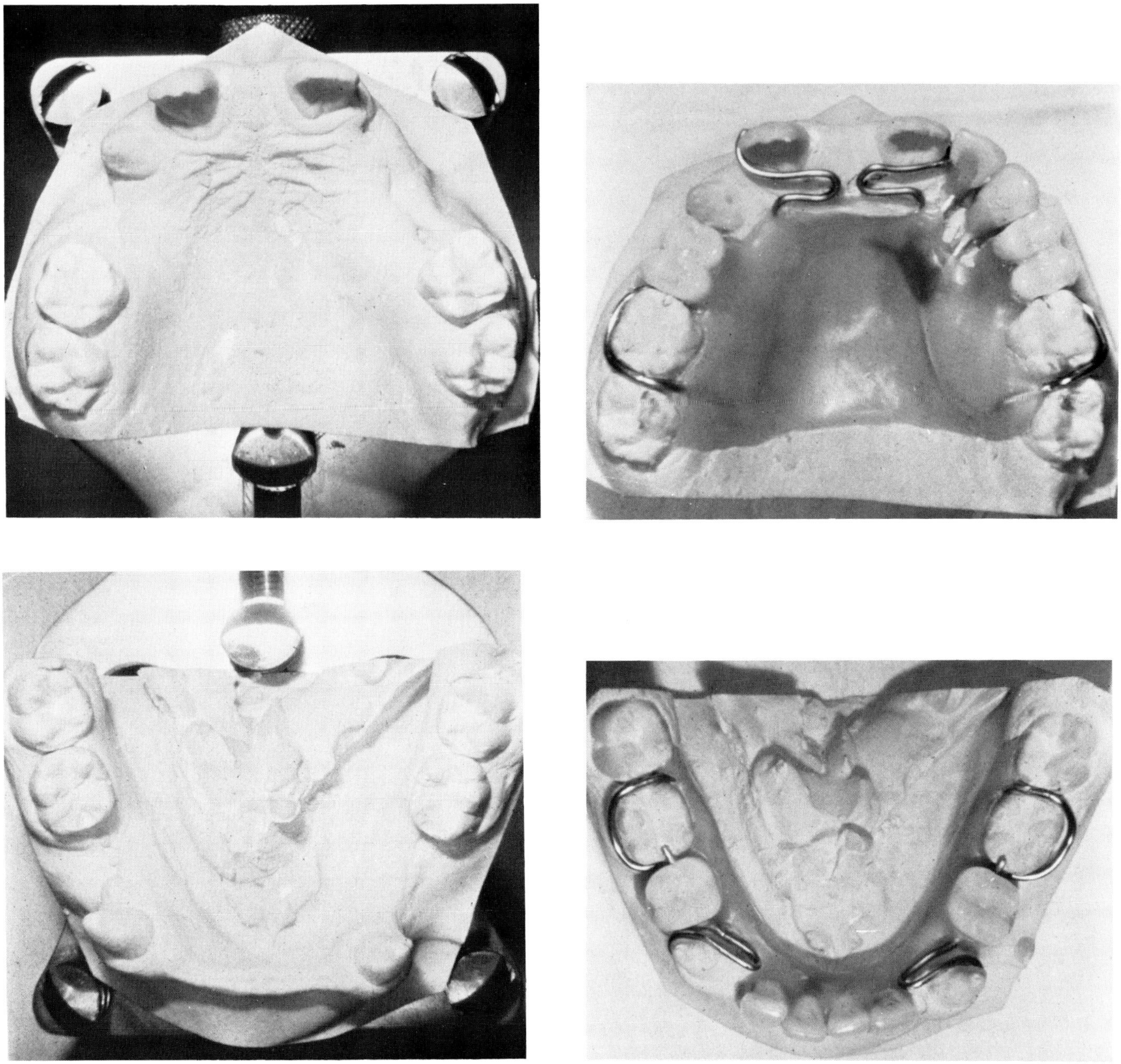

M-2

Fig. 8–7 *continued.* *M-2.* Simple orthodontic appliances were fabricated that doubled as treatment partial dentures. Note upper lateral and canine processed on wires to allow movement as central incisors are drawn together.

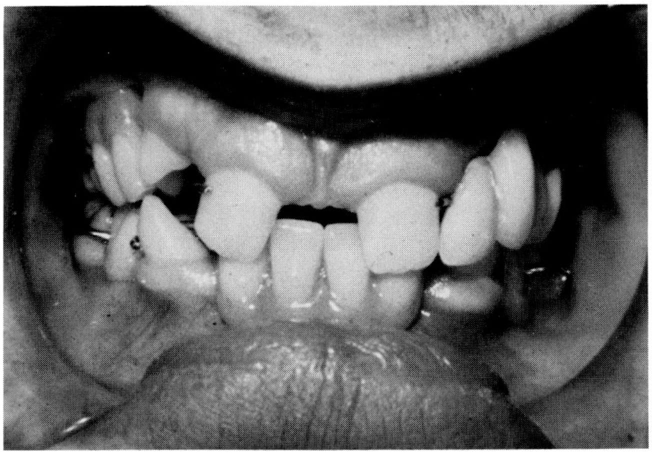

1 mo.

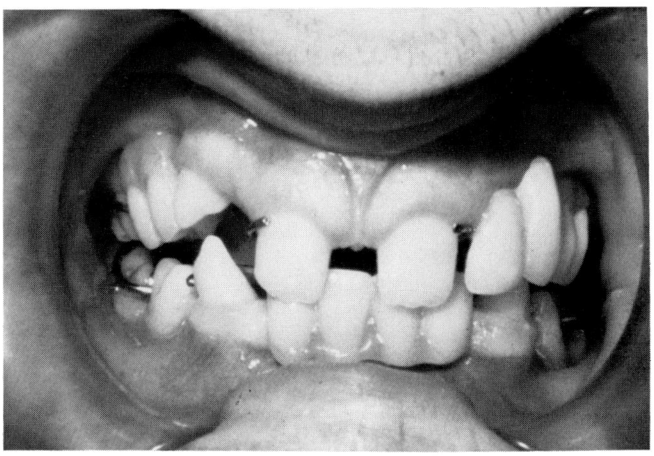

6 mo.

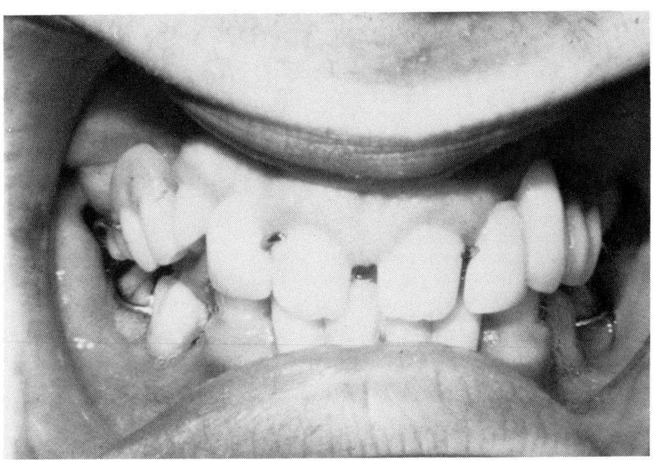

9 mo.

M-3

Fig. 8–7 *continued.* *M-3.* Clinical views of orthodontic progress over 10 months. Note at nine months that another lateral incisor has been added to the appliance. The *psychologic benefits* of having teeth on the appliances *cannot be underestimated.*

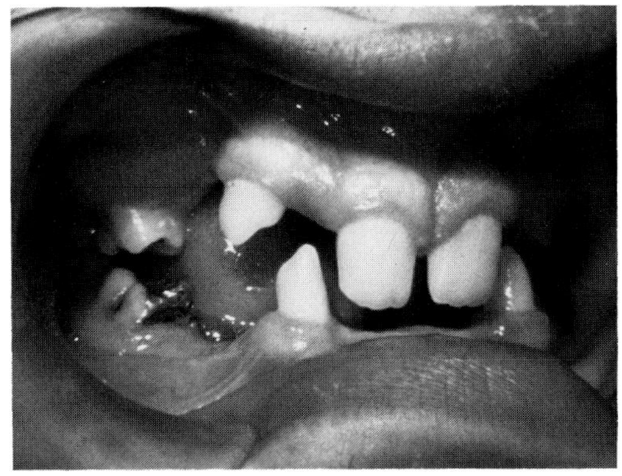

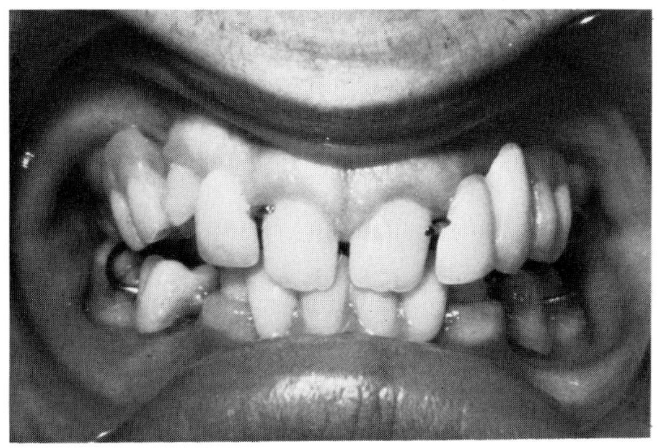

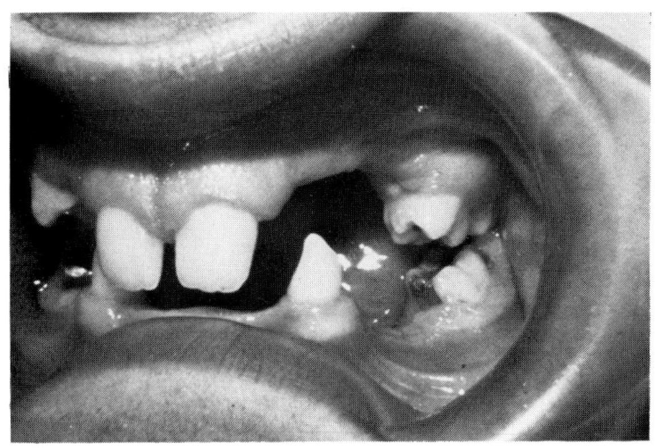

M-4

Fig. 8–7 *continued.* *M-4.* Appliances served as retainers for 3 months, and these clinical views show the situation after teeth had stabilized. While still a complex case, fairly simple orthodontic treatment has greatly simplified it.

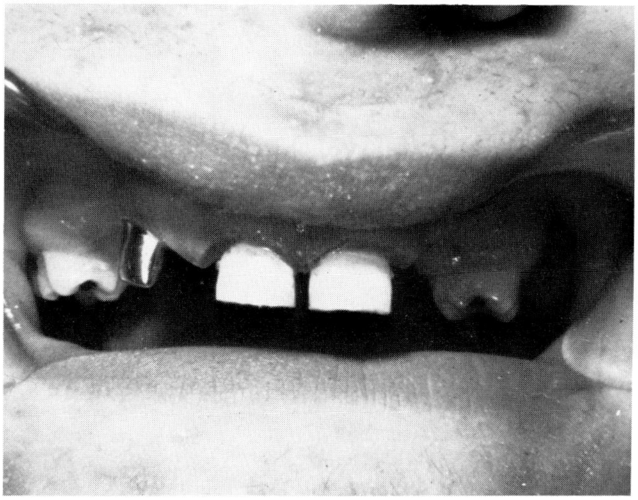

M-5

Fig. 8–7 *continued.* *M-5.* Further simplification was accomplished by shortening the central incisors. Endodontic therapy was done, the gingiva was electrosurgically resected, and the teeth reduced 5 to 6 mm in length. Note the coping placed on upper right canine. Most important, observe the plane of occlusion that has been established in the maxilla.

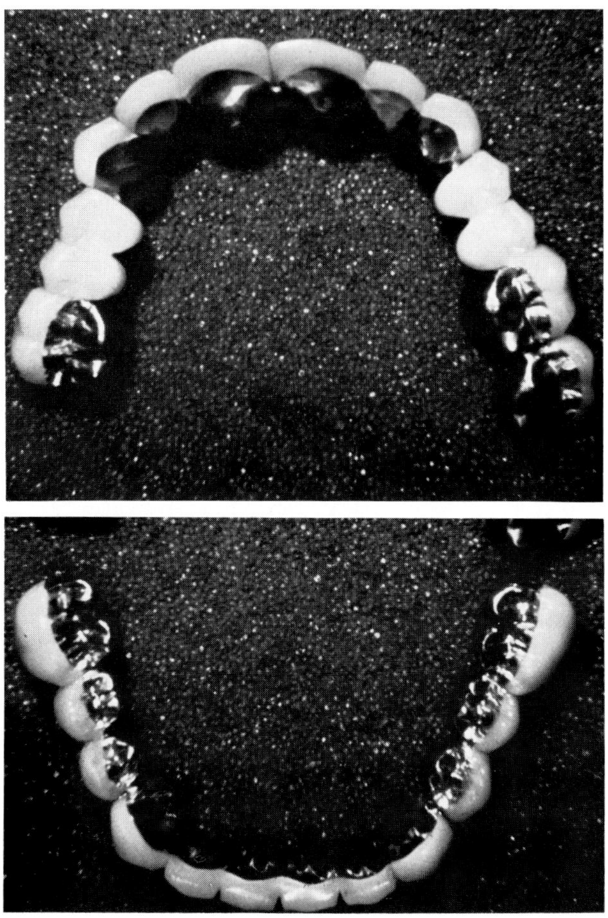

M-6

Fig. 8–7 *continued.* *M-6.* Upper and lower fixed bridges were fabricated using all the key teeth available. Occlusion was designed gnathologically and carried out on fully adjustable articulator (TMJ, using molded articular analogs).

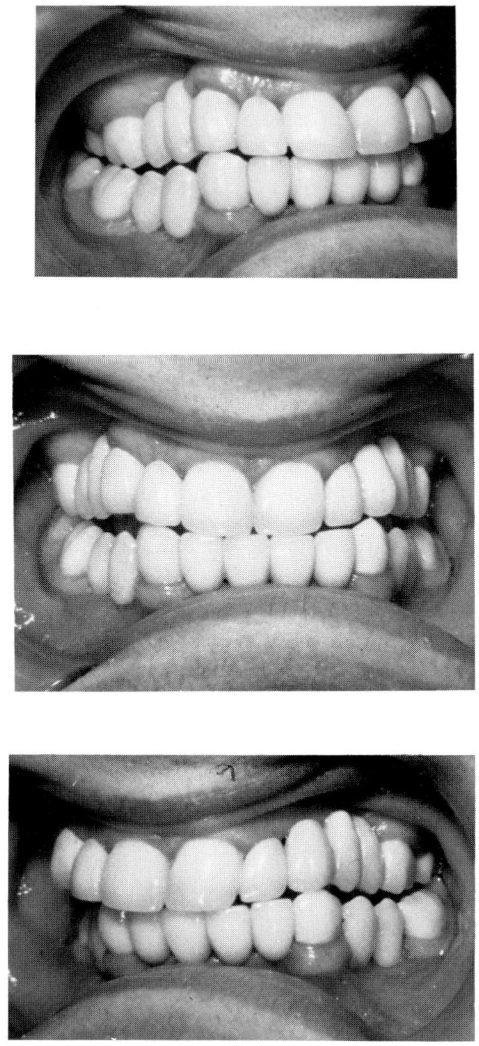

M-7

Fig. 8–7 *continued.* *M-7.* Clinical view of 3-year follow-up illustrating esthetic result and anterior group function guidance.

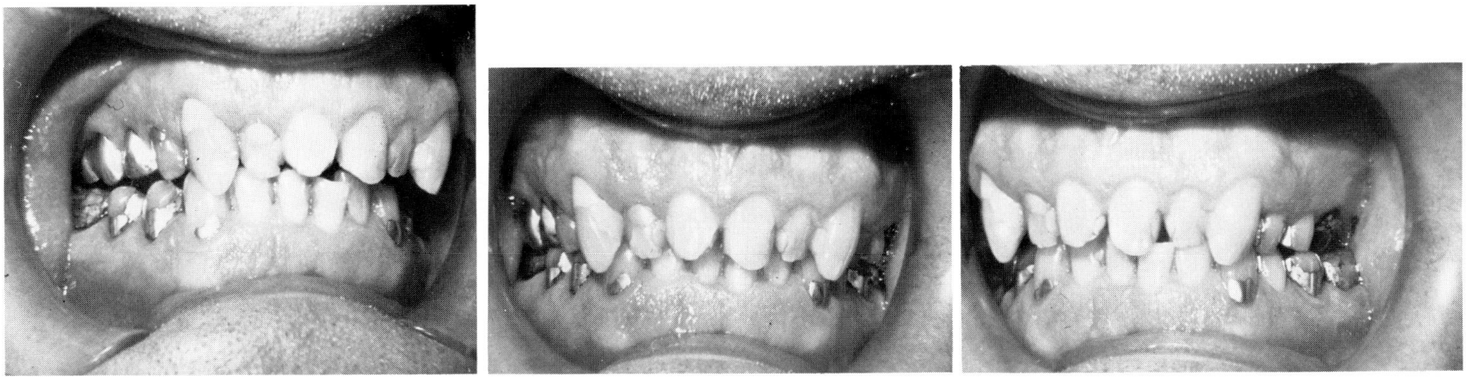

A

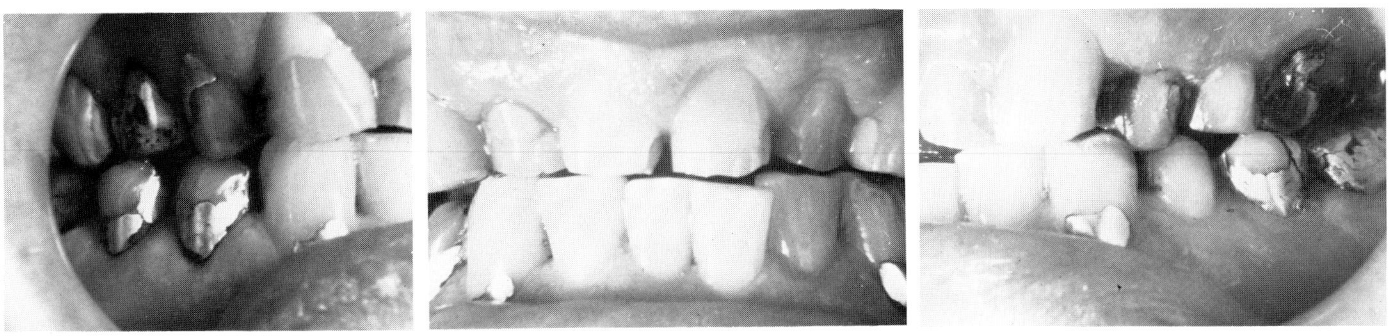

B

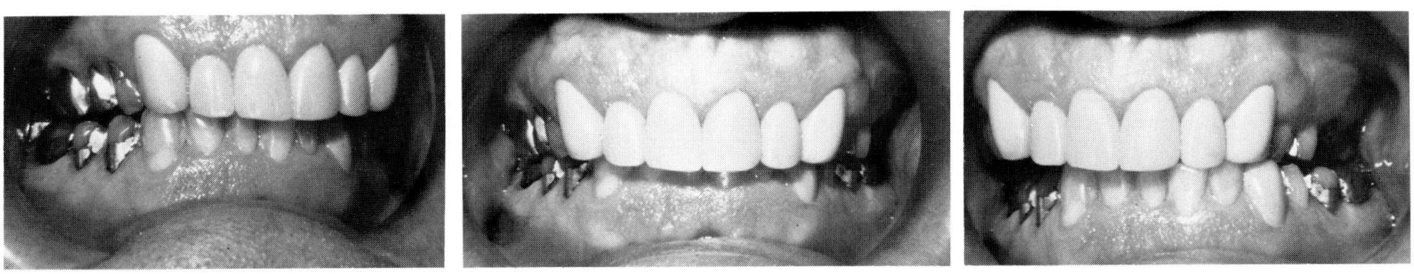

C

Fig. 8–8. Establishment of anterior guidance.

A, Canine guidance is available in this badly debilitated dentition, but caries and abrasion have compromised the incisors.

B, The first step in preparing the upper anterior teeth is the reduction of incisal height. This is done and observed in lateral excursion so that anteriors function together. This planning in the preparation stage facilitates creation of anterior group function in the porcelain-fused-to-gold restorations.

C, Crowns of equal metal thickness and equal porcelain thickness require only minimal fine tuning in the mouth to create a smooth anterior group function.

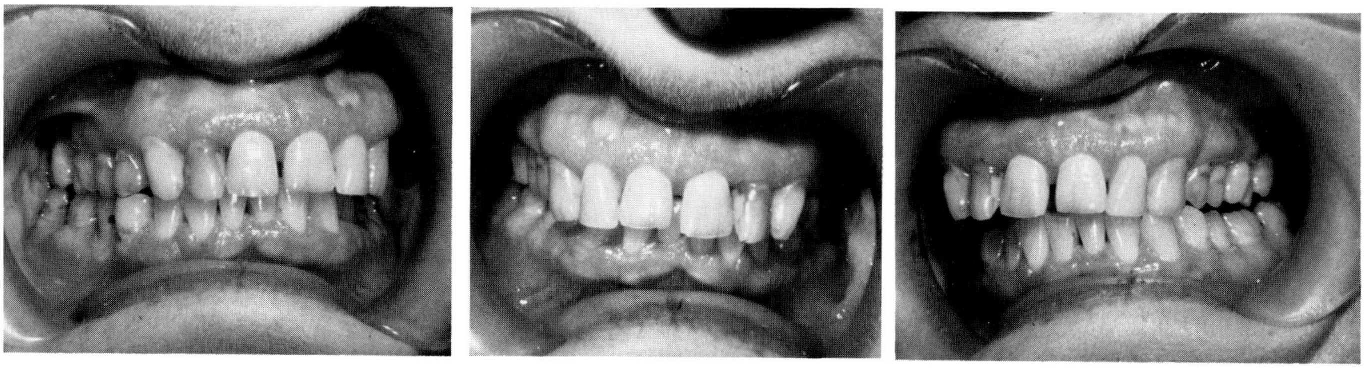

D

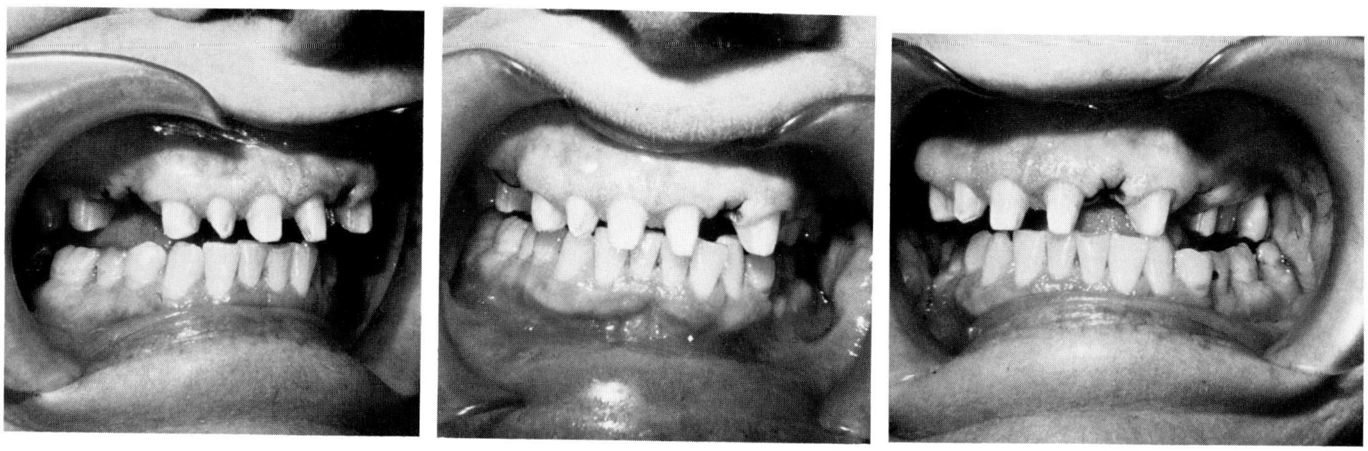

E

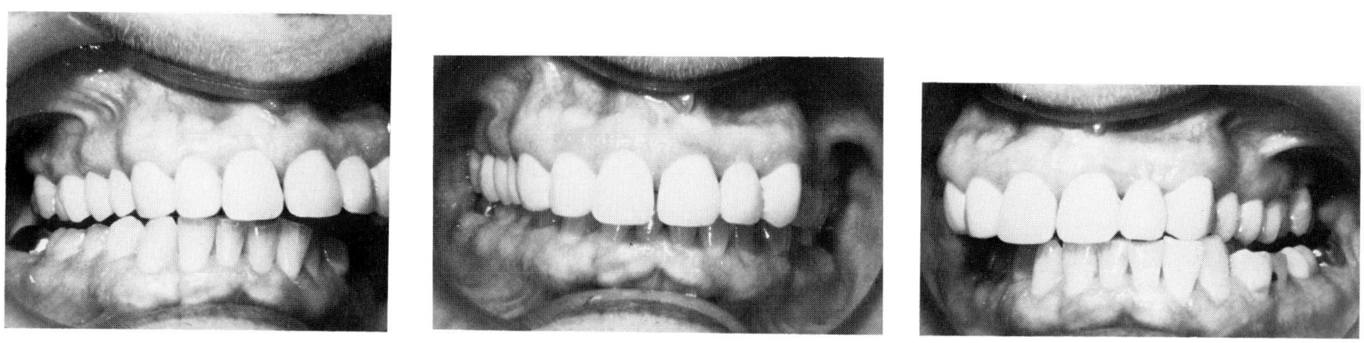

F

Fig. 8–8 *continued.* *D,* This postperiodontal surgery case will require extraction of four upper teeth in which bone loss is related strongly to lateral stresses.

E, Teeth are prepared (and extractions performed) so that anterior teeth have *uniform clearance* in lateral excursion.

F, The reconstructed dentition is then easily built into a therapeutic occlusion, with anterior group function allowing disocclusion of posteriors.

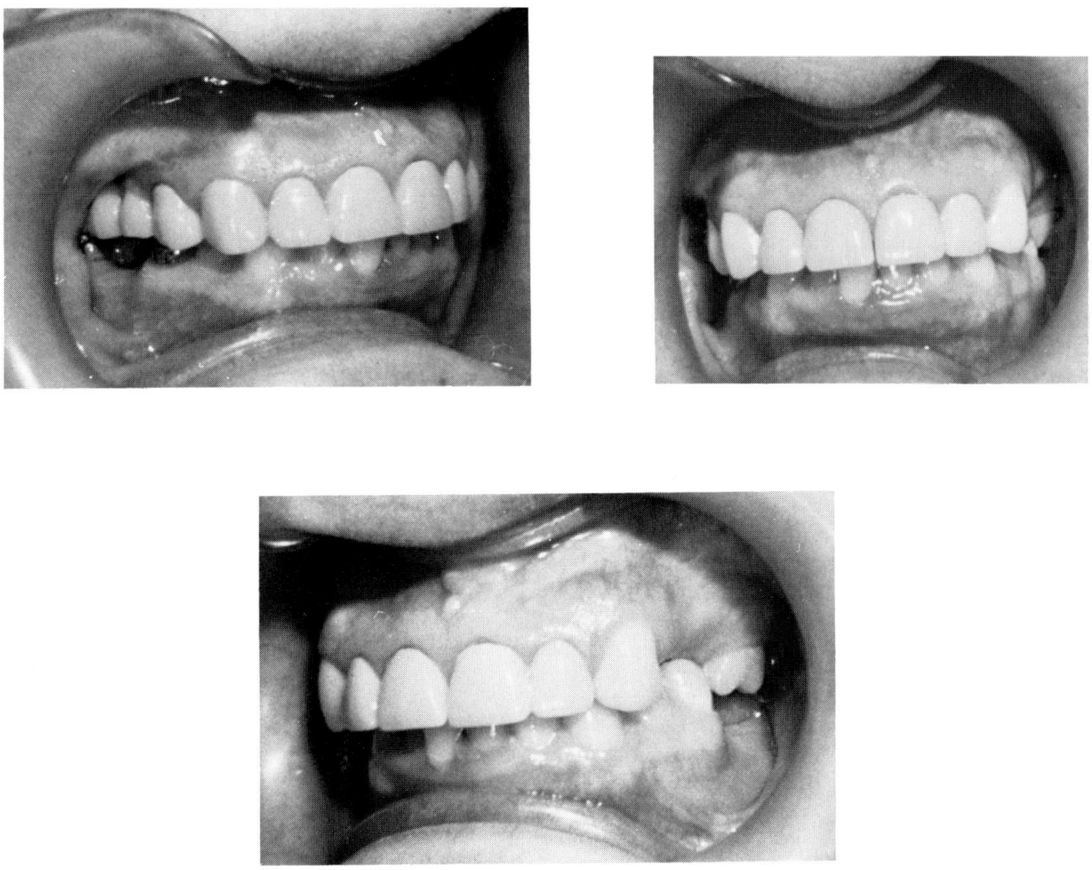

Fig. 8–9. Extensive restorative dentistry done on maxillary arch; this failed due to collapsed vertical dimension that was not considered in restorations.

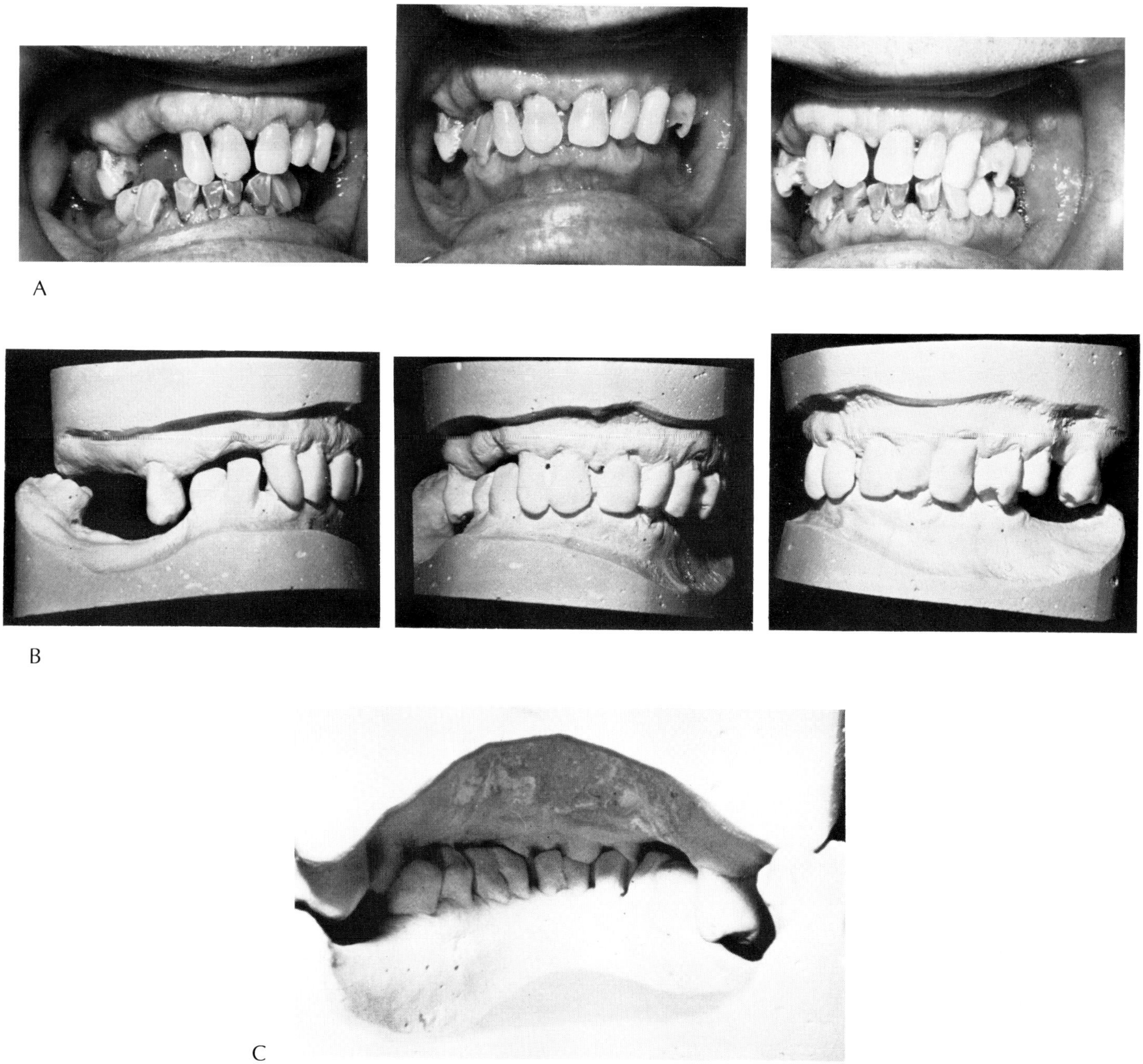

Fig. 8–10. Restoration of lost vertical dimension.

A, This 54-year-old male engineer was seen originally following a coronary episode. His physician recommended he have "needed dental treatment done" prior to catheterization. Obviously, only the most pressing treatment was done, due to the tremendous occlusal problems present.

B, Diagnostic casts further illustrate the loss of vertical dimension owing to tremendous abrasion of the teeth, the Class II relationship, and the loss of posterior support.

C, Viewed from the posterior, the lower anterior teeth can be seen seated in fossas worn into the lingual aspect of upper anteriors.

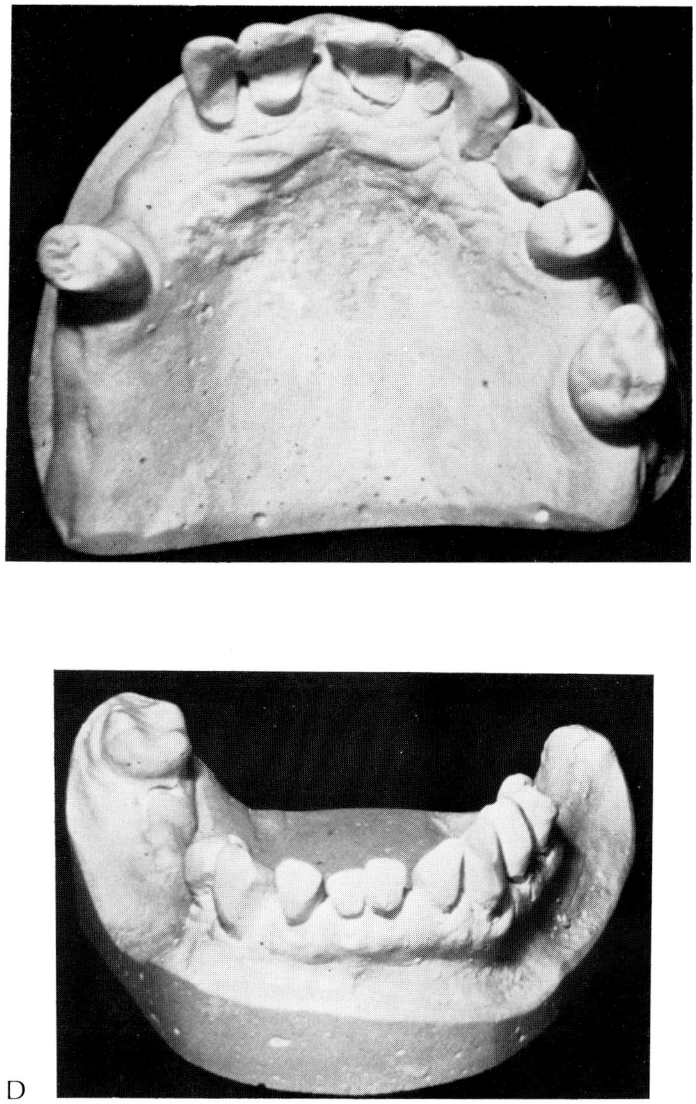

D

Fig. 8–10 *continued.* *D*, Prosthetic reconstruction will obviously require extensive treatment and the restoration of lost vertical dimension.

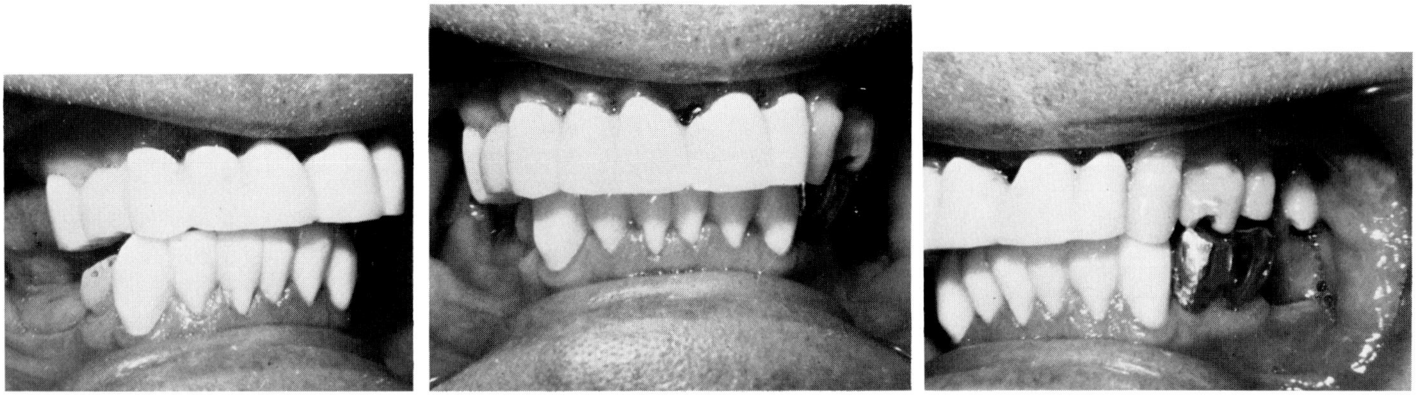

E

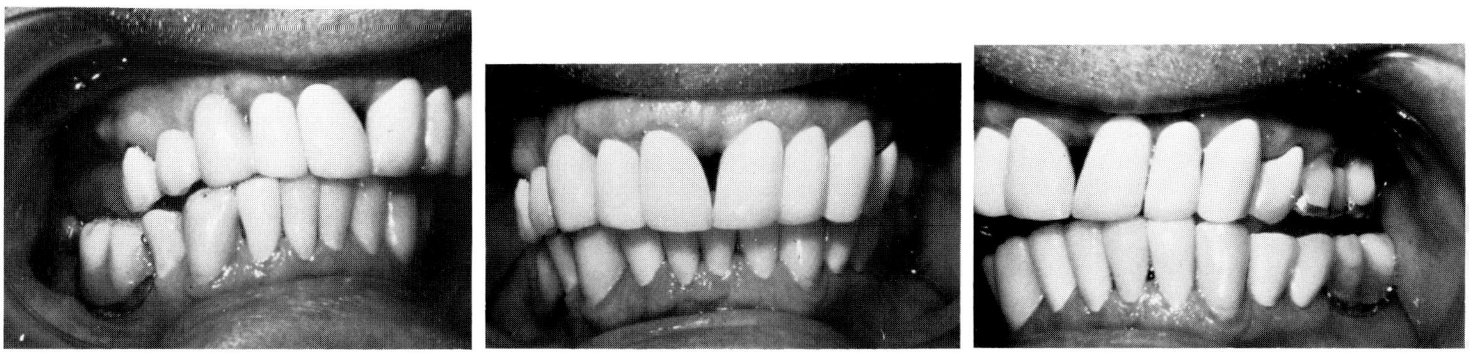

F

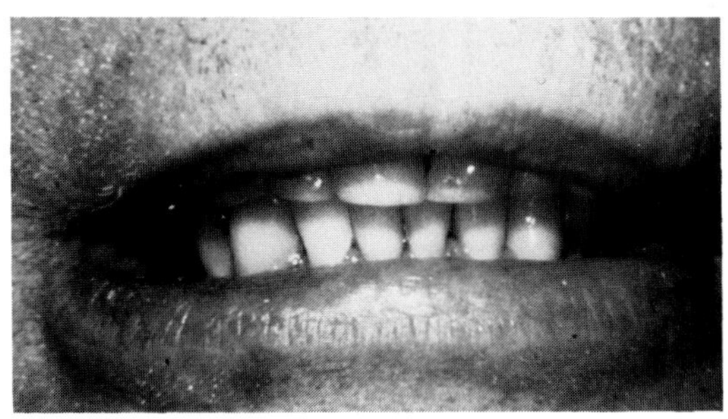

G

Fig. 8–10 *continued.* *E,* Acrylic splints were fabricated, one arch at a time, increasing the vertical dimension sufficiently to place fixed and removable prostheses. Some teeth were shortened considerably where supereruption had probably occurred (e.g. upper right premolar). Cast gold temporary crowns were fabricated for more positive occlusal support at the new vertical dimension (lower left premolars). The splints were employed for a period of 4 months, during which time periodontal surgery was performed in the maxilla. Throughout the 4 months, the patient was closely monitored for comfort and function and for any signs of TMJ or muscle dysfunction at the regained vertical dimension.

F, With good functional response and periodontal healing, preparations were refined as needed and definitive restorations placed. This 5-year follow-up shows the fixed prostheses on the upper arch, ending at the upper right second premolar and lower crowns, some splinted as abutments for a cast-gold base (mucostatic) semiprecision attachment removable partial denture.

G, Despite the extreme length of the upper anterior teeth, esthetic results were quite good, owing to the long upper lip.

lomandibular relationship. Furthermore, the restorations must generally be carried out at once, adding to the complexity of the treatment. The clinical examples in Figure 8–10 will illustrate some possible approaches to the problem of restoring lost vertical dimension.

REFERENCES

1. Clark, J.W., et al.: Clinical Dentistry. Hagerstown, Harper and Row, 1979.
2. Cohn, L.A.: Integrating treatment procedures in occluso-rehabilitation. J. Prosthet. Dent., *7*:511–528, 1957.
3. Eich, F.A.: The role of removable partial dentures in the destruction of the natural dentition. Dent. Clin. North Am., *6*:717–732, 1962.
4. Evans, C.A., et al.: Indications for orthodontic-prosthodontic collaboration in dental treatment. J. Am. Dent. Assoc., *99*:825–830, 1979.
5. Geiger, A., and Hirschfeld, L.: Minor Tooth Movement in General Practice. 3rd ed. St. Louis, C.V. Mosby, 1974.
6. Grieder, A., and Cinotti, W.R.: Periodontal Prosthesis. St. Louis, C.V. Mosby, 1968.
7. Hyman, S., and Schlossberg, A.: Treatment planning. *In* Adult Tooth Movement in General Dentistry. Edited by A. Schlossberg. Philadelphia, W.B. Saunders, 1975.
8. McCracken, W.L.: Partial Denture Construction. St. Louis, C.V. Mosby, 1960.
9. Mitchell, P.: Selection of abutment teeth. *In* Clinical Dentistry. Vol. 4. Edited by J.W. Clark. Hagerstown, Harper and Row, 1979.
10. Muir, J.D., and Read, R.T.: Tooth Movement with Removable Appliances. St. Louis, C.V. Mosby, 1979.
11. Newman, G.V.: Treatment of compromised teeth: A multidisciplinary approach. Am. J. Ortho., *76*:530–537, 1979.
12. Peterson, R.J., et al.: Periodontal considerations for the overdenture. J. Nebr. Dent. Assoc., *55*:15–20, 1978.
13. Schluger, S., Youdelis, R.A., and Page, R.C.: Periodontal Disease: Basic Phenomena, Clinical Management, and Occlusal and Restorative Interrelationships. Philadelphia, Lea & Febiger, 1977.
14. Seide, L.J.: A Dynamic Approach to Restorative Dentistry: The Application of Interdisciplinary Techniques and Management Consideration. Philadelphia, W.B. Saunders, 1980.
15. Steiner, J.C.: Guidelines for selecting teeth to be treated with endodontic therapy. Dent. Clin. North Am., *13*:769–783, 1969.
16. Swoope, C.C.: Prosthodontic considerations in tooth removal. Dent. Clin. North Am., *13*:857–870, 1969.
17. Taintor, J.F. et al.: Endodontic considerations for the overdenture. J. Nebr. Dent. Assoc., *55*:11–14, 1978.
18. Tylman, S.D., and Tylman, S.G.: Theory and Practice of Crown and Bridge Prosthodontics. St. Louis, C.V. Mosby, 1960.
19. Wagenberg, B.D., Eskow, R.N., and Langer, B.: Orthodontic procedures that improve the periodontal prognosis. J.A.D.A., *100*(3):370–373, 1980.
20. Wie, H., et al.: Evaluation of endosseous implant abutments as a base for fixed prosthetic appliances—a preliminary clinical study. J. Oral. Rehabil., *6*:353–363, 1979.

CHAPTER 9

Establishing the Prognosis

The human organism is wonderfully resilient, surviving not only the ravages of dental disease, but dental treatment as well!

In essence, the prognosis is a prediction of the future and at best, an educated guess. For this reason, it is often ignored or glossed over by the dentist. Effective dental treatment planning, however, which strives to develop the most rational, cost-effective approach for the individual patient, requires that a likely prognosis be established. Most patients would like to know the longevity of a given treatment proposal, and the dentist must be prepared to answer those questions intelligently, avoiding answers such as "it will last as long as you care for your teeth properly"; although this may be true, most often it is not. Perhaps the dentist fears that a costly and extensive course of treatment will not be accepted by the patient if he cannot absolutely guarantee its permanence. Patients deserve (and sometimes demand) a more realistic assessment of their oral and dental future and will often proceed with extensive treatment even if that future is bleak. They do so, however, knowing what the score is and acting on the good information provided by the dentist.

What kind of information can the dentist provide when predicting the future? All too often, dentists feel compelled to express the projected life of some restoration or prosthesis in years; this is generally foolhardy, unless one has a crystal ball. The prognosis should outline, in general terms, the future outlook based on factors we can observe and discuss with the patient. We must define what we consider to be the end point. Taking, for example, a single silver-amalgam restoration placed on a molar tooth, we can attempt to establish a prognosis. We might say that such a restoration can be expected to provide good function, comfort, and cleansibility, and that in itself is a prognosis. If we attempt to affix some time factor to the treatment, we must ask whether we are predicting the useful life of that particular restoration or of the tooth itself. Dental treatment is, after all, a means to an end. The patient must understand that lifetime retention of teeth does not necessarily imply lifetime retention of any given dental restoration, but that various dental treatments, restorations, and prostheses might enhance the outlook for a lifelong dentition.

If we must predict the useful life of a specific component of treatment, such as the single silver-amalgam restoration just cited, we must consider and discuss with the patient the various ways in which the restoration's end point might be reached.

First of all, the restoration's end point might be brought about by *technical failure*. If the restoration has insufficient retention, gross open margins, or is in such hyperocclusion that it must be removed or ground through for relief, the end point is immediate and hence, is the dentist's responsibility. Any prognosis should assume that the attending dentist will perform with competence and integrity in this regard. Competence implies that treatment that meets minimum standards of clinical acceptability will be rendered. Integrity demands that, should the treatment fall short of such standards for any reason, it would be corrected before the treatment is considered complete.

Assuming that all standards have been met in placing the amalgam restoration, the restoration can be lost due to *early mechanical failure*—breakage of either the material or the surrounding tooth structure—and such mishaps can occur even to sound, unrestored teeth. Obviously, the patient should be made aware of this potentiality, especially if the amalgam restoration in question is large or extensive, and the remaining tooth walls relatively thin. Indeed, the dentist must apprise the patient when a casting would better restore a given tooth, so that an informed choice based on relative cost and prognosis can be made.

The end point of a restoration can also be achieved by *uncontrolled dental disease*. If the restoration in question was placed to restore a carious lesion, recurrent caries at a margin or elsewhere on the tooth may bring about the end point for that restoration. Likewise, should severe periodontal disease result in the loss of the entire tooth, the restoration would no longer be of much service. The patient's responsibility is obvious; however, it is first the dentist's responsibility to apprise the patient of the situation and to provide the patient with the necessary counselling and mechanical training to control his dental disease (see Chap. 3).

The goal of every restorative dentist is to see his restoration reach an end point *after years of rigorous and constant service*. We must accept, and the patient must be made to understand, that the delicate, miniature mechanisms we place in the mouth must withstand tremendous forces and a hostile environment in which constant moisture, bacterial action, and dramatic temperature changes never cease. Consider that, in a period of 1 year, our amalgam restoration must withstand well over 1000 mastication sessions (assuming three meals and/or snacks per day) and around a half a million bracing occlusal contacts during swallowing (assuming 1200 to 2000 swallows per day). Temperature gradients from 0° F (hard ice cream from the deep freeze) to 200 ° F (hot coffee) may alternate as our patient has dessert, whereupon any organized plaque will immediately begin dumping acids on and around our amalgam within seconds of the ice cream entering the mouth. When a 10-year-old amalgam restoration breaks or is to be replaced due to marginal ditching, surface roughness, corrosion, or wear, we must consider the 11,000 mastication sessions and 5 million swallowing contacts it has survived and marvel with the patient at this minor miracle of dental science, rather than explain to an irate patient why the permanent filling must now be replaced.

Just when, under the best conditions, any given restoration or prosthesis is likely to wear out depends on many factors, which will be discussed shortly.

Finally, the endpoint of a restoration may be reached when *the restored tooth (if deciduous) exfoliates or when the patient dies*. Without being macabre, lifetime restorations are easiest to achieve on terminally ill patients. Conversely, the young, healthy patient must appreciate the likelihood of outliving a number of successive dental restorations no matter how well executed they were.

With this as a background, we can return to the problem of predicting the useful life of a given restoration, If, with the patient, we hypothetically rule out the end points caused by incompetence, accident, disease, or death, we can concentrate on estimating the time it will take a restoration to wear out. We may then wish to give the patient a time, in years, at which we would consider the treatment a "success." Physicians, for example, when assessing treatment of malignancy, consider 5 years without recurrence to be a cure. It is possible, in the dental setting, to make conservative estimates of the minimum, useful life of a restoration with the expectation that its actual service may be considerably longer. Indeed, if a course of treatment is carried out and the patient remains healthy and effectively restored for 5 years, the prognosis for continued health and function is excellent.

Finally, in establishing a prognosis, it may be neither necessary nor desirable to attach a specific life span to the treatment and/or restorations; rather, we should attempt to relate the likely effects of the proposed or completed treatment on the long-term goals established prior to treatment planning and to rate the apparent chances of the treatment achieving those goals. For example, if the long-term goal is retention of all the teeth, a given course of treatment might result in a poor, fair, good, or excellent prognosis for achieving that goal independent of the useful life of any given component of the treatment. The prognosis can and must be continually reassessed and updated. Observation over time is the most useful predictive tool, and a dismal prognosis may turn bright, or a good prognosis become dismal as time passes.

FACTORS IN THE PROGNOSIS

In establishing a prognosis, many factors must be considered that will enhance or hinder the final outcome. These plusses and minuses must be considered for each patient, because no two people are alike, and seemingly identical treatment done for seemingly identical problems may present completely opposite prognoses based on individual factors. I will discuss certain factors that should be considered highly significant in establishing the prognosis.

Patient Behavior

Patient behavior is at once the most significant and least controllable factor in the dental prognosis. As discussed in Chapters 2 and 3, the ability and willingness to control plaque determines whether oral health will be maintained, or whether caries and/or periodontal disease processes will continue unabated. The maintenance of a healthful, relatively noncariogenic diet is also totally the patient's responsibility. Home-use fluoride regimens, the proper use and maintenance of dental appliances (such as night guards and removable partial dentures), and the curtailment of potentially harmful, conscious oral habits are just some of the areas that are under the sole control of the patient.

The periodic recall visit to the dentist, an essential element in any comprehensive, long-term oral-health strategy, is also dependent on patient commitment and cooperation. The most sophisticated, computerized recall system, using both phone and mail reminders, will not ensure a patient's return to the dental office.

It is essential, then, that the dentist involve the patient intellectually (see Chap. 2) from the first day of their relationship and emphasize the patient's vital role in establishing and maintaining his oral health. Assuming that the dentist has discharged that responsibility effectively, we may attempt to predict patient behavior based on a number of criteria, including past experience, present behavior, and future commitment.

Past Experience

What level of health maintenance was being achieved when the patient was first seen? Was the patient brushing regularly and using floss? Did the patient admit high frequency of sugar intake? Had the patient sought regular preventive care, at least annually, or merely when symptoms arose?

While we must not prejudge behavior on the basis of past experience, we must realize that some habit patterns are difficult to change, and relapse into old habits is always a possibility. Especially significant is the regularity of preventive maintenance visits. We can reinforce plaque control and good dietary habits only if the patient returns on a regular, periodic basis. Likewise, small problems can be dealt with simply if they are diagnosed in early stages. Simple mechanical maintenance—smoothing a chipped tooth or restoration or adjusting an appliance—is possible on a regular recall regimen and can greatly enhance the prognosis.

A track record of poor oral-health maintenance and/or sporadic dental care detracts from the prognosis, while a history of daily home care and regular recall visits enhances it.

Present Behavior

Behavioral change, while difficult, is not impossible. Often the most satisfying moments in dentistry arise from the realization that, with our assistance, a patient has effectively exchanged oral disease for oral health, making those adjustments in lifestyle that will ensure freedom from major dental problems and greatly enhance the prognosis of any treatment or restoration. If our course of dental treatment is unhurried, we have the opportunity to observe and encourage such new behavior as novelty develops into habit. Such gradual and apparently sustained changes in behavior bode well for the overall prognosis. On the other hand, if the patient is unwilling or unable to achieve effective health maintenance while undergoing dental treatment, the prognosis may be very poor. If the dentist must push the plaque aside to place a restoration, it is unlikely that the restoration will succeed; hence, the overall prognosis is dismal.

Future Commitment

Assuming that present behavior is at least reasonably effective in maintaining oral health, we must assess the strength of the patient's future commitment to that end. If, for example, a patient has grudgingly accepted plaque control as a prerequisite to the desired dental treatment, the strength of the future commitment might be very dubious, and the overall prognosis will be guarded. A discussion with the patient about the need for periodic recall visits may reveal enthusiasm and commitment or apathy and resistance, and the effect on the prognosis can be assessed accordingly.

In our own dedication to oral health for ourselves and our patients, we may, in effect, coerce the patient into commitments he cannot or will not keep. Indeed, if we create standards of plaque control, dietary discipline, or frequency of recall visits that the patient is not prepared to accept, we may ensure failure. Being incapable of achieving what for him are unrealistic goals, the patient's tendency is to give up entirely, to quit trying, and to not return to the dental office.

The future commitment must be the patient's rational assessment of what he feels capable of doing, even if it is less than ideal. It might be better for a patient to commit to every-other-day flossing and usually succeed, than to commit to daily flossing and generally fail and become discouraged. Annual recalls visits, if they are kept by the patient, are preferable to 6-month checkups if the latter are rejected by the patient and several years go by before he returns. Having established a reasonable future commitment, the overall influence on the prognosis can be assessed.

Host Resistance

Host resistance is the innate resistance to injury or disease, regardless of behavior, that is unique to each individual. Why, in the presence of bacterial plaque, some individuals remain caries free, with little or no gingival inflammation or loss of attachment, we do not know. Why, even with relatively good maintenance, other individuals succumb rapidly and dramatically to oral disease, deteriorating almost before our very eyes, we do not fully understand. We must, in rationally establishing a prognosis, accept the fact that some patients will survive with or without us, and others will be forever on the brink of debilitation and disease despite our best efforts on their behalf. Although we do not understand the reasons for this, we can at least assess host resistance using two clinical yardsticks, each requiring a good history and each related to the other.

Apparent Progress Rate of Existing Disease

If we have the opportunity to observe a particular patient over a period of years, we can assess the progress rate of oral disease rather well. For example, the patient who, in 6 months to a year, develops multiple carious lesions has a much more rapid rate of disease than one who develops a similar number of lesions over 3 to 5 years. If we follow two periodontally involved patients over time, we might see one whose pocket depths increase and bone levels decrease noticeably from year to year and another who, while initially presenting with a similar condition, might progress very little in the same time.

Often, however, we do not have the luxury of such continual surveillance and must employ a history to assess the progress rate of existing disease. A patient presenting with many carious lesions who reports having had regular dental care (checkups and treatment) on at least an annual basis shows a greater disease-progress rate than another patient who also has a number of carious lesions but who has not had dental care for 5 or 10 years. Obviously, the size and extent of the lesions as a function of time are also significant.

The net effect of the progress rate is that the prognosis is good for patients whose disease rate is apparently slow and not as good for those patients whose disease rate has been rapid. While striking changes in oral health and disease are possible after treatment and behavior modification, the innate host resistance must be taken into account when establishing the prognosis.

Age vs. Level of Disease

This criterion, while similar to the first, differs in that it dwells less on the rate of existing disease states than on the progress of oral disease over the patient's lifetime. This criterion has long been employed in assessing the periodontal outlook and has been described in various terms. One of those terms is "bone factor," the amount of bone loss relative to the patient's age. Given a typical case of periodontal disease with pockets and bone loss, the prognosis may be dismal if the patient is in his twenties, poor if in his thirties, fair if in his forties, good if in his fifties, excellent if in his sixties, and the patient may require little or no treatment if he is in his seventies. This is due to the fact that periodontal disease often starts early in life and progresses slowly over long periods of time. If, for example, a patient exhibits 20% horizontal bone loss around the first permanent molars at age 55, we must, in assessing the prognosis, realize that the loss may have occurred over a period of nearly 50 years. The prognosis is better when a given disease level is seen at older ages (assuming a reasonably healthy patient) and is worse when that level is reached earlier in life.

This criterion is more applicable to periodontal disease than caries, but it could be applied to either in some cases. A history is necessary, but it may be misleading, since periodontal disease may be present for some time and go unnoticed by the patient and undiagnosed by the dentist.

Physiologic Environment

Just as significant in the prognosis as patient behavior and innate host resistance is the oral environment that bears on the treatment we have rendered. In this discussion of physiologic environment, we can consider local biologic factors, mechanical factors, and general systemic factors.

Local Biologic Factors

Local biologic factors include the patient's musculature, oral habits, and periodontal status.

Heavy, well-developed muscles of mastication and perioral groups may create a worse prognosis, because they may put greater stresses on the teeth, the periodontium, and any restorations or prostheses we may have placed. A normal or a delicate musculature may improve the prognosis.

Clenching, grinding (bruxism), or uncontrolled tongue or lip habits worsen the prognosis, whereas the absence of such habits improves it. Indeed, the size and tonus of the oral and perioral musculature are often related to parafunctional muscle activity, such as bruxism. The prognosis may be bolstered through muscle retraining, protective appliances, and extra strength designed into restorations and prostheses.

Following definitive therapy, the resulting periodontal status bears heavily on the prognosis. Approximate bone level, cleansibility of all sulcular areas (assuming pocket elimination will be carried out as necessary), and integrity of the gingival attachment must be considered. A periodontal result that promises reasonably good bone levels, readily cleansible architecture, and intact, attached gingivae offers support to the prognosis. The prognosis deteriorates if any or all of these factors are lacking.

Even in the absence of frank periodontal disease, the nature of the periodontium affects the prognosis. The patient with copious bone support, and a broad band of attached gingiva will have a more favorable long-term prognosis than one with thin, friable tissues, narrow, attached gingiva, and prominent roots belying thin bone coverage.

Mechanical Factors

In terms of pure mechanical advantage or disadvantage, we can relate the prognosis to the number and position of key teeth in the dental arches (see Chap. 8). Mechanically, an intact dental arch with many key teeth will have a better prognosis than a restored arch with few or no real key teeth. A three-unit fixed bridge with two sound abutments and one pontic is mechanically more stable than a five- or six-unit bridge with the same two abutments.

Occlusal relationships also affect the mechanical factors. A normal healthy Class I occlusion may produce fewer mechanical stresses on dentition and restorations than a Class II malocclusion with deep anterior overbite.

Obviously, this factor is closely related to the biologic factors just discussed in terms of the potential stresses to be applied. In addition to the musculature, oral habits, and periodontal status of the patient, we can also consider the great difference in mechanical stress when one arch is edentulous. This is an advantage for the arch with teeth (whether restored or replaced) as less force is generated; at the same time, it is a disadvantage to the edentulous arch since greater forces may be applied to the ridge under a full prosthesis when it is opposed by natural dentition. The net effect on the prognosis often depends upon which arch is edentulous. An upper full denture may do very well against lower restored dentition, while a lower full denture often presents great mechanical problems, difficulties and stresses to the ridge tissues, when it is opposed by upper natural dentition.

Whatever the situation, greater mechanical stresses on teeth, soft tissues, restorations, and prostheses generally lessen the chances of a good prognosis, while a mechanical environment that is more harmonious and nonstressful enhances them.

Systemic Factors

The general systemic health and well-being of the patient influences the oral environment and thereby, the prognosis of dental treatment.

A healthy, well-adjusted individual may have a better dental prognosis than a debilitated, neurotic individual. Systemic diseases and disorders are often reflected in the oral cavity by lowered resistance to disease, impaired healing processes, and lessened ability to maintain a plaque-free mouth. Problems such as diabetes, thyroid disorders, rheumatoid arthritis, Parkinson's disease, and various malignancies are but a few of the systemic problems that detract from a good prognosis. Heavy smoking generally will also lessen the chances of a good prognosis. On the other hand, a history of good health or of rapid and full recovery from past diseases may improve the prognosis.

Quality of Treatment

Obviously, the quality of treatment bears heavily on its prognosis and should be considered in two categories: the type of treatment approach selected, and the care, skill, and judgment applied in its execution. Both of these factors depend upon the joint decisions and actions of dentist and patient.

Selected Treatment Approach

The prognosis is often in direct relation to the cost or quality of the selected treatment approach. Typically, we might consider the prognosis in an operative dentistry treatment plan to be better if cast gold restorations are employed, but less favorable if large silver amalgams are placed instead, and this is generally true. Quality and durability of materials play an important role in prognosis. Glazed porcelain facings will generally outlast acrylic, cast onlays will generally outlast pin-retained amalgams, and cast-gold crowns will generally outlast stainless-steel shell crowns. However, there may be situations in which the "quality" treatment has a poorer prognosis than an alternative approach. Using a continuous, full-arch fixed bridge to retain five or six periodontally weakened teeth is a risky procedure, and the prognosis would likely be better (in terms of long-term use) with a full denture or an overdenture.

The patient and dentist must often select a treatment approach that satisfies certain criteria (cost, esthetics, comfort, longevity) but may sacrifice others. The selection of a course of treatment based on the patient's goals, desires, finances, and lifestyle (see Chap. 2) will influence the prognosis both in terms of the useful life of the restorations and prostheses employed and in the overall retention of teeth.

Level of Execution

The care, skill, and judgment applied in dental treatment will vary greatly among different dentists, and at given times and situations, will vary for the individual dentist. Many factors influence the dentist's level of execution. Obviously, no two dentists possess the same native ability or the same standards of excellence, quality of judgment, or concern for the patient's well-being. Clinical results will vary greatly among dentists, and the prognosis will reflect the relative level of a dentist's performance. Just as significant are the day-to-day variations in execution of any given dentist. Assuming that every dentist has some optimal performance level, that performance can be compromised by fatigue (last patient of a long day), emotional distress (marital crisis), physical discomfort (prodromal symptoms of head cold, incipient diarrhea), or any number of other impairments.

Working conditions also greatly affect execution levels, especially those inherent to the given patient. A patient may be willing and able to cooperate fully and have a readily accessible oral cavity of good size. Another patient may consciously or unconsciously resist treatment procedures, have a small mouth or a large tongue, gag easily, and make even the simplest dental procedure a monumental task.

The net effect of all these factors is an execution level that may vary from being barely acceptable to being undeniably excellent, and the prognosis is likely to reflect the level of execution. The dentist's critical self-assessment is essential in establishing a prognosis, as is an objective, nonjudgmental evaluation of the patient's treatability.

The factors discussed here are not necessarily the only ones bearing on the prognosis of dental treatment, nor can each factor be given equal or consistent weight when assessing its long-term effects. A single negative factor might result in failure of the entire effort, but long-term success might be achieved even in the face of many negative factors. Assessing the factors is still critical, however, both in establishing a prognosis for and with the patient and in identifying potential threats to the treatment plan. Anticipation of future problems allows us to plan for them and hence, to protect the overall prognosis.

PLANNING FOR FAILURE

It can be said that the prudent practitioner always hopes for success but plans for failure. By carefully assessing the factors that influence the prognosis, we can identify possible sources of failure. We must then attempt to design into the treatment plan some "escape routes," alternative approaches that can be used without having to redo or start from scratch. Indeed, the ability to recover from such failures often allows the dentist to propose and the patient to accept some rather high-risk treatment approaches that, if successful, will provide optimal comfort, function, and esthetics even if for a limited period of time. When and if some of the components fail, the alternative approach can be implemented with a minimum of time, money, and trauma to the patient. This is treatment planning at its most sophisticated; it must be done with great caution and full patient involvement, and if applied judiciously, it is an important tool in dental treatment planning. Several strategies in planning for failure—some rather simple, some fairly grandiose—will be discussed.

Provisional Splinting of Questionable Teeth

Following periodontal therapy, we often encounter teeth with marked bone loss and extreme mobility. Provisional splinting with acrylic temporary bridges or multitooth splints may allow better evaluation prior to definitive restoration (Fig. 9–1). Such splinting, by reducing occlusal stresses (especially lateral stresses), may allow consolidation of the periodontium over several months or longer. Periodic removal of the splint allows evaluation of the gingival attachment by probing and mobility testing. Similar results can be obtained by wire ligature and acrylic extracoronal splinting, but there are some limitations in terms of effective hygiene and ease of removal for evaluation.

In some cases, interim intracoronal splinting can be done with the use of "A" splints, which are cast or twisted-wire arches laid directly into grooves cut mesio-occlusal-distal in large posterior alloys. The splints are luted into the grooves with a liquid mix of composite resin. Alternatively, the teeth can be prepared and based, and the splint placed into the prepared teeth with composite alone (after acid-etching). Effective hygiene can be a problem in this application, and repair and maintenance can be very time consuming.

Long-Term Splinting

Long-term splinting of mobile or periodontally compromised teeth has many applications. Some authors question whether splinting is indicated for posttreatment mobility—that is, whether mobility is a problem as such. A typical example of such splinting is the application of wire ligatures and acrylic to mobile lower anteriors after periodontal therapy. Without a doubt, the teaming of such teeth may make

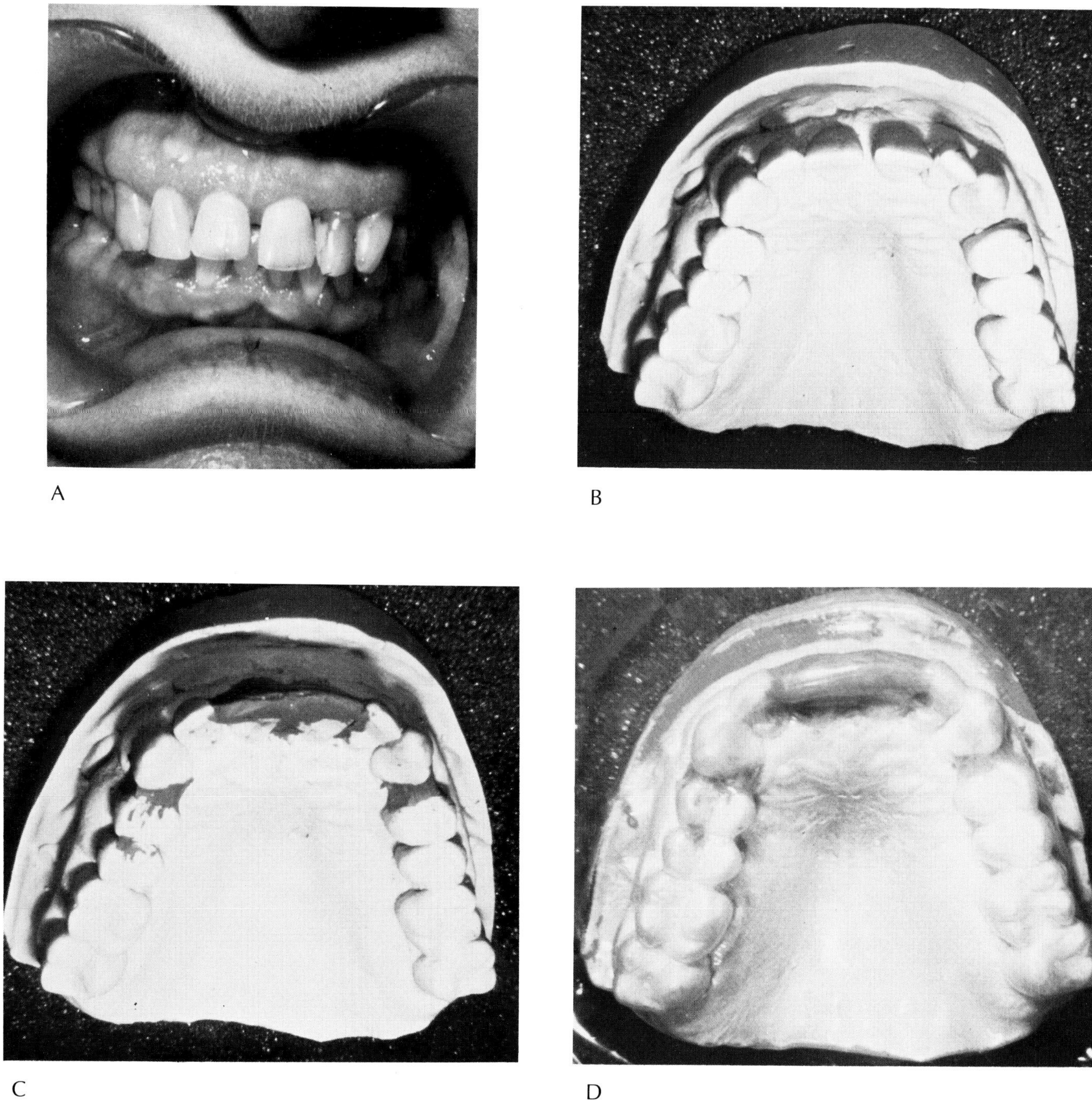

Fig. 9–1. Provisional splinting. *A*, This 52-year-old nurse had severe periodontal involvement, and extraction of a number of maxillary teeth was planned. *B*, Maxillary diagnostic cast. *C*, Open proximal areas blocked out. *D*, Thin celluloid "shim" is vacuformed over model.

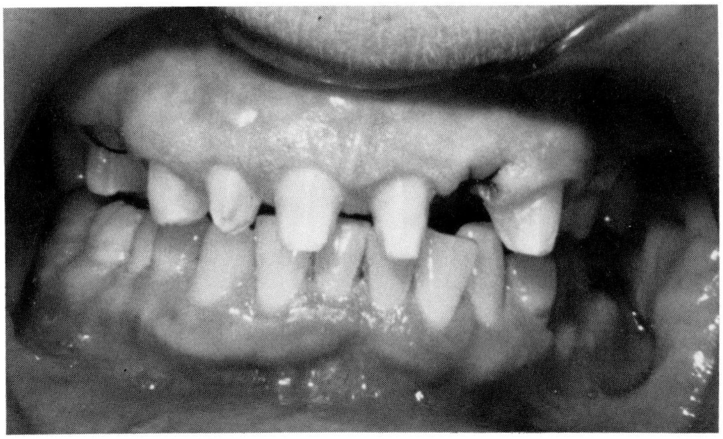

E

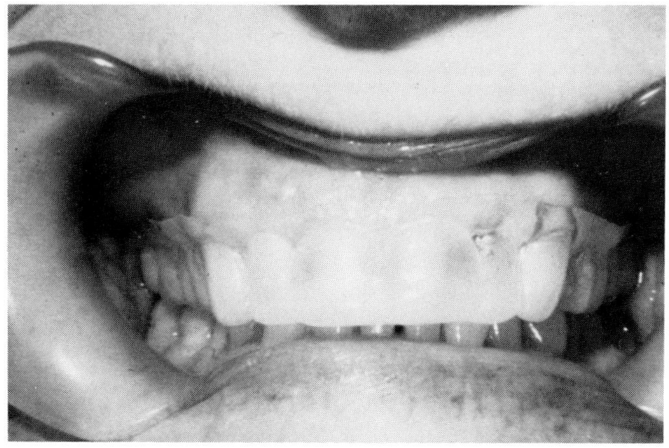

F

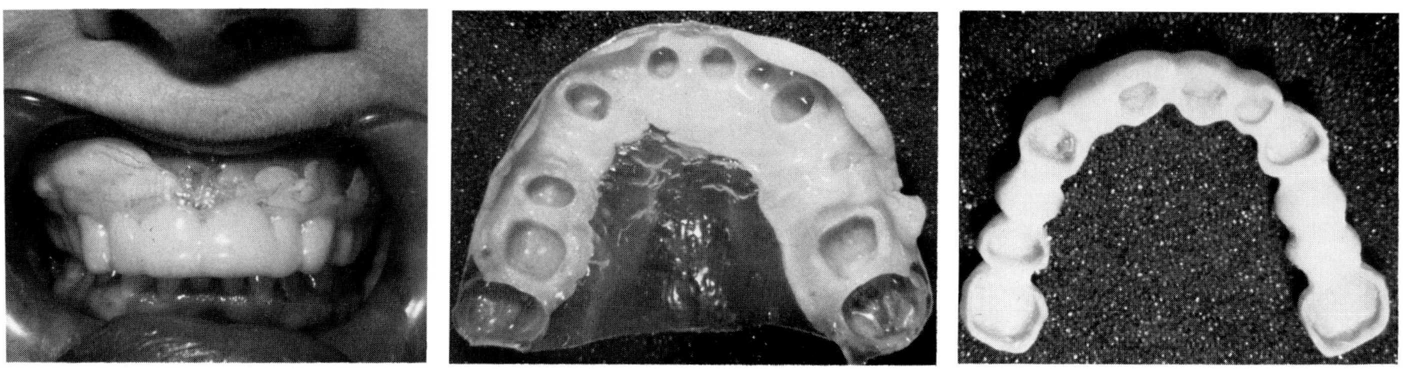

G

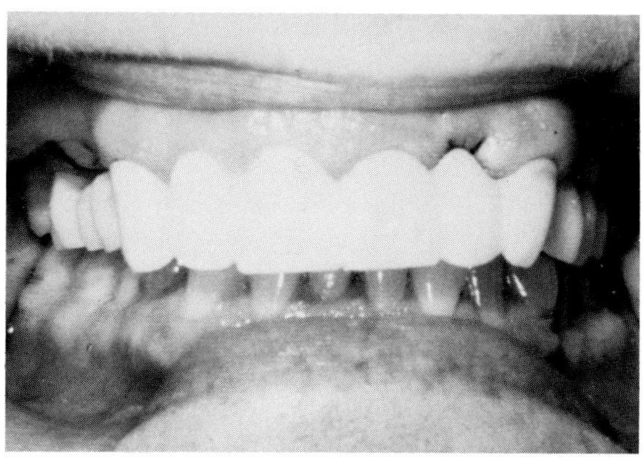

H

Fig. 9–1 *continued.* *E*, Maxillary teeth prepared and extractions done. *F*, Vacu-formed "shim" placed over preparations to verify sufficient reduction. *G*, Cold-cure temporary bridge acrylic fills shim and is placed over prepared teeth (left). It is then removed, trimmed, and can be marginally relined for subgingival adaptation. *H*, Provisional splint in mouth.

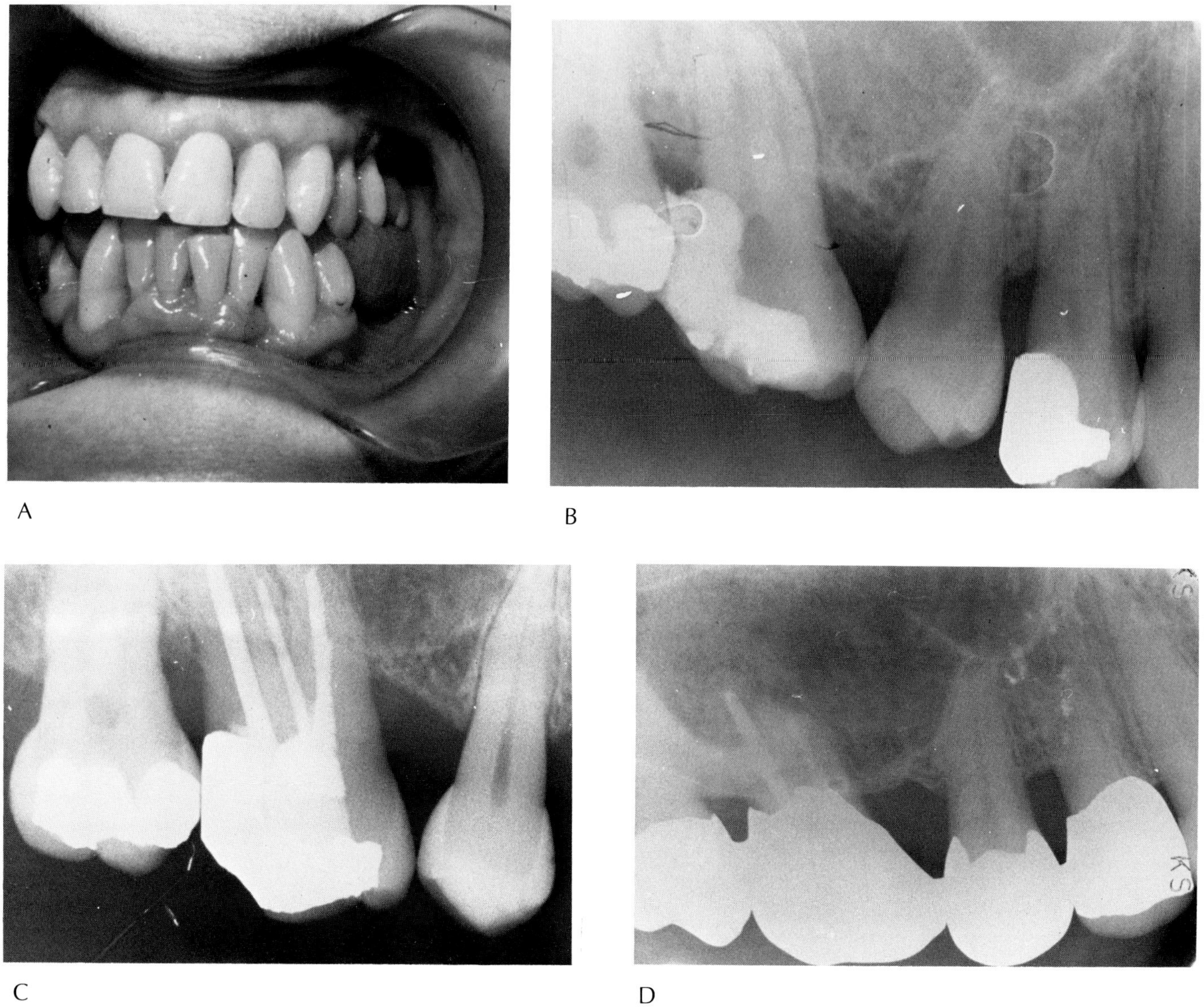

Fig. 9–2. Fixed splinting.
A, Severe periodontal involvement 6 weeks post surgery. Many teeth were mobile, especially upper molar.
B, Both endodontically and periodontally compromised, upper second molar (first molar missing) had questionable prognosis.
C, Endodontic therapy was carried out, followed by periodontal surgery. Splinting was indicated.
D, Five-year follow-up radiograph shows good bone leveling. Multiple tooth splint exhibits no mobility.

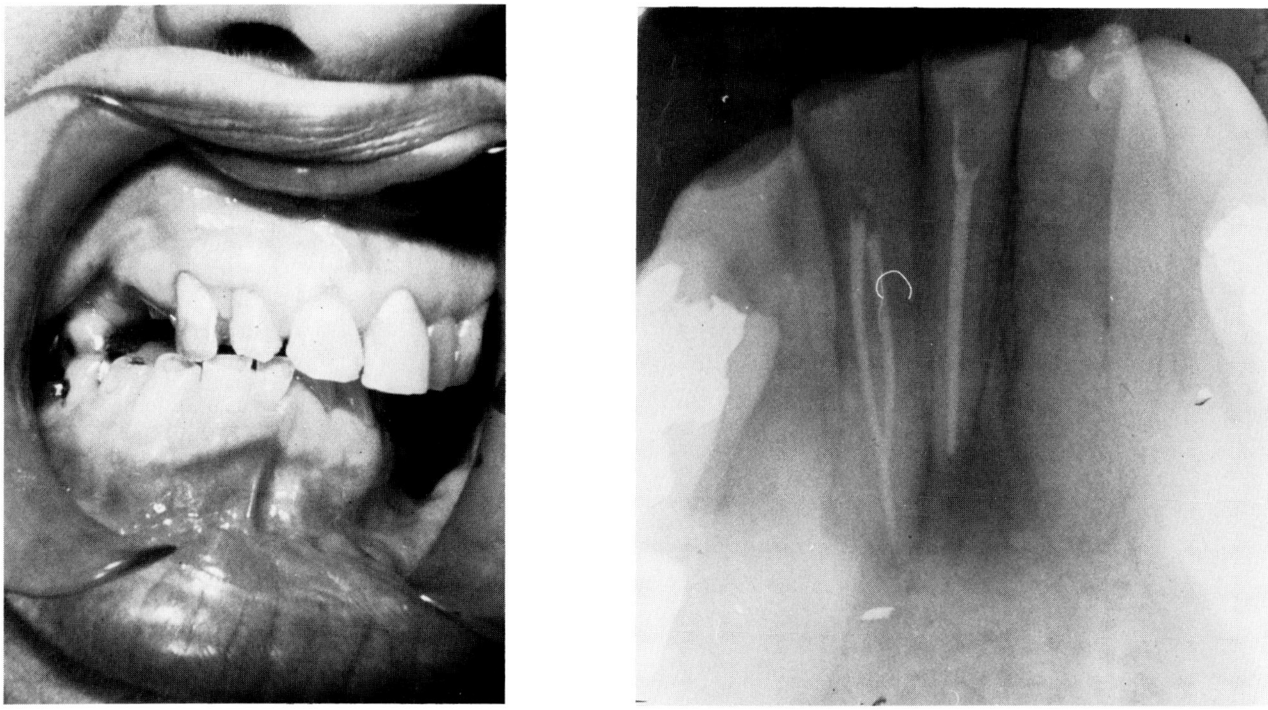

E

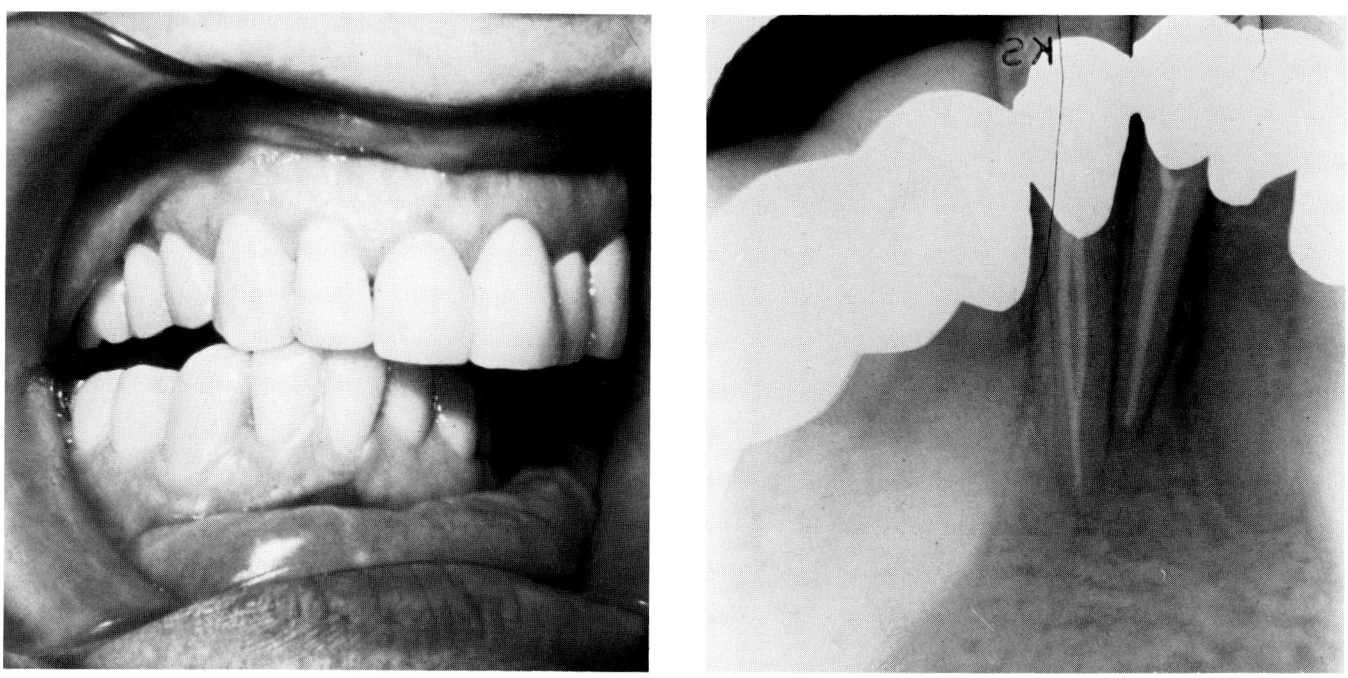

F

Fig. 9–2 *continued.* *E*, Lower anterior teeth incur heavy lateral functional forces, show severe wear, and have been endodontically treated.

F, Five-year follow-up demonstrates multitooth splinting to gain mechanical advantage under heavy functional forces; no mobility present.

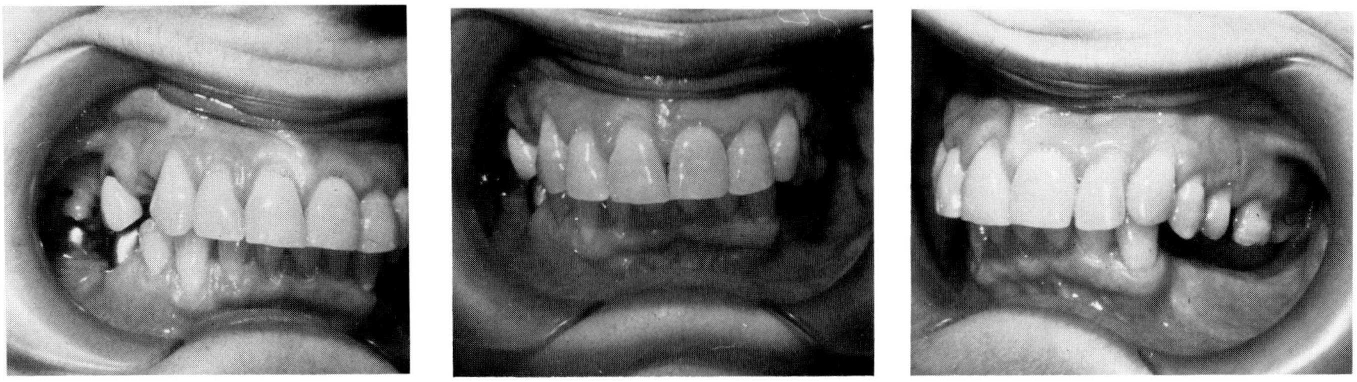

G

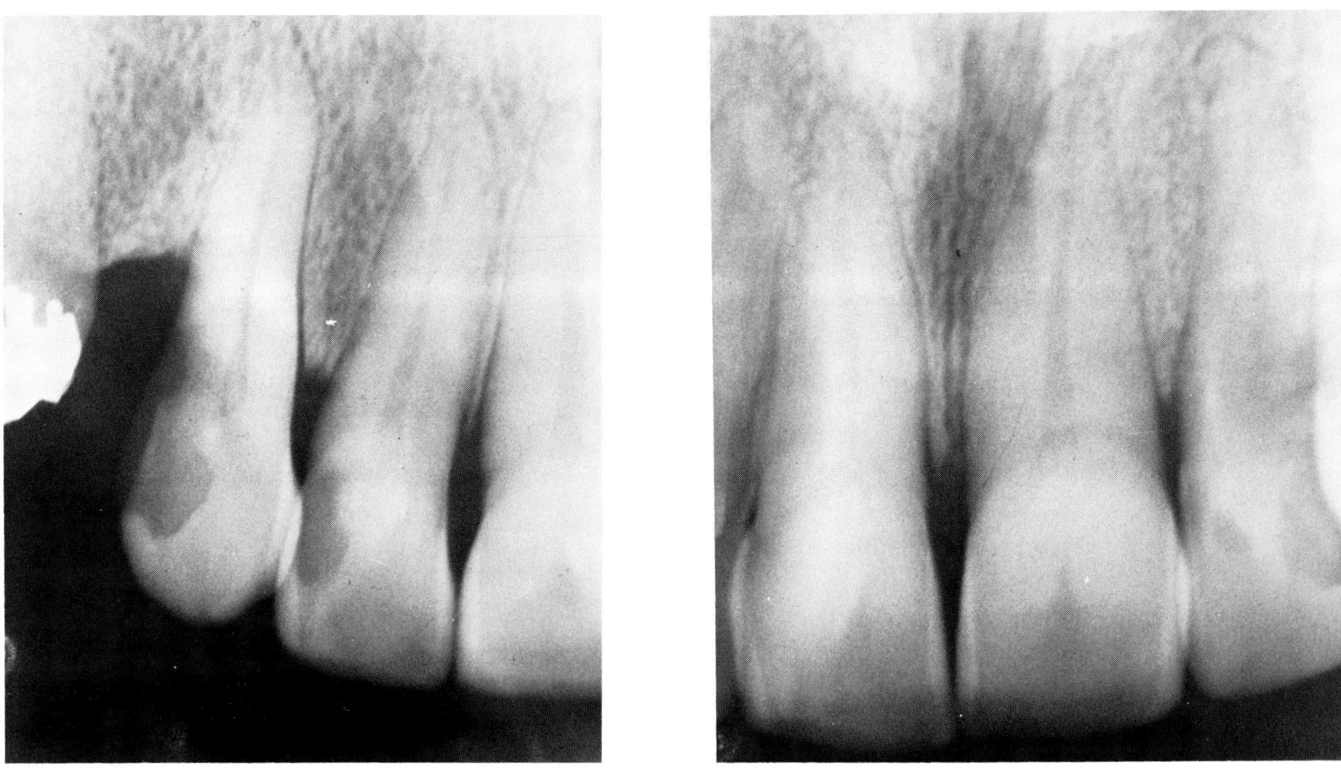

H

Fig. 9–2 *continued.* *G*, This 48-year-old woman exhibited Class II to III mobility on upper anterior teeth with loss of vertical dimension.

H, Radiographs of upper anterior.

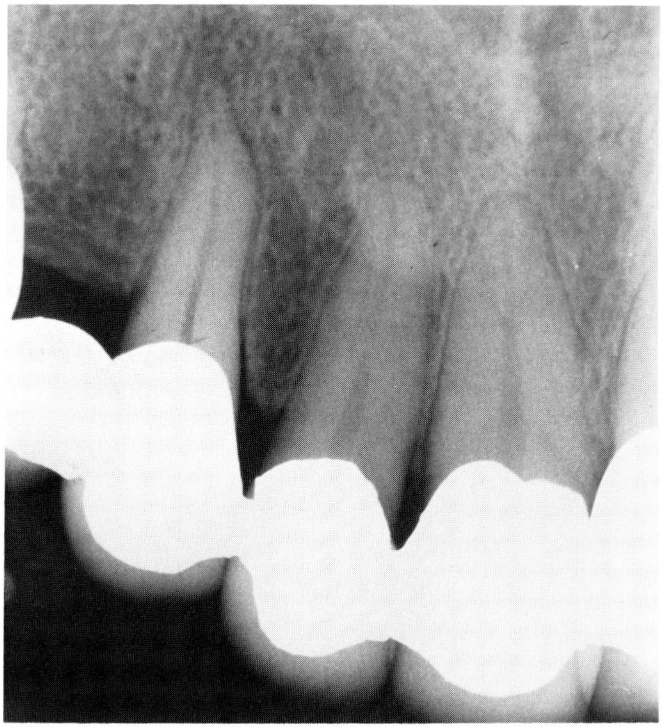

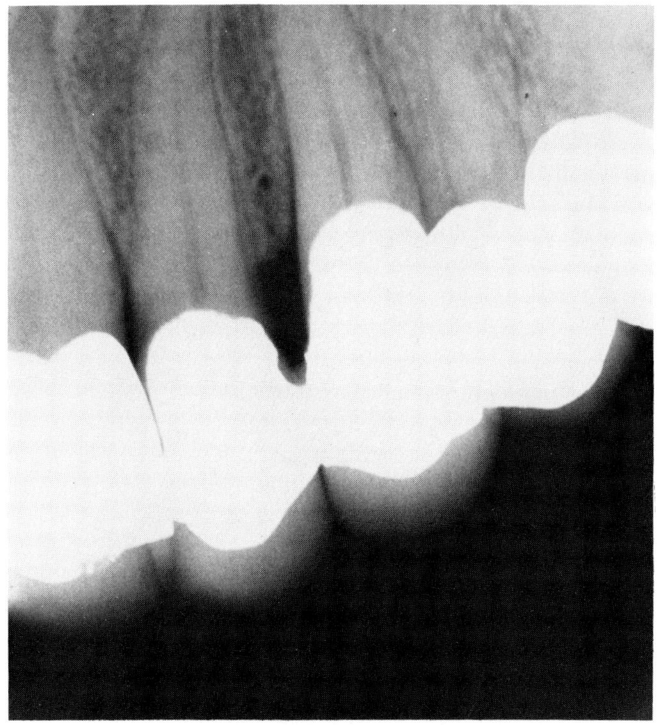

I

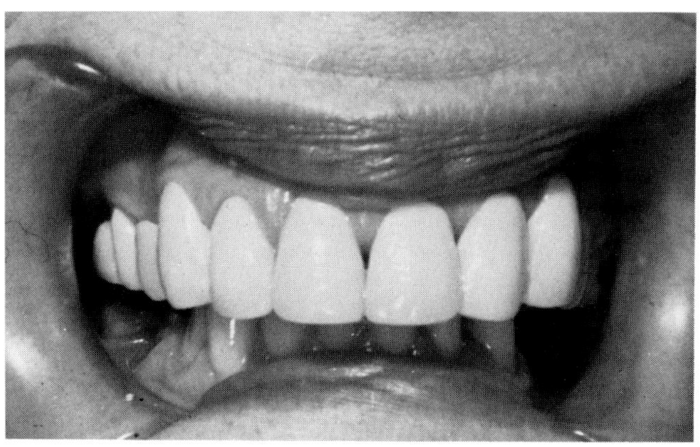

J

Fig. 9–2 *continued.* *I*, Vertical dimension was regained by posterior restoration and orthodontic retraction of upper anterior teeth. These radiographs demonstrate multitooth splinting of the area on 8-year follow-up.
J, Clinical view, 8-year follow-up. Anterior teeth are stable and well maintained.

them less mobile, especially if weaker teeth can be splinted to stronger ones. However, such splints may complicate plaque removal (since areas are less accessible to brush and especially floss), and periodic loosening of the splint can be a major maintenance problem for the dentist and his patient. A fixed splint, such as that utilizing cast restorations (pin ledge, three-quarter crowns, or full crowns), will provide better stability at much higher cost; yet if the teeth have been compromised periodontally, moved orthodontically, and perhaps worn or restored so as to warrant definitive restoration in any situation, fixed splints may be both necessary and reasonable (Fig. 9–2). This application is even more effective when tripodization is employed—that is, when an angle (in effect, a "tripod") is created in multiple splints or long fixed bridges (Fig. 9–3).

Stability is then assured in the anteroposterior and lateral directions. Extending this principle, we see cross-arch splinting, which provides an even broader base for the tripod or may even create a four-point base (Fig. 9–4).

Splinting as a hedge against failure is best exemplified by the use of double or multiple abutments in fixed or removable prosthetics. A typical prosthetic situation is an edentulous lower posterior with the mandibular first premolar being the terminal abutment tooth. This tooth often has the smallest, shortest root of any posterior tooth, yet removable partial dentures are attached to it routinely. The result is often mobility of the tooth and early loss.

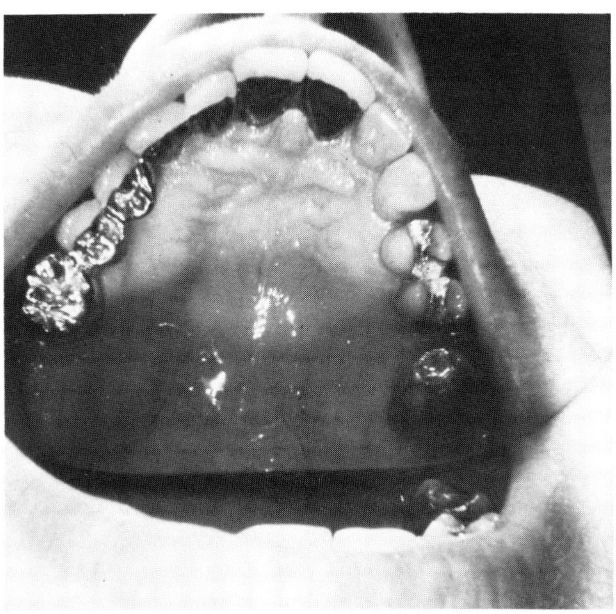

Fig. 9–3. Fixed bridge illustrating a "tripod" splint.

Adjacent to the first premolar is the canine tooth, which is often the most stable tooth in the mouth. Good judgment sometimes calls for the removal of the first premolar (see Chap. 8) if it is compromised. Often, however, it is a sound tooth, but simply ill-suited as a lone abutment. Crowning the first premolar and canine and splinting them together creates an entirely different support structure. In effect, we can create root surface and length that is equivalent to that of a lower first molar; such a unit can easily withstand the rigors of a lower removable partial denture. Splinted abutments may also be used to accommodate semiprecision or precision attachments by virtue of their great stability, especially as compared to individual, unsplinted, abutment teeth (Fig. 9–5).

Provisional Cementation of Fixed Prostheses

Fixed prosthetic devices require a major investment of time and effort, not to mention money, and once they are cemented with a permanent luting agent, they cannot be readily removed intact. When placing fixed bridges over teeth that have been compromised pulpally, periodontally, or mechanically, one assumes a considerable measure of risk should any of the abutment teeth fail. This risk increases with the severity of the previous problem and with the complexity (length, number of units) of the bridge.

Many clinicians attempt to temper this risk through provisional cementation—that is, by placing the appliance on the teeth with a nonsetting or temporary cement that permits subsequent removal of the appliance. The advantages of this strategy are obvious and many, both in assessing the abutment teeth over time as to endodontic and periodontal status and in evaluating the form and function of the prosthesis. Defective solder joints, porcelain fractures, and unforeseen occlusal or esthetic problems can be rectified fairly easily if the fixed prosthesis can be removed.

Unfortunately, provisional cementation has a number of disadvantages that limit its use. The primary disadvantage is that, being removable, it is subject to accidental displacement through mastication of sticky foods or through failure of the cement seal. Since cements must be selected and applied carefully to ensure removal (inability to remove a prosthesis placed with temporary cement is another major problem), loss of cement integrity must be anticipated. Accidental displacement raises the possibility of aspiration, ingestion, loss, or damage of the prosthesis. Cement leakage can lead to pulpal irritation and, over time, caries under the retainer. Therefore, under the best of circumstances, provisional cementation requires periodic inspections, removal, and recemen-

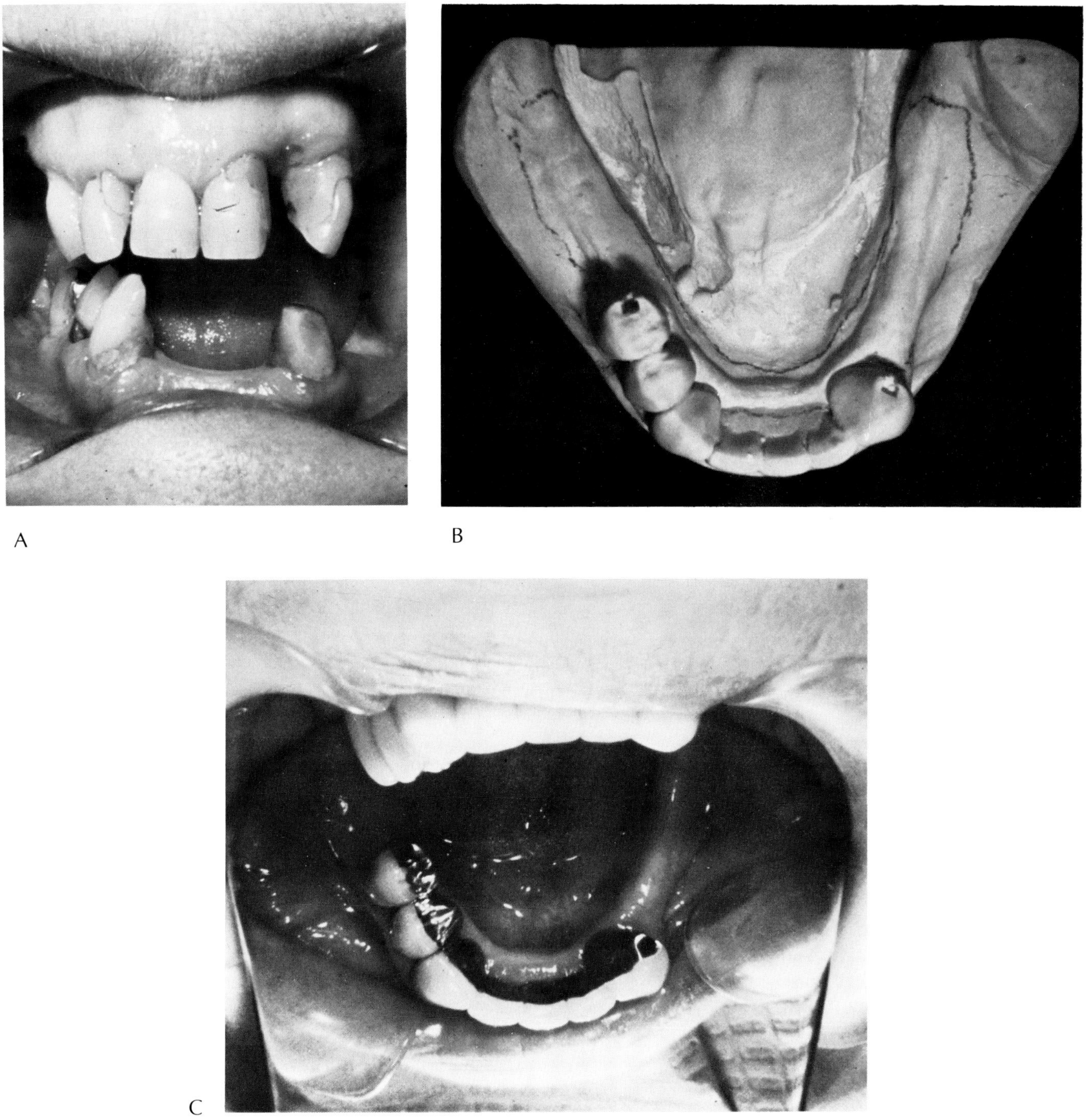

A B C

Fig. 9–4. *A*, Treatment plan calls for anterior fixed bridges (splints) and posterior removable partial dentures. *B*, Diagnostic cast showing cross-arch splinting in lower arch (note attachments for removable appliance). *C*, Clinical view.

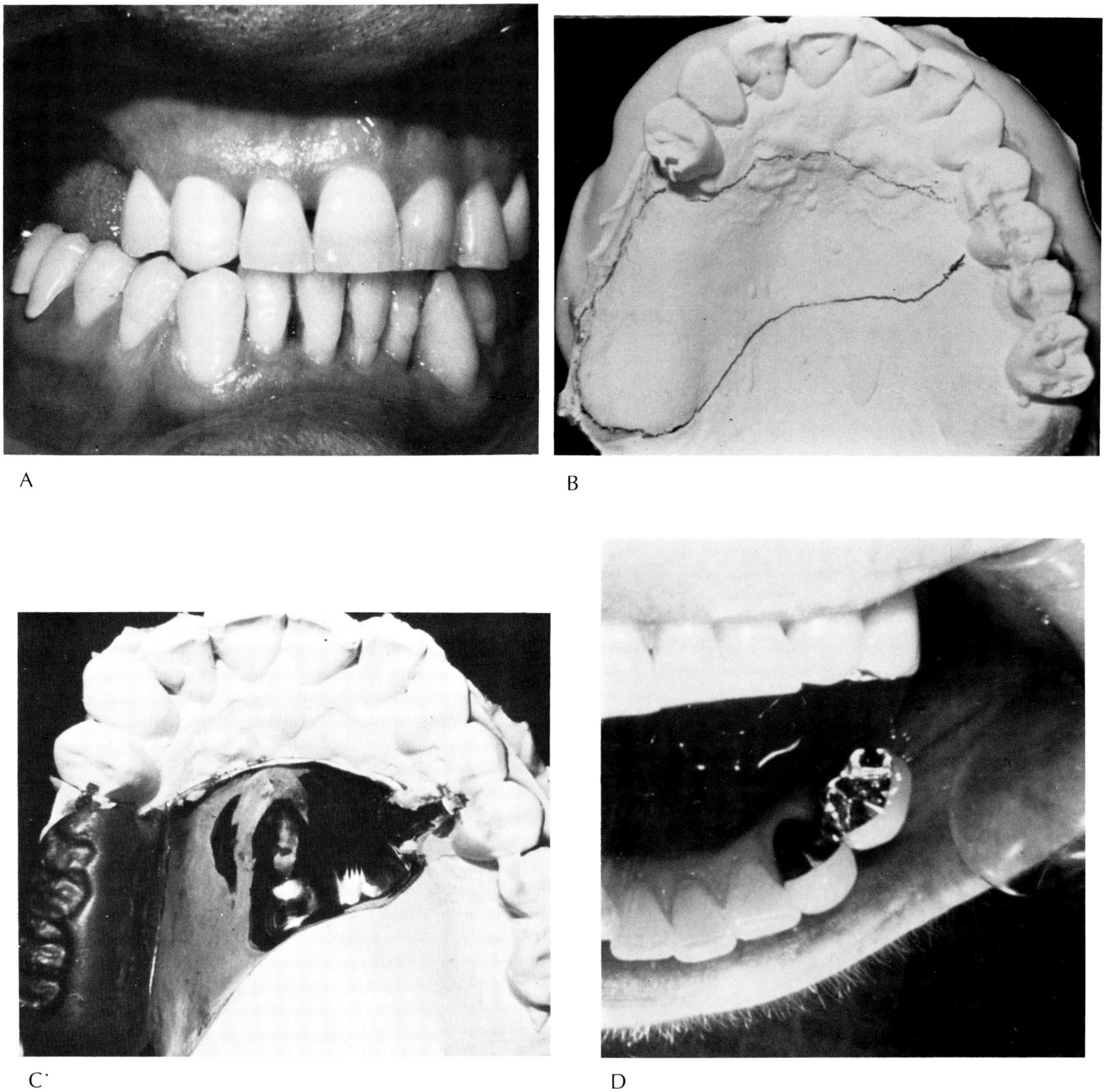

Fig. 9–5. *A*, Following periodontal therapy, upper removable partial will be fabricated. *B*, Design on diagnostic cast illustrates use of attachments in fixed bridge pontic (left side), and in double abutment splint (right side). *C*, Cast-gold base (mucostatic) with attachments soldered; wax bite for articulation prior to setting teeth. *D*, Double-abutment castings, first premolar/canine.

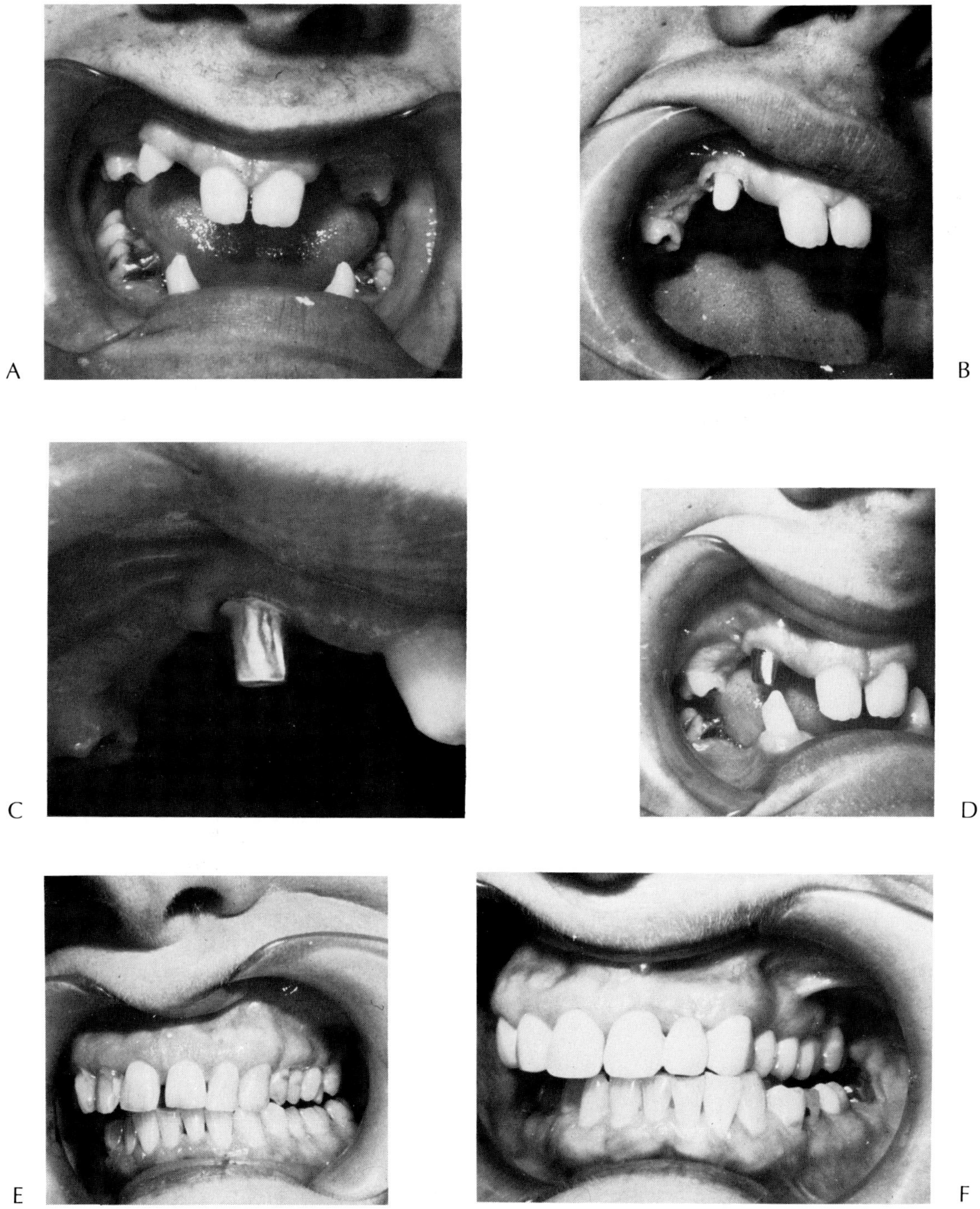

Fig. 9–6. Telescope technique with provisional cementations. *A*, Upper right canine in this reconstruction case was nonparallel and out of the plane of occlusion. *B*, Tooth prepared with full shoulder preparation, with bevel at gingiva. *C*, Cast-gold coping in place that is designed to be parallel with other potential abutments. *D*, Canine is now a usable abutment. *E*, Extensive fixed bridges were planned for this periodontally involved maxillary arch. *F*, Two six-unit anterior/posterior bridges were placed from central incisor to first molar on each side and cemented temporarily. Bridges were evaluated and removed periodically (every 3 months) to assess occlusion and periodontal status. One year from initial insertion the bridges were cemented permanently.

tation. Although it is a valuable tool in planning for failure, the logistics and risks involved generally limit the length of time one should employ it. Generally, some target date should be set (3, 6, or 9 months), at which time the prosthesis will be permanently cemented if all factors are positive.

An alternate approach that allows provisional cementation over an indefinite period is the use of telescope crowns. In this technique, abutment teeth are over-prepared to allow a thin cast coping to be placed with some permanent cement, over which the fixed prosthesis is constructed. This allows periodic removal without the risk of pulpal irritation or caries under the crowns. Indeed, sometimes no cement is used between coping and telescope, and some mechanical retention is employed instead.

Advantages of the telescope system are flexibility, the potential for recovery should an abutment tooth be lost, and the added potential to correct for nonparallel abutment teeth in the coping, thereby allowing a mutual insertion path without orthodontic alignment and/or endodontic treatment and core build-up of the nonparallel tooth (Fig. 9–6). When the prosthesis can be removed by the patient, oral hygiene is greatly facilitated, since threading of floss under pontics and solder joints is eliminated.

Disadvantages of the telescope include the rather severe preparations that must be made if one is to avoid overcontour of the superstructure prosthesis, and the same potential for accidental or inadvertent loss as in any removable prosthesis. In addition, the significantly greater cost and complexity of a telescope system can render it impractical for many patients.

Endodontic Recovery

Any tooth that has been subjected to the rigors of dental disease and/or treatment may be compromised pulpally. Even virgin teeth may have received traumatic blows at some time and although they are asymptomatic, they may be pulpally compromised. In planning for failure, we must always ask ourselves what can be done if this or that tooth should fail pulpally. This is particularly important when we are involving teeth in multiple-abutment fixed prostheses or using them as removable partial-denture abutments. The major factors to consider are the likelihood of pulpal problems, the feasibility of endodontic therapy should such problems arise, and the significance of the tooth to the overall treatment plan.

Careful assessment of clinical and radiographic findings may reveal pulpal abnormalities in otherwise asymptomatic teeth. Pulp chambers that are larger than expected (compared with other teeth in the mouth) or smaller, or that are occluded with pulp stones might suggest an abnormal pulpal status. Discolored teeth and teeth with a questionable periapical appearance might also be suspect. Electronic pulp testing might reveal nonresponsive teeth that are otherwise asymptomatic. Indeed, it is likely that many quiet and functional teeth are compromised pulpally and no one knows it. Even if we recognize a possible abnormality in pulpal appearance or reaction, we may choose to simply watch and re-evaluate it periodically. If the tooth in question is not involved in an overall treatment plan, does not require extensive restoration, and could be treated or even removed and replaced without affecting other restorations and/or appliances, it is often better left alone.

If teeth such as those just discussed are involved directly or indirectly in overall dental treatment, the feasibility of future endodontic therapy must be considered. Involvement in overall treatment could necessitate cast restoration of the tooth. Proximity to a fixed or removable prosthesis may mean that loss of the tooth would require extensive modification or complete replacement of the prosthesis. One must then envision the need for successful endodontic therapy and look at pulp and root morphology, clinical access, and the feasibility of surgical endodontics and apical treatment, should they become necessary. The obvious example here would be the contrast between an upper central incisor with a straight root and an apparently normal pulpal configuration that generally lends itself to conventional endodontics or surgical approaches and a lower first premolar that often exhibits unusual root morphology, multiple canals, and such apical proximity to mandibular and mental canals and mental foramen as may complicate or prevent a surgical approach.

Prophylactic endodontic therapy may be indicated in cases in which pulpal status is in question, involvement in the overall treatment plan unavoidable, and feasibility of treatment in doubt. If such endodontic therapy cannot be successfully completed, the tooth can be removed and the treatment plan developed accordingly.

Pulpal failure of a bridge abutment tooth that also retains a precision-attachment removable partial denture is obviously more significant than if that same tooth were merely part of a three-unit fixed bridge. Similarly, the pulpal failure of a three-unit bridge abutment is more significant than that of a single crowned tooth that, if lost, could be readily replaced without affecting other crowns or fixed or removable appliances in the mouth. Thus, in certain situations, a questionable tooth absolutely requires prophylactic endodontic treatment; in other situations, the same tooth might simply be watched for future signs or symptoms, all based on its relationship to the overall situation.

Finally, a word should be said about planning for failure, because while endodontic therapy can be, and often is, successfully performed on teeth with cast restorations, it is not always easy. The use of metal, rather than porcelain over metal on occlusal and lingual surfaces may greatly facilitate later access to the pulp, as well as subsequent repair and restoration of the opening. Likewise, the prudent clinician will control the thickness of the casting over the occlusal surface so that, should entry to the pulp be required, he does not face the prospect of boring through 5 mm of cast alloy.

Design Flexibility in Prosthetic Appliances

Having accepted the concept that components in the stomatognathic system can fail despite our best efforts, it makes good sense to anticipate and when possible, to prepare for that failure so as to salvage as much of our previous treatment efforts as possible. Designing flexibility into prosthetic appliances is one way of doing this, and a number of examples follow that embrace this concept. This is in no way an exhaustive listing of all possible options, but it is a challenge to the practitioner to seek out, in the literature and through his own ingenuity, creative solutions to the problem of potential failure.

Partial-Denture Design Flexibility

In many cases, anterior abutments should be planned and designed as though posterior abutments were not present. Should a posterior abutment be lost at a later time, the framework can then be adapted to the distal extension situation without being totally remade. This is especially true when distal abutment teeth are questionable to begin with. There is much to recommend retention of such teeth due to the greater stability and retention of a tripodal or four-point system, provided that the appliance can be readily modified (Fig. 9–7).

Alternate abutment teeth can be selected in some partial-denture designs so that, should the terminal tooth fail, the framework lends itself readily to adaptation. Great caution must be exercised here, however, as partial dentures all too often act as slow extraction devices, and the patient perceives a gradual and costly serial extraction process. Questionable teeth should not generally be employed as abutments, especially not as terminal abutments in partial-denture applications. However, in cases in which all or nearly all remaining teeth are questionable and the partial denture is employed in a holding action, planning for alternate abutments makes great sense. We have seen abuses of this approach, such as a full denture that embodied a partial denture framework modified no less than six times in a 5-year period as teeth were lost. In such cases, the cost/benefit ratio should be carefully considered, as well as other options, such as overdenture appliances. Indeed, if longevity will be limited by periodontal disease (as it most often is), the practitioner must also consider the effect on the residual ridge of progressive bone loss resulting from attempts to maintain hopeless teeth. Good clinical judgment and patient involvement are, as always, essential.

Partial-denture design should often be carried out even when partial dentures are not being placed. If questionable teeth are in posterior segments of the mouth (furcation involvements) and cast restorations are being placed elsewhere in the arch, those cast restorations can be surveyed and modified to serve as direct or indirect retainers for a hypothetical partial denture, should that become necessary. A fixed bridge can be fabricated with a semiprecision attachment (keyway or similar apparatus) built into the pontic that can be filled in with acrylic and kept in reserve, if posterior teeth are lost on the opposite side of the arch (Fig. 9–8).

Fixed bridgework may be employed using questionable distal abutment teeth if anterior abutments are designed as partial-denture abutments. Should the distal abutments fail, the fixed bridge can be sectioned at the anterior abutment and a distal-extension partial denture placed using the already surveyed and designed retainer. If cast restorations on the opposite side have also been placed with partial-denture design built in, the shift from all fixed to partial removable appliances can be made readily and with minimal backtracking. This presents obvious economies in time and money, and provides a psychologic cushion to the patient desperately hoping to preserve as many teeth for as long as possible (Fig. 9–9).

Fixed-Bridge Design Flexibility

Fixed bridgework, unless it is cemented provisionally, is the most difficult to modify; therefore, "escape routes" must be planned very carefully. Using nonrigid connectors, keyways of various types, to allow subsequent construction of partial dentures with the anterior female as the attachment site is risky at best. Indeed, lack of rigidity may contribute to the anticipated failure or at the very least, may

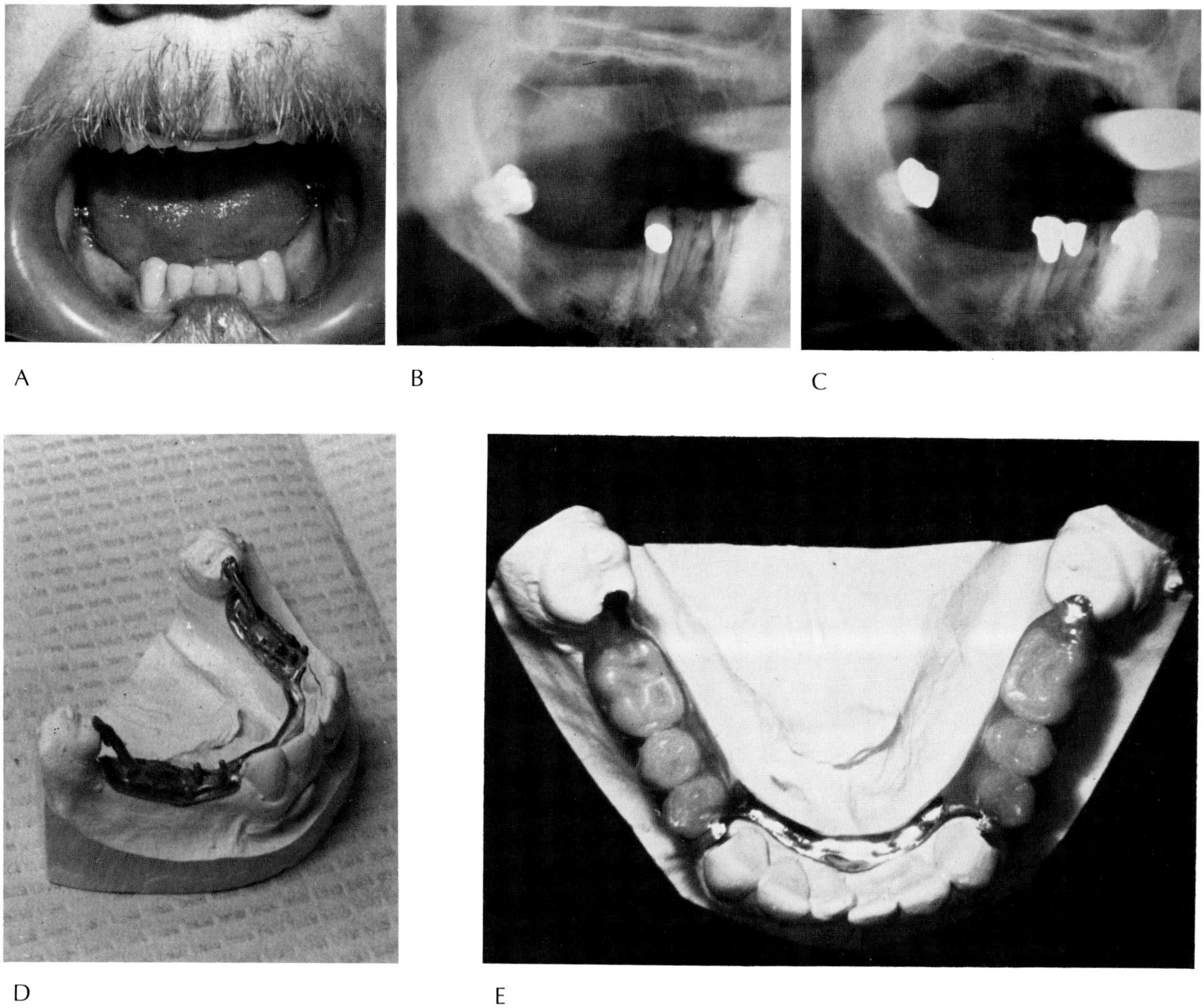

Fig. 9–7. Partial denture design flexibility. *A*, This patient has full maxillary denture, six lower anterior teeth, and two lower third molars that are severely tipped mesial and lingual. *B*, Radiograph shows lower situation; opposite side is similar. *C*, Radiograph shows double abutment crowns for precision-attachment lower removable partial denture. Third molar has also been crowned and has mesial guide plane and rest designed into it. *D*, Cast-gold base (mucostatic) frame sitting on model shows how third molars are being utilized. *E*, Occlusal view of finished appliance. Distal rests on third molars could simply be removed if either or both distal abutments are lost.

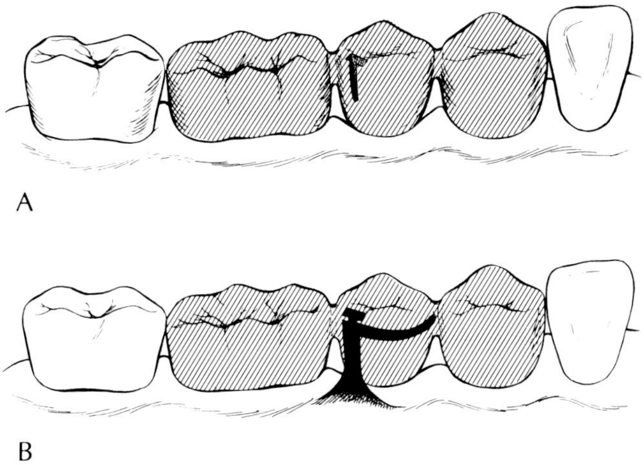

Fig. 9–8. *A*, Diagram of fixed bridge with female attachment designed into pontic. This can be filled with acrylic and kept in reserve. *B*, Semiprecision attachment of removable partial denture made subsequent to fixed bridge.

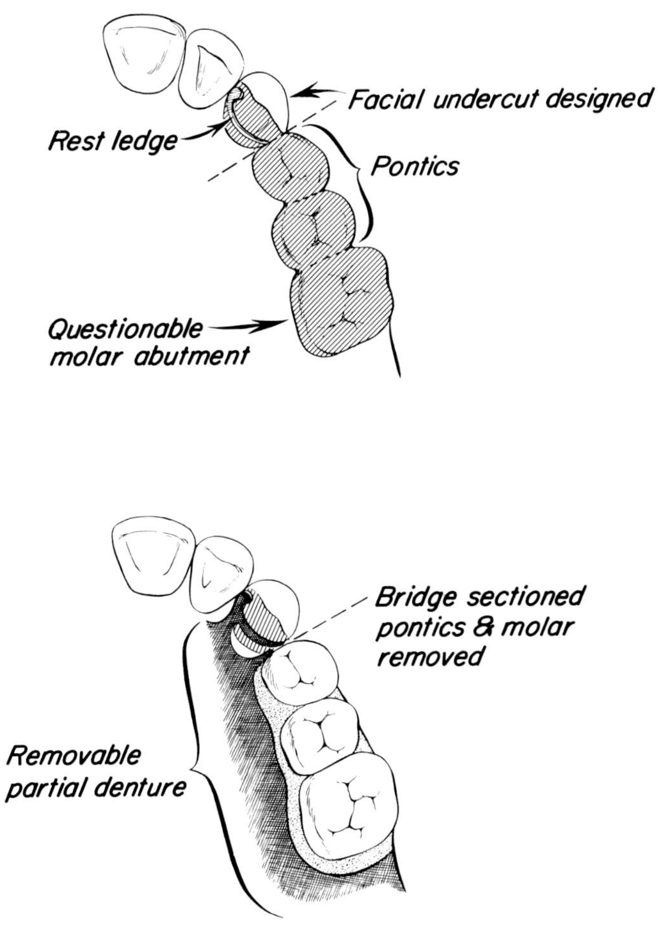

Fig. 9–9. Fixed bridge with anterior abutment designed for removable partial denture should questionable distal abutment fail.

sacrifice some of the inherent advantages of the rigid fixed bridge. Likewise, unless the attachment in question is in an extremely stable tooth or in a multiple abutment, if may not be suitable for use in a distal-extension situation. Merely being able to change the design of an appliance is not enough. The altered appliance must be stable and functional to be of practical value.

Splinted teeth, when used as anterior piers of a fixed bridge with questionable distal abutment, can allow subsequent modification into a cantilever design if certain criteria are met. First, the abutments used must be of sufficient strength and stability to support the cantilever design. Second, the retainers must generally be full-coverage crowns, and the preparations must be carried out to gain maximum length and relative parallelism. This consideration would not be nearly as critical in a noncantilever mode. Third, the pontic must be designed for easy sectioning either at the solder joint of the distal abutment or through the pontic itself. The advantage of a two premolar pontic over a molar configuration becomes obvious here, as it allows for the modification. Last, the resulting cantilever fixed bridge must provide the necessary function given the overall dentition in question. For example, a lower cantilever may occlude fully with a shortened upper arch, or it may result in loss of second-molar function, which might or might not be acceptable. In a Class III relationship opposing an upper full denture, the lower cantilever may be obviously insufficient in posterior support and function, and a removable partial denture be indicated instead (Fig. 9–10).

Another approach to flexibility in fixed-bridge design is the anticipation, when placing a cast crown or retainer, of a future adjacent prosthesis. In this application, a nonrigid, keyway-type attachment, while admittedly not ideal, may greatly enhance the stability of the subsequent appliance. The examples in Figure 9–11 will illustrate some typical applications of this approach.

Role of the Dental Laboratory

It is obvious that in any complex treatment plan—especially in one attempting to "plan for failure"—the laboratory procedures involved take on tremendous importance. The best approach to the laboratory phase is for the restorative dentist to carry out some or all of the key procedures himself or to employ a technician. When this is not practical, close communication is necessary between the dentist and a commercial laboratory. Not all commercial laboratories are prepared to carry out sophisticated techniques effectively, and care must be taken in choos-

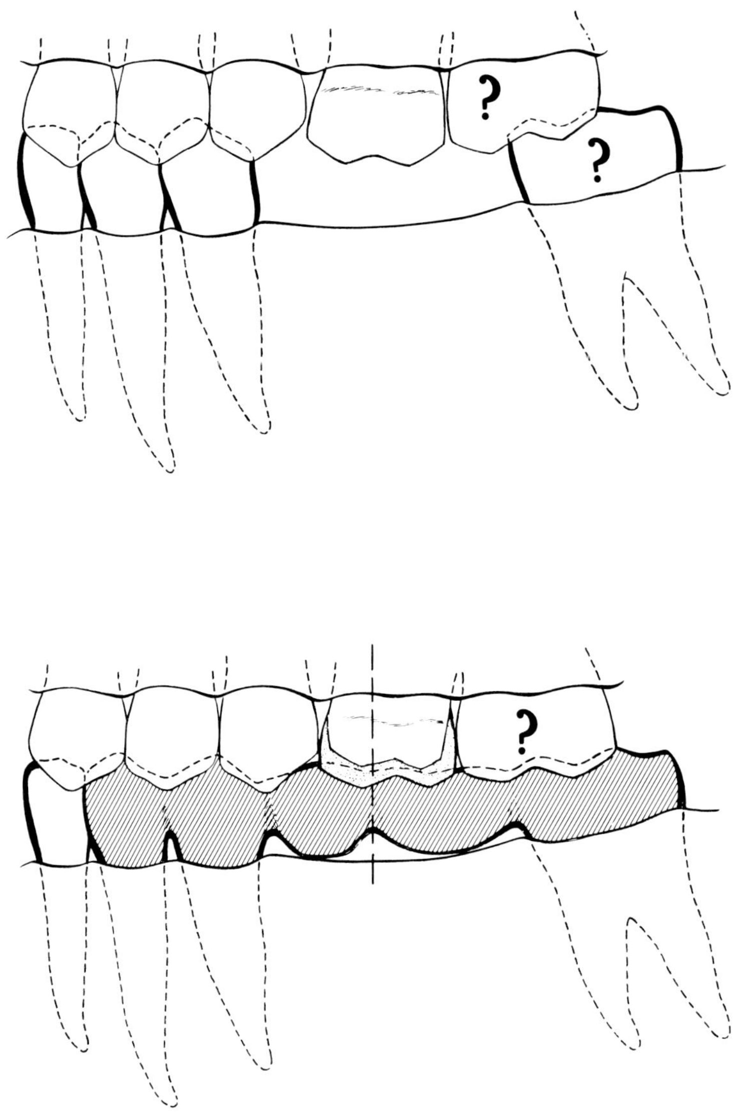

A

Fig. 9–10. Modification of fixed bridge into cantilever. *A*, Diagrammatic representation. Second molars are questionable and upper first molar is supererupted (top). Double abutment in anterior and pontic design allow for potential sectioning of bridge should distal abutment fail (bottom).

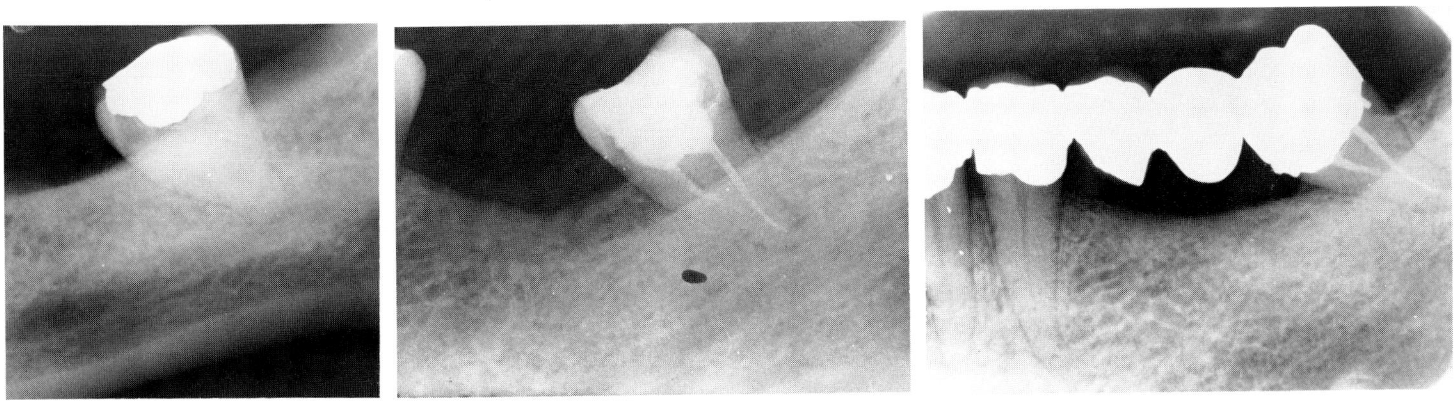

B

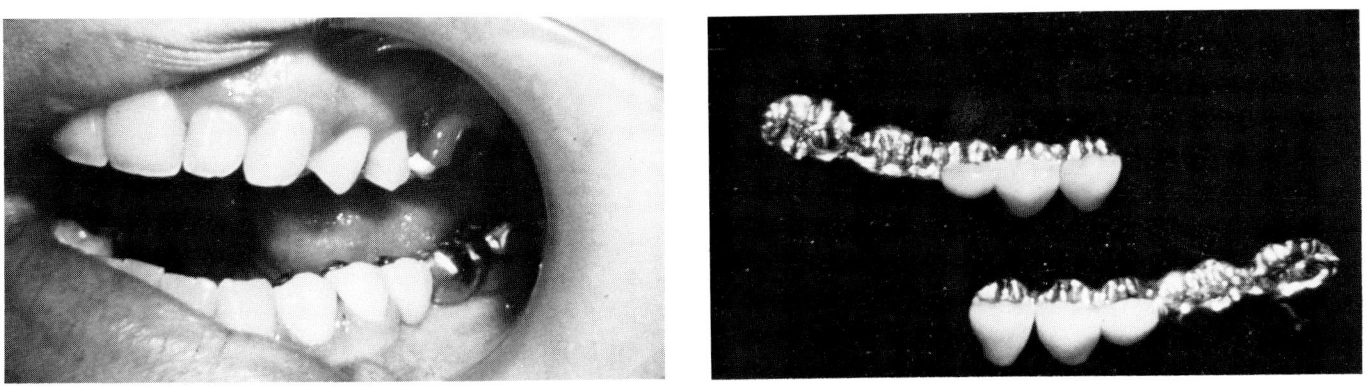

C

Fig. 9–10 *continued.* *B*, Radiographs of actual example. Carious and pulpally involved lower third molar with poor root structure is treated endodontically (center) and utilized as abutment (right). This radiograph is a 5-year follow-up, and the third molar is doing well, but conversion to cantilever is readily done if need be. *C*, Clinical view of another potential cantilever (left) and two more such bridges about to be inserted in the same mouth (right).

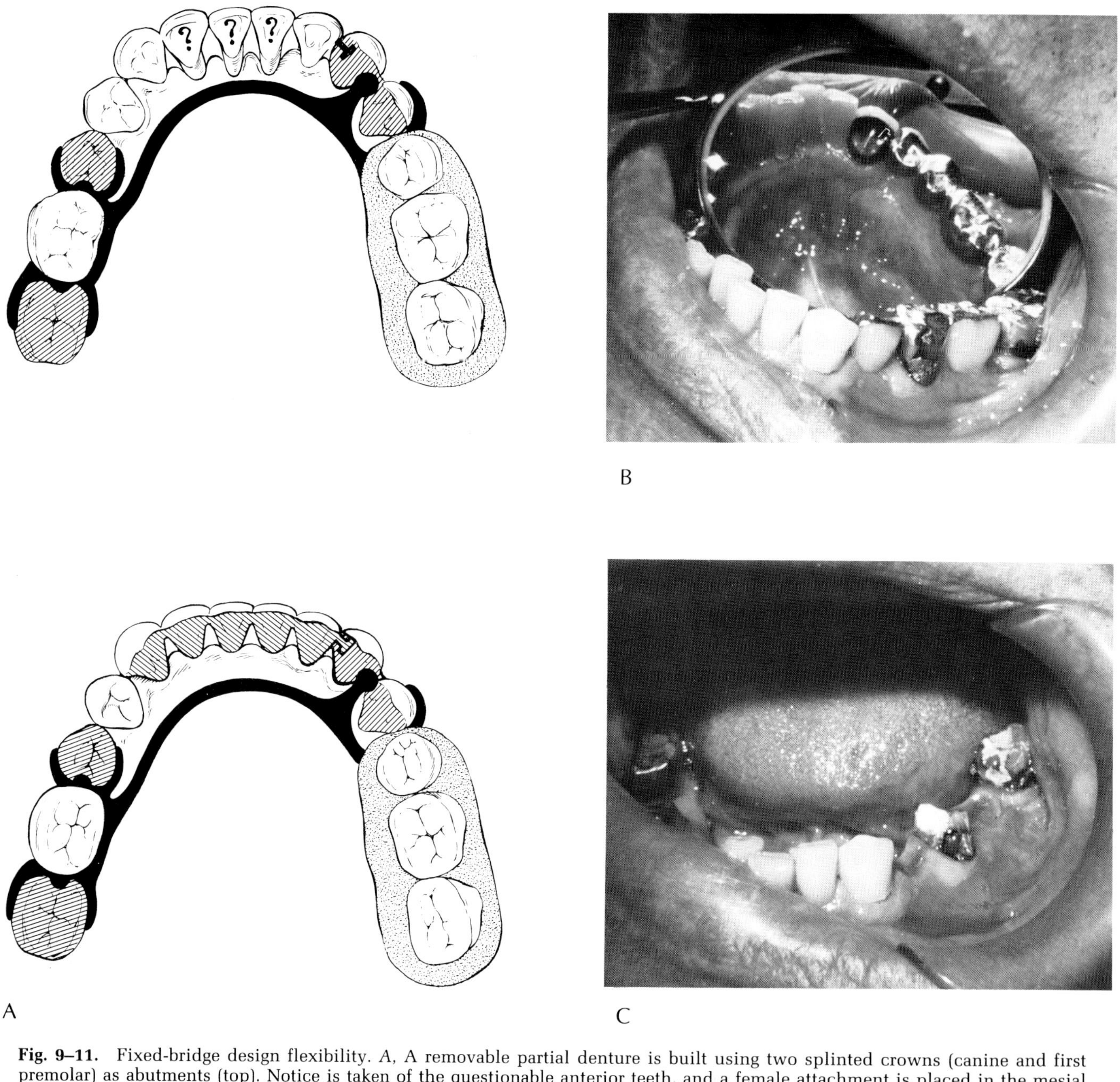

Fig. 9–11. Fixed-bridge design flexibility. *A,* A removable partial denture is built using two splinted crowns (canine and first premolar) as abutments (top). Notice is taken of the questionable anterior teeth, and a female attachment is placed in the mesial aspect of the canine. If questionable teeth are later removed (bottom), the remaining lateral incisor can be greatly aided as a retainer by nonrigid connection to the canine. This also precludes having to remove the crowns previously placed. *B,* Clinical view of lower canine crown that was placed in 1979 with distal female attachment (highlighted in white) anticipating replacement of old fixed bridge. *C,* Bridge removed in 1981 can be replaced with male attachment linking into canine crown.

ing the lab. Once a laboratory or specific technician is selected, face-to-face discussions about techniques and goals are often helpful, along with detailed written directions, sketches, diagnostic wax-ups, and verbal clarification.

The dentist cannot do these things effectively unless he has a working familiarity with the laboratory procedures he is prescribing. The dentist who knows laboratory technology is a better clinical dentist, for many lab procedures can be readily simplified (or horribly complicated) by the clinical approach, design, and preparation format used. The dentist who attempts to employ sophisticated restorative and prosthetic approaches without an understanding of the laboratory procedures is tempting failure.

Compromise Treatment

The most difficult and frustrating problem faced in diagnosis and treatment planning is the need to carry out compromise treatment in the face of inevitable failure. Often, the patient's financial picture will not allow necessary definitive restorative treatment, or else the prognosis is so clouded by a number of factors that costly and extensive treatment is contraindicated. Total edentulation and full removable prostheses may be an alternative, yet that approach is not without cost. Furthermore, removal of all teeth may simply not be necessary or justified at the time. The patient may be better served with an incomplete and somewhat debilitated natural dentition than with full dentures. The dentist is then left with a dilemma: he is unable to justify removing the teeth and unable to replace or restore them properly. The only course available in many cases is patchwork dentistry, the placement of add-on and wrap-around silver amalgam, composite resins, and/or various types of shell crowns in an attempt to hold off the inevitable. When the situation requires it, patchwork is the treatment of choice and needs no apology. Patchwork, however, does not justify sloppiness or negligence. One need not make a dismal prognosis worse by failure to remove caries, by improper occlusion, contour, or contacts, or by rough, noncleansible margins or surfaces. Good quality patchwork can prolong the useful life of a terminal dentition and postpone total edentulation.

Techniques and strategies in this area of treatment planning are numerous. Their application requires that two criteria be met. First, the cost/benefit ratio must be considered—that is, can the time and money to be invested be justified in light of the prognosis? For example, one would not likely place a massive, multisurface silver amalgam on a periodontally condemned molar that has already had acute periodontal episodes. On the other hand, a similarly involved molar with severe periodontal breakdown but no history of acute symptoms might provide a number of years of useful service, and the amalgam restoration would be well worth the effort. Second, and related to the first point, is that the patient must know, understand, and accept this type of treatment approach for what it is—a temporary holding action, or patchwork.

If the preceding criteria are met, a number of compromise treatment strategies are possible. The following are examples of a few such strategies:

1. *Recovery from gross overhang.* Large overhanging margins on silver amalgams often require complete replacement of the restoration. In some cases, a fine needle-shaped diamond point can be used to recontour interproximally (a tissue curettage is performed simultaneously) and smoothing can be done with a similar-configuration multiflute finishing bur and/or abrasive strips (Fig. 9–12 A). Difficulty of access sometimes makes this approach impossible, however, and another strategy is to cut away the entire mesial aspect of the overhanging restoration with a slice approach, and then replace just the proximal with silver amalgam, cutting a retentive box into the remaining alloy. If the existing restoration is large, but otherwise well-condensed and contoured, the modification can be done quickly and without anesthetic in most cases (since cutting is primarily done on and in the restorative material) (Fig. 9–12 B).
2. *Recovery from open contact.* The same strategy can apply when an existing restoration lacks proximal contact. By cutting a retentive box into the existing restoration in the contact area and by placing a band and wedge, the restoration can be built out to proper interproximal configuration and contact; this can be done without removing and replacing the entire restoration and without using anesthesia (Fig. 9–12 C).
3. *Pin-retained crown build-ups.* When there is insufficient tooth structure to hold a restoration, retentive pins must often be employed. When entire coronal build-ups are performed and retained with such pins, the term "patchwork" can be applied; yet a sound root that would ideally require endodontic therapy to allow dowel and core and crown restoration might well be retained on an interim basis simply with a pin-retained build-up. Failure of such a restoration would then signal for removal and perhaps replacement by addition to an existing partial-denture frame (Fig. 9–13).
4. *Transitional prostheses.* When applied appropriately, the wrought wire and acrylic temporary partial denture can provide an esthetic service, if not a

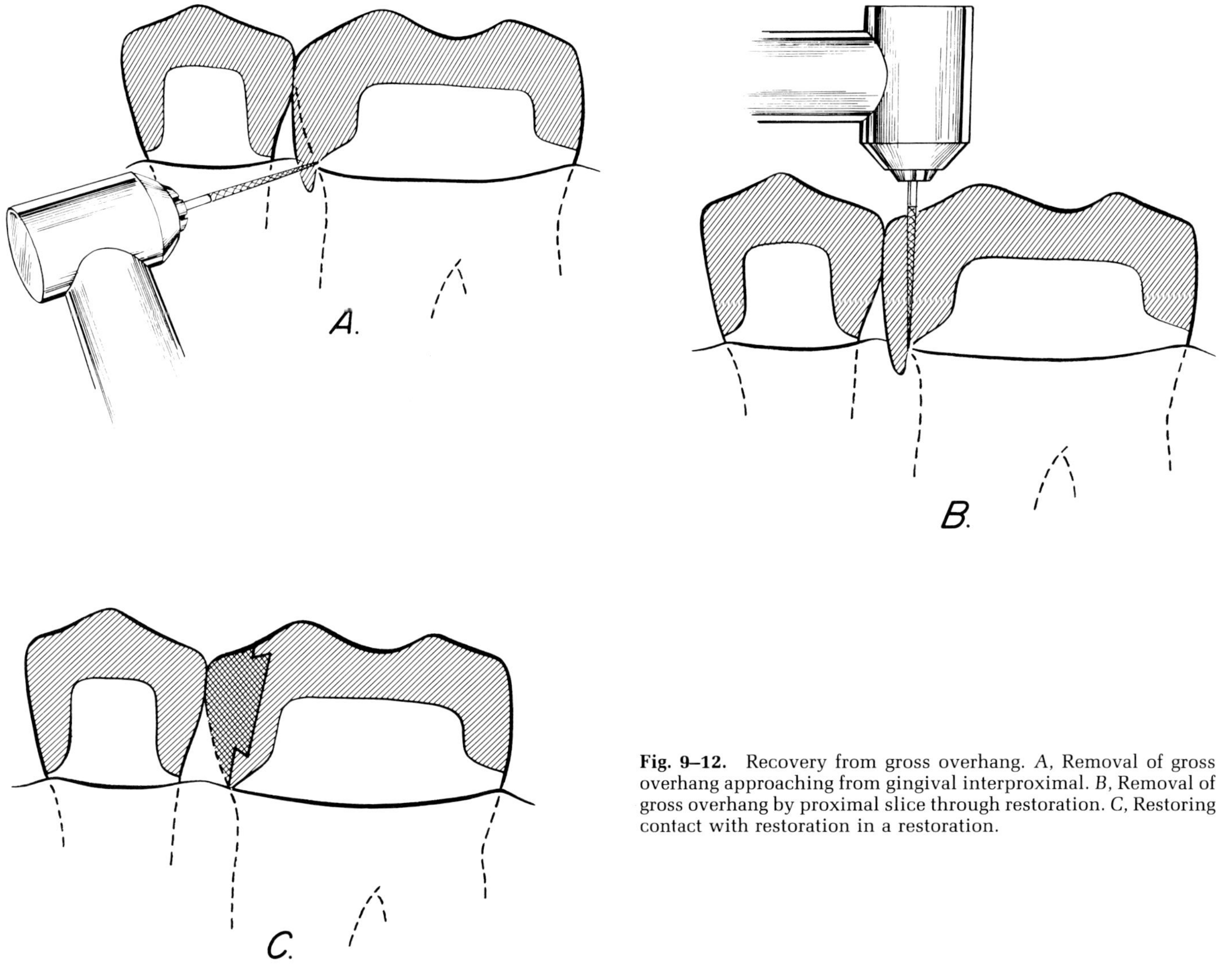

Fig. 9–12. Recovery from gross overhang. *A*, Removal of gross overhang approaching from gingival interproximal. *B*, Removal of gross overhang by proximal slice through restoration. *C*, Restoring contact with restoration in a restoration.

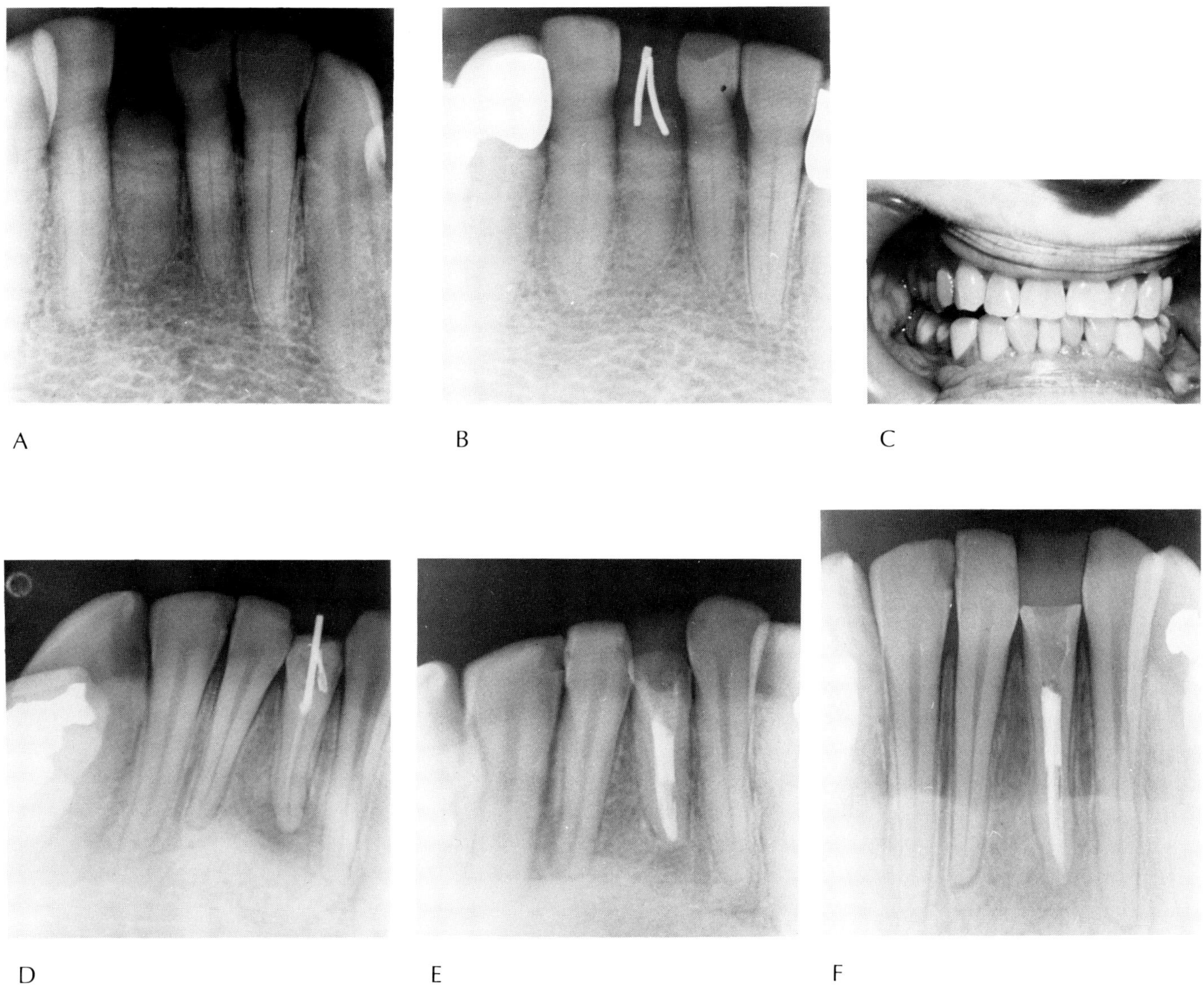

Fig. 9–13. Pin-retained crown build-ups. *A*, Coronal fracture, but tooth is still vital. Patient wanted cast-gold base partial with double crown abutments (but could not afford endodontics as well as dowel and core and porcelain-veneer crown). *B*, Threaded pins were placed in dentin and composite resin crown build-up carried out. *C*, Clinical view after 3 years shows build-up doing well. *D*, Apical lesion on lower anterior with some kind of previous pulpal treatment. *E*, Endodontic therapy carried out, but patient financially unable to proceed with dowel and core and porcelain-veneer crown. Composite build-up is employed as holding measure. *F*, Six years later, composite crown is still providing good service and esthetics.

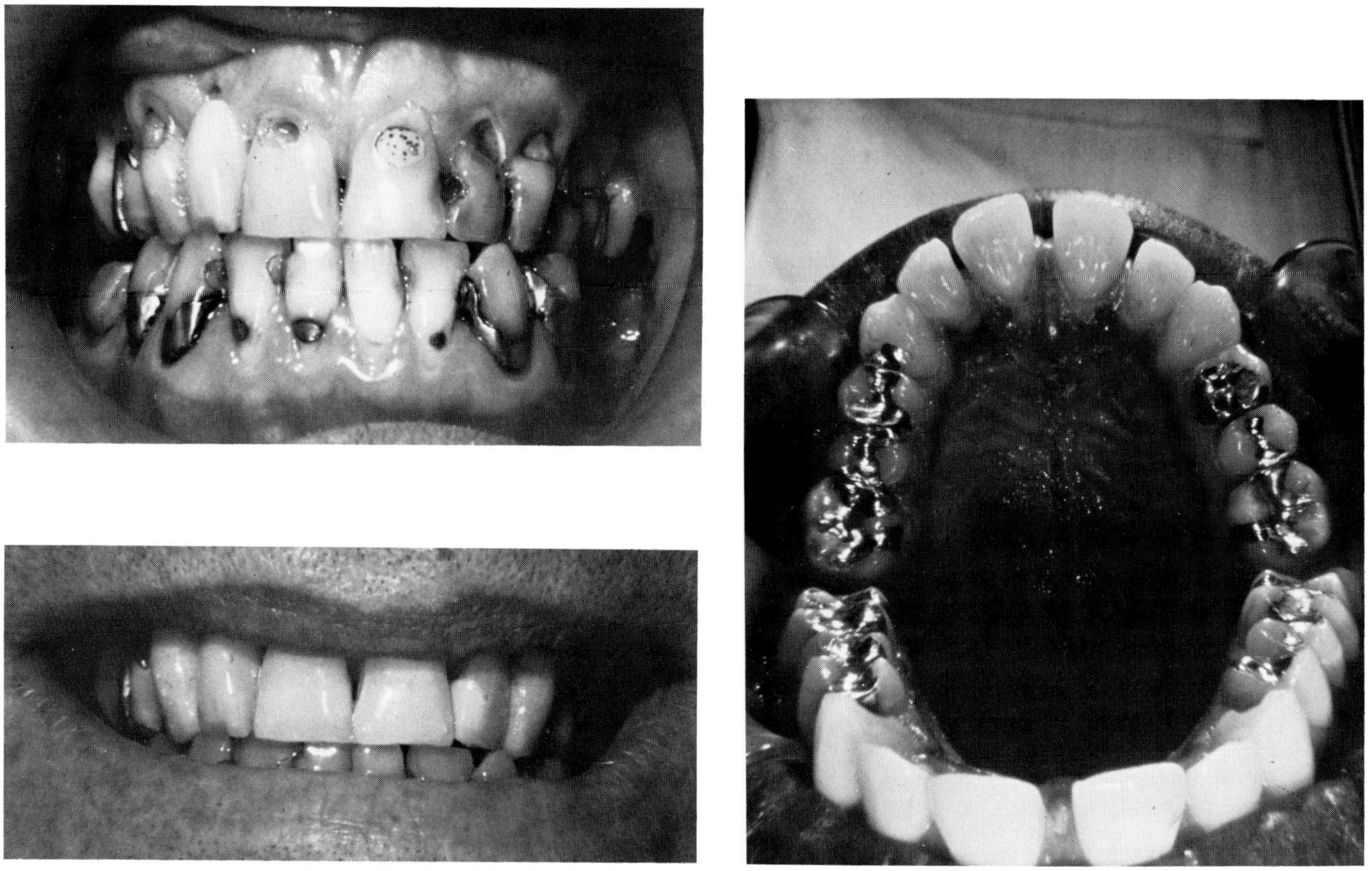

A B

Fig. 9–14. Compromise treatment. *A*, Severely debilitated dentition; crowns and fixed bridgework indicated (top). Due to financial limitations, restoration with composite resin was carried out as compromise treatment (bottom). *B*, Extensive restoration with silver amalgam. Although many of the teeth would be better restored with castings, no one need be ashamed of this kind of "patchwork."

highly functional one, in the terminal dentition. Once again, the patient must appreciate the transitory nature of the appliance. An immediate overdenture utilizing vital-pulpotomy treatment on the retained roots was described earlier in the text. When such roots are unsuitable for long-term service, the overdenture becomes a transitional prosthesis, anticipating later removal of the roots and relining of the prosthesis. In the interim however, the greater stability and proprioception of the overdenture may have made the transition from natural teeth to full removable prosthesis easier. We have even seen full dentures built around a single remaining tooth, for whatever retentive, stabilization, or psychologic benefits might be gained, prior to its inevitable transition to a full prosthesis.

Compromise treatment is difficult, frustrating, and often less rewarding personally or financially. It is, however, a service that some patients desperately need and deeply appreciate. Applied indiscriminately, it can be poor dentistry; applied when it is indicated, it can be a legitimate tool and a source of pride for the dentist who does it well (Fig. 9–14).

REFERENCES

1. Going, R.E., and Jendresen, M.D.: Failures related to materials used in restorative dentistry. Dent. Clin. North Am., *16*:71–86, 1972.
2. Green, E.: Prognosis for occlusal therapy. *In* Clinical Dentistry. Vol. 2. Edited by J.W. Clark. Hagerstown, Harper and Row, 1979.
3. McCracken, W.L: Partial Denture Construction. St. Louis, C.V. Mosby, 1960.
4. Newman, G.V.: Treatment of compromised teeth: A multidisciplinary approach. Am. J. Ortho., *76*:530–537, 1979.
5. Reuter, J.E.: Contingency planning in crown and bridgework design. Dent. Update, *5*:169–179, 1978.
6. Swenson, M.G., and Stout, C.J.: Complete Dentures. St. Louis, C.V. Mosby, 1975.
7. Tylman, S.D., and Tylman, S.G: Theory and Practice of Crown and Bridge Prosthodontics. St. Louis, C.V. Mosby, 1960.

Index

Numerals in *italics* indicate figures, "t" indicates tables.

Abnormality, analyzation of, in diagnosis, 93
  description of, in diagnosis, 93
  recognition of, in diagnosis, 93
Abrasion, causes of, 103, *103*
  dysfunction in, 103
  gingival, 103, *103*, 104
Abutment(s), alternate teeth for, in partial denture design, 221, *222*
  splinted, 216, *218*
Acid-etch bonded composite resin, in misshapen teeth, 108
Acid-etch bonded sealant system, 30
Acrylic jig, anterior, in centric relation recording, *66*, 67
Alignment, definition of, 114
  normal, 114
    deviations from potential pathology in, 114
  pathologic, examples of, 114
Allergies, recording of, in adult examination, 36
Angle system, in classification of occlusal relationships, 56
Anterior guidance, establishment of, in simplification of treatment, 189, *197–198*
Antibiotics, prophylactic, in systemic treatment, 135
Appliances. See *Prosthesis(es).*
Array, normal, 113
  of less than 28 permanent teeth, as pathologic, 114
  pathologic, typical findings in, 114
  pathology in, from too many teeth, 113
Arthrography, of temporomandibular joint, 119
Articulator(s), mounting of diagnostic casts on, 64, *64*
  relating diagnostic casts and one another and, 64–67, *64*, *65*, *66*
Ascorbic acid test, lingual, 61
Attitudes, of dentists, toward patients, 5
Audio-visual aids, 14–16, *15*, *16*

Bacteriologic cultures, 60
Balancing-side contacts, observation of, 58
Bases for casts. See *Cast(s), diagnostic.*
Behavior of patient, as factor in prognosis, 205–206
Behavioral disease, as factor in dental problems, 6
Biologic factors, local, in prognosis, 207–208
Biopsy, of oral lesions, 60
Bite plane therapy, for achieving full retrusion, 57
  flexibility in, 136
  in myofascial pain/dysfunction syndromes, 110
Bite-wing film, standard, *40*, *42*
  vertical, in bone loss, *42*, 44
Bleaching, in intrinsic stains, 107–108
Blood pressure, obtaining of, in adult examination, 46
Blood tests, 60
Bone, crestal, assessment of, in adult examination, 44
  level, determination of, 165
  pathology, assessment of, in adult examination, 44
Bridge, fixed, design flexibility in, 221–223, *224*, *225*, *226*
    modification of, into cantilever, 223, *224–225*
    with anterior abutment for removable partial denture, 221, *223*
    with semiprecision attachment, in partial denture design, 221, *223*
  simple fixed, simple and complex cases of, compared, 160–162, *162*
Bruxism, results of, *102*
  treatment of, etiology as influence on, 103
Bulimia, erosion in, 103–104
Business information, in adult examination, 35
  in dental records, 71

Calculus, assessment of, in adult examination, 49
Cancer, oral, early detection of, 30
Canine guidance, pure, 115
Cantilever, modification of fixed bridge into, 223, *224–225*
Capitation payment systems, 25
Caries, charting of, in adult examination, 52
  clinical evidence of, 52
  control, assessment of, for phasing of treatment, 146
    phasing of treatment by, 145–147
  deep excavation of, and placement of sedative intermediate restoration (IRM), during restoration, *149*
    for maintenance of pulpal health, 148–149
  elimination of, for healthy oral environment, 129
    in caries control, 146
  factors contributing to, 95
  fluoride and, 49
  in lack of or failure of marginal seal of restoration, 106
  incidence of, 6
    and distribution of, *98*, 99
  radiographic evidence of, 52
  sucrose and, 49
Case(s), complex. See *Complex case(s).*

Case(s) *continued*
 simple, and complex case, in same situation with same teeth involved, compared, 160–162, *162*
  examples of, 160, *161*
Cast(s), diagnostic, 62, *62*
  articulation of, 64–67, *64, 65, 66*
  base(s) for, arbitrary, 62
   orthodontically trimmed, 62–63, *62*
  base formers for, 63, *63*
  high accuracy, 62, *62*
  "immediate," 61–62, *61*
  mounting of, on articulator(s), 64, *64*
  relating of, 63–64, *64*
  split, 63, *63*
Cementation, provisional, disadvantages of, 216
 of fixed prostheses, 216–220, *219*
Centric relation (CR), and centric occlusion, in normal model, 115
 as reference point, 57, 115
 clinical significance of, 115
 definitions of, 114–115
 discrepancy in, disorders associated with, 57
 full, bite plane for, 57
 location of, 56–57, *56, 57*
 tolerance to, 57
Centric-relation interocclusal record, with arbitrary hinge location and transfer, 64, *64*
Centric-relation records, with actual hinge-axis location and pantographic or analog records, 64–67
 with actual hinge-axis location and transfer, 64, *65*
Chart(s), dental. See also *Record system(s).*
  commercial, selection of, 72
  in dental diagnosis, 108, *109*
  in dental records, 71
  entries on, describing same procedure, 71, *72*
Checklist, for patient history, 17
Cheeks, abnormal, 121
 normal, 121
Clenching, results of, *102*
Clinical examination, in adult examination, 46
 record and chart of, *73*
Clinical findings, description of, in diagnosis, 92
Communication, basic, 8–12
 between dentist and third-party administrator, 159
 in urgency-based treatment, 125
 of dentist with patient, 5
 photographs in, 16
 processes in, 8–9
  conceptual model of, *10*
 setting for, 11–12
Complex case(s), and simple case, in same situation with same teeth involved, compared, 160–162, *162*
 management of, 160–203
 multiple problems in, 160
 planning of, approaches to, 162–166
  key tooth in, creating of, 165–166
   identification of, 162–165
  tooth inventory in, 166
 simplification of treatment in. See *Treatment(s), simplification of.*
 subtle in appearance, *163–164*
Composite resin, acid-etch bonded, in misshapen teeth, 108
 as compromise treatment, 227–231, *230*
Condylar guidance, and tooth guidance, 116, *117*
 in dynamic occlusion, 116
 in lateral excursion, 116
Condyles, movements of, roughness in, in temporomandibular joint abnormalities, 120
Consent of patient, forms for, 87–91, *88, 89, 90, 91*
Consent statement(s), compared, 90–91, *91*
 treatment agreement with, 90, *90*
Contact(s), balancing-side, 116
  in lateral excursion, 118
  observation of, 58
 faulty, in dental restorations, 106
 improper, in defective restorations, 52–53
 open, recovery from, 227, *228*
Contours, axial, improper, in overbulking of restorations, 106
 improper, in defective restorations, 53
 natural, in gingival third, 106
Corrective treatment, examples of, 136
Cost of treatment, as concern of patient, 23
 presentation of, to patient, 7
Cost/benefit considerations, in defective restoration, 106
Cost/benefit ratio, in compromise treatment, 227
Cost-effectiveness criteria, in extractions, 183–184
Courteousness, in control of fear, 22
"Cracked" tooth. See *Fracture(s), nonseparation.*
Crown(s), abnormal morphology of, 101
 build-ups, pin-retained, 227, *229*
 cast, in nonseparation fracture, 105
  placement of, in anticipation of adjacent prosthesis, 223, *226*
 clinical, assessment of, in adult examination, 44
 shortening of, for stability of key teeth, 165
 telescope, in provisional cementation technique, *219*, 220
Crown/root ratio, 165
Cultures, bacteriologic, 60
Cytology, of oral lesions, 60

Data gathering, and records, 35–91
Demonstration material, effective use of, 16
Dental aids, specific, 60
Dental diagnosis. See *Diagnosis(es), dental.*
Dental examination, findings in, approaches for verbalizing, 20–21
 in adult examination, 51–53
Dental health, importance of knowledge of, 17
Dental history, in adult examination, 35–36
 in custom record system, *77*
 interview following, 17
Dental laboratory, role of, in complex treatment plan, 223–227
Dental problems, discovery of, by patient, treatment approach in, 23
Dental records. See *Record(s), dental.*
Dental team member, questions of, during examination, 20–21
"Dentalese," 8, 19–20
Dentifrice, fluoridated, 29
Dentist(s), and patient, sharing of goals by 1, 6–7, *6*
 attitudes of, toward patients, 5
 conveying feelings to patient, 1
Dentist-patient relationship, in third-party involvement, 157
Dentistry, as practice of occlusion, 55
Dentition. See *Tooth(Teeth).*
Denture, partial, design flexibility in, 221, *222, 223*
Diagnosis(es), 92–123
 analyzation of abnormality in, 93
 definition of, 92
 dental, dental chart in, 108, *109*
  disease in, 95–101, *98, 100*
  disfigurement in, 107–110
  dysfunction in, 101–107
  in multifactorial diagnosis, 95–110
  medical model of diagnosis in, 92–93
  written summary in, 108–110
 description of abnormality in, 93
 functional. See *Functional diagnosis.*
 general systemic, examples of, 94
  influence of, on dental disorders, 94
   on dental treatment, 94
 in treatment planning, 4
 knowledge of normal for, 93
 labels in, as misleading, 92
 medical model of, 92
  supplementing of, with other approaches, 93
  uses of, in dental diagnosis, 92–93
 multifactorial. See *Multifactorial diagnosis(es).*
 periodontal. See *Periodontal diagnosis.*
 radiographic, problems in, 44
 recognition of deviations from norm in, 93
Diagnosis(es), soft-tissue. See *Soft-tissue diagnosis(es).*
Diagnostic casts. See *Cast(s), diagnostic.*
Diagnostic tools, quality of, 53, *53*
Diagnostic wax-ups, 67, *68–69*

Diastema(s), patient perception of, 56
Diet, as factor in dental disease, *27*
as factor in dental problems, 6
control of, in caries control, 146
3-day food inventory and, *81–82*
Dietary history, in custom record system, *77*
Diplomacy, and restraint, as important for dentist, 24
Disclosing stains, 61
Disease(s), dental, factors contributing to, 26–27
in dental diagnosis, 95–101, *98*, *100*
level of, age versus, as factor in host resistance, 207
oral, systemic treatment of, 135
progress rate of, as factor in host resistance, 207
systemic, as criteria for clinical urgency, 125
as factor in prognosis, 208
prevention of, by premedication, 135
recording of, in adult examination, 36
treatment of, 135
Disfigurement, in dental diagnosis, 107–110, *108*
Displays, 15–16, *16*
Drainage, in pulpal disease, 99
Dysfunction, in dental diagnosis, 101–107

Edentulous space, as factor in prognosis, 208
assessment of, as possible cause of deterioration, 188
questions to consider in, 188
Education of patient, in dental health needs, 24
in prevention, 26–27, 28
Electric vitality tester, for pulpal evaluation, 54–55, *55*
Emergency radiographs, 36
Emergency/investigative treatment, steps in, 135
Enamel, defects in, 101
facets on, significance of, 118
Endodontic implants, for stability of key teeth, 165
Endodontic therapy, for healthy oral environment, 129
in periodontal lesions of pulpal pathology, *100*, 101
insufficient, discovery of, assessment of clinical urgency in, 126–127
on teeth with cast restorations, 221
prophylactic, 220–221
treatment pending resolutions of lesions of, 149, *150–151*
Environment, for communication. See *Setting, communication.*
in control of fear, 22
physiologic, as factor in prognosis, 207–208
Erosion, causes of, 103
dysfunction in, 103
Esthetics, dental, judgments of, as personal, 56
loss of, as impetus for seeking treatment, 124
as primary felt need, communication in, 125
treatment in, 125
Examination(s), adult, clinical examination in, 46
data gathering in, 35–67
dental history in, 35–36
medical history in, 36, *37–39*
modifications of, in special situations, 67
radiographic survey in, 36–46, *40–43*
socio-economic status assessment in, 35
dental, findings in, approaches for verbalizing of, 20–21
in adult examination, 51–53
involvement of patient in, 16–21
oral-cancer, 46–53, *48*, *51*
special, record of, 78, *79–82*
Excursion(s), lateral, balancing-side contacts in, 118
condylar guidance factors in, 116
movement of teeth in, 118
posterior tooth guidance in, 118
wear patterns in, 118
Exploratory procedures, in emergency/investigative treatment, 135
Extraction(s), ethical questions in, 183
factors to consider prior to, 183
in pulpal disease, 99
indications for, 183–184
second opinion prior to, 182, *182*
strategic, in simplification of treatment, 166–185

Faceting, causes of, 101
significance of, 118
Failure, planning for, design of alternate approaches in, 209–231
Fear, control of, courteous treatment in, 22
environment in, 22
for dental treatment, 21–22
professionalism in, 22
referral in, 22
skilled hygiene treatment in, 22
verbal reassurance in, 22
dealing directly with, 12
Feedback, as continuous, 9
eliciting of "message-received" signal in, 9
interpretation of, by effective listening, 11
prevention of communication problems with, 10
quality of, conversations illustrating, 10
repetition of information received in, 9–10
Fees, as concern of patient, 23
for specific procedures, forms detailing, *137*, *138*
written review of, to be signed by patient, *89*, 90
Films. See specific types of films.
Fluoride(s), 28–32
daily supplements of, 29
dental caries and, 49
forms of, 29
in dentifrice, 29
in drinking water, 29
level, in water, determination of, 60
therapy, in caries control, 146
topical, home-use, 30
patients warranting, 30
professionally applied, 29–30
Food inventory, 3-day, form for, *81–82*
Form(s), 3-day food inventory, *81–82*
treatment planning, *137*, *138*
Fracture(s), dysfunction in, 104–105
major, treatment of, 104
nonseparation, cast crown restoration in, 105
diagnosis and treatment of, 104
diagnostic measures in, 104
signs of, 105
symptoms of, 104
treatment of, 104–105
separation, treatment of, 104
Fremitus, 118
Functional diagnosis, 110–121
as difficult to make, 110
clinical approach in, 110
comparison of findings and documented norms in, 110
definition of normal stomatognathic system in, 110–111
in absence of pathology, 113
of existing prostheses or appliances, 121
of myofunctional status, 120–121
of occlusion, 113–119
of temporomandibular joint, 119–120
Functional disorders, correction of, for healthy oral environment, 129–130
priority for, 130
Functional evaluation, in adult examination, 55–59
in dental records, 71
Furcation involvement, *97*

Gingiva, abrasion of, 103, *103*, 104
normal, *96*
Gingivitis, 95, *96*
Glucose tolerance test, 60
Goals, sharing of, by patient and dentist, 1, 6–7, *6*
Gross interferences, definition of, 58
examples of, 58
Group function, anterior, 115–116
anteroposterior, 116
Guidance, anterior, establishment of, in simplification of treatment, 189, *197–198*
Guidance patterns, temporomandibular joint, in dynamic occlusion, 116
tooth, 115–116
and potential pathologic signs in dynamic occlusion, 118
condyles and, 116, *117*
posterior, in lateral excursions, 118
in protrusion, 118

Habits, oral, as factor in prognosis, 207
Handicapped patient, plaque control by, 27
Hawley-type removable appliance, in interoceptive orthodontics, *31*
Head, and neck, observations of, in adult examination, 46, 47
Health, oral, level of, phasing of treatment by, 145
Health history(ies), in adult examination, 36, *37–39*
Health maintenance payment systems, 25
Hinge position. See *Centric relation (CR).*
History(ies), dental, in adult examination, 35–36
  in custom record system, *77*
  interview following, 17
 dietary, in custom record system, *77*
 health, in adult examination, 36, *37–39*
 medical, in adult examination, 36, *37–39*
  in custom record system, *77*
  interview following, 17
 patient, form for, 17
  in dental records, 71
  verbal, disadvantages of, 18
  well-designed, for effective interview, 19
Host resistance, assessment of, age vs. level of disease in, 207
  progress rate of existing disease in, 207
 definition of, 206–207
Hostile patient, interview of, 17–18
Hygiene, oral. See *Oral hygiene.*
Hygiene treatment, skilled, in control of fear, 22
Hyperemia, transient pulpal, 99

Ideas, accurate expression of, 8
Implants, dental, 166
Information, about patient, dentist gathering, 1, 4
 conveying of, by displays, 15–16, *16*
  by posters, 14–15, 3215
 for patient, in maintenance of healthy oral environment, 206
  in prognosis, 204
  in treatment planning, 7
  on treatment options, 138, *138*
 received, repetition of, in good feedback, 9–10
Informed consent, forms for, 87–91, *88, 89, 90, 91*
Instructional aids, 61
Instrument(s), concealing of, during communication, 12
 diagnostic, quality of, 53, *53*
Insurance programs, dental, phasing of treatment in, 155–158
 payment of dental treatment by, 23–24, 25
Interferences, gross, definition of, 58
 examples of, 58
Interview, following medical/dental history, 17
 benefits of, 17
 format of, 18
 of hostile patient, 17–18
Interview record, 78, *78*
Intraoral mirror, 19, *19*
Introductory letter, 13–14, *13*
Investigative treatment, in urgent dental or oral threats, 126
Involvement of patient, in examination, 16–21
 in stepwise process, 1
 reasons for, 6
 techniques for, 7–25

Jargon, dental, 8, 19–20
Jig, anterior acrylic, in centric relation recording, 66, 67
Joint, temporomandibular. See *Temporomandibular joint (TMJ).*
Judgment, clinical, based on observed pathology, 53–54
  based on predicted patient behavior, 54

Key-tooth concept, in complex treatment situation, 162–166

Labels, in diagnosis, as misleading, 92
Laboratory, dental, role of, in complex treatment plan, 223–227
Laboratory aids, 60–61
Language, clear, as important, 8, 90–91
  for interview, 19–20
Legal aspects of dental records, 86–87
Lesions, biopsy of, 60
 noting of, in adult examination, 46, 47
Letter, introductory, 13–14, *13*
 preappointment, 12–13, *12*
 review of treatment plan and fees, *89, 90*
Lip(s), abnormal, 121
 assessment of, in adult examination, 47
 habits, observation of, 59
 normal, 121
Listening, effective, 10–11
 factors influencing, 11
Lymph system, examination of, in adult examination, 47

Maintenance program(s), as individualized, 134
 following establishment of healthy oral environment, 133–134
Maintenance treatment, commencement of, 136
 examples of, 136
Malformation, dysfunction in, characteristics of teeth in, 101
Malocclusion, severe, periodontal maintenance in, 148
Mandible, movements of. See *Excursion(s).*
Mastication, difficulties in, 121
 normal, 121
Maxillomandibular relationship, and occlusal stability, 114
 centric relation position in. See *Centric relation (CR).*
Mechanical factors, in prognosis, 208
Medical aids, systemic, 60–61
Medical history, in adult examination, 36, *37–39*
 in custom record system, *77*
 interview following, 17
Message, connotative, importance of understanding, 11
 decoding of, 8–9
 encoding of, 8
 transmitting of, 8
Microscopy, phase contrast, 61
Mirror, intraoral, 19, *19*
Misshapen teeth, treatment of, 108
Mobility, tooth, charting of, 54
Models, study. See *Cast(s), diagnostic.*
Molars, occlusal relationship of, classification of, 56
 third, partially erupted, treatment of, assessment of clinical urgency in, 126
  removal of, in preventive therapy, 32
  unerupted, problems associated with, 113–114
Morphology, improper, diagnostic factors in, 106
  in defective restorations, 106
  significance of, assessment of, 106
Motivation, and reinforcement, in prevention, 27–28
 encouragement in, 28
 lack of, by patient, plaque control in, 27
Motivational aids, 61
Mouth, cancer of, early detection of, 30
 concept of, as environment, 128
 floor of, palpation of, in adult examination, 47
Mucosa, assessment of, in adult examination, 47
Multifactorial diagnosis(es), 93–121
 brief, examples of, *122*
 dental diagnosis in, 95–110
 establishment of, 122
 functional diagnosis in, 110–121
 general systemic diagnosis in, 94
 goal of, 122
 major factors in, 93–94
 periodontal diagnosis in, 95
 soft-tissue diagnosis in, 94
Muscles, as factor in prognosis, 207
Myofascial pain/dysfunction syndrome(s), bite-plane therapy in, 110
 temporomandibular joint and, 120
Myofunctional analysis, 59
Myofunctional status, awareness of, 120
 clinical normality in, 120–121
 functional diagnosis of, 120–121

Neck, head and, observations of, in adult examination, 46, 47

Needs, hierarchy of, dental treatment and, 24
Needs, of patient, satisfaction of, in treatment plan, 23

Occlusal films, *43*
Occlusal relationships, dynamic, 58–59
gross interferences with, 58
space for prostheses and, 58
static, 56–57
Occlusal traumatism, primary, as cause of tooth mobility, 54
in periodontal disease, 118–119
secondary, as cause of tooth mobility, 54
in periodontal disease, 119
Occlusal wear, as form of dysfunction, 101
etiology of, as influence on treatment, 103
severe, causes of, 103
types of, 101–103
Occlusal/temporomandibular joint patient questionnaire, *79–80*
Occlusion, abnormal, without pathologic symptoms, case history illustrating, *111*, 113
alignment and, 114
array and, 113–114
Class II, healthy, case history illustrating, *112*, 113
dentistry as practice of, 55
dynamic, condylar guidance in, 116
description of, 115
guidance of temporomandibular joint in, 116
guidance patterns in, 115–116
potential pathology in, signs of, 118
faulty, in defective restoration, 106–107
functional diagnosis of, 113–119
maxillomandibular relationship and, 114
static, potential pathology in, signs of, 115
status of, as factor in prognosis, 208
Office, appearance of, as factor in control of fear, 22
Oral disease, systemic treatment of, 135
Oral environment, and restorations, maintenance of, 133–134
healthy, establishment of, 128–130, *130–131*
maintenance of, 133–134
Oral habits, as factor in prognosis, 207
Oral health, level of, phasing of treatment by, 145
Oral health progress record (OHPR), 78–83
purposes of, 83
sample of use of, 83, *85*
scoring graph of, 83, *84*
scoring system for, criteria for, 83, 83t
Oral health theory, during treatment, 133
Oral hygiene, during treatment, as factor in prognosis, 206
evaluation of, in adult examination, 47
good, in past, as enhancing prognosis, 206
Oral-cancer examination, 46–53, *48*, *51*
Orthodontic therapy, in preventive therapy, 30, *31*
phasing of treatment by result of, 154, *155–156*
sequence of, in establishment of healthy oral environment, 129–130
Overdenture(s), advantages of, 185
as intermediate treatment option, 184–185
as transitional prosthesis, 231
factors precluding use of, 185
Overhang(s), gross, recovery from, 227, *228*
in dental restorations, 106

Pain, as impetus for seeking treatment, 124
relief of, in emergency/investigative treatment, 135
Palate, hard, assessment of, in adult examination, 47
soft, assessment of, in adult examination, 47
Pamphlet, preprinted, 14, *14–15*
Panographic films, 36–44, *40*
Patient(s), age of, versus level of disease, as factor in host resistance, 207
and dentist, sharing of goals by, 1, 6–7, *6*
behavior, as factor in prognosis, 205–206
-dentist relationship, in third-party involvement, 157
felt need of, flexibility of treatment sequence to accommodate, 132, 136
future commitment of, as factor in prognosis, 206
role of, in dental treatment planning, 5–25
in maintenance of healthy oral environment, 205–206
Patient history. See *History, patient.*
Patient interview record, 78, *78*
Patient-oriented treatment planning, 1–32
Pay, ability to, as continuum, 24
Percussion, in assessment of pulpal status, 55
Periapical film, as occlusal film, *43*
full-mouth, *41*
standard, *40*
Periapical lesion, asymptomatic, assessment of clinical urgency in, 126
Periodontal diagnosis, as specific, 95
evaluation of oral-hygiene status in, 95
examples of, 95, *96*
in multifactorial diagnosis, 95
Periodontal disease, and pulpal disease, relationship of, 100–101, *100*
attitudes toward, 50
early recognition of, 51
incidence of, 6, 49
lack of effectiveness in treating, 49–50
occlusal influence on, 118–119
referral to periodontal specialist in, 50
signs of, 51
treatment of, possible solutions to, 50–51
Periodontal evaluation, in adult examination, 49–51, *51*
scope of, 51
Periodontal probe, calibrated, 51, *51*
Periodontal therapy, for healthy oral environment, 128–129
for stability of key teeth, 165
phasing of treatment by result of, 149–154, *152–154*
Periodontitis, acute, 95, *96*, *97*
chronic, 95, *96*
Periodontium, conditions threatening integrity of, as criteria for clinical urgency, 125–126
maintenance of, environment factors in mouth influencing, 148
for phasing of treatment, 147–148
hypothetical treatment plan based on, 148
in severe malocclusion, 148
indices of, 147
normal healthy, *51*
status of, as factor in prognosis, 207–208
Personal profile, in adult examination, 35
Pharynx, assessment of, in adult examination, 47
Phase contrast microscopy, 61
Phasing of treatment, 143–159. See also *Treatment model, phased plan.*
by caries control, 145–146
plan for 45-year-old man, 147
plan for 14-year-old girl, 146–147
by level of oral health, 145
by periodontal maintenance, 147–148
hypothetical treatment plan based on, 148
by quadrant, 145
case history illustrating, 145
by result of deep excavations of carious lesions, 148–149, *149*
by result of endodontic therapy, 149, *150–151*
by result of orthodontic treatment, 154, *155–156*
by result of periodontal surgery, 149–154, *152–154*
by success or failure of preceding steps, 148–155
commitment of time and effort by dentist in, 159
continual reassessment in, factors for consideration in, 159
development of plan for, 159
in third-party relationships. See *Third-party payment plan(s), phasing of treatment in.*
patient commitment for, 159

Photographs, in communication, 16
in diagnosis and treatment planning, 67
Physician, referral to, for medical laboratory tests, 60–61
Physiologic environment, as factor in prognosis, 207–208
Pitting, congenital, accumulated stain in, *108*
Plaque, as cause of caries and periodontal disease, 26
control, in caries control, 146
in periodontal maintenance, 147–148
mechanical, by patient, 26–27
handicapped patient and, 27
training patient in, 27
unmotivated patient and, 27
definition of, 26
evaluating and recording of, in adult examination, 48–49, *48*
factors contributing to, 6
Posters, 14–15, *15*
Praise, in reinforcement process, 28
Preappointment letter, 12–13, *12*
Preparatory treatment, examples of, 135
Prepayment plans, dental, phasing of treatment in, 155–158
Prevention, as continuing process, 28
as critical in all phases of dentistry, 26
aspects of, in dental treatment, 28–32
education of patient in, 26–27
motivation and reinforcement in, 27–28
training patient in plaque control for, 27
understanding and effectiveness in, patient in, 26
Preventive dentistry, 26–32
Preventive therapy, early detection of oral cancer in, 30
for healthy oral environment, 128
orthodontics in, 30, *31*
prosthetic appliances in, 30–32
removal of third molars in, 32
restorative dentistry in, 30–32
sealants in, 30
Priorities of patient, factors influencing, 24
Probe, periodontal, calibrated, 51, *51*
Professionalism, in control of fear, 22
Prognosis, as requirement in treatment planning, 204
establishment of, 204–231
host resistance as factor in, 206–207
information provided by dentist in, 204
patient behavior influencing, 205–206
physiologic environment influencing, 207–208
prediction of useful life of restorations in, 204, 205
quality of treatment influencing, 208–209
Projection systems, in communication, 16
Prosthesis(es), age of, assessment of, 59
clinical, diagnostic wax-ups for, 67, *68–69*
condition and fit of, evaluation of, 59–60
design flexibility in, 221–223, *222*, *223*
existing, evaluation of, 59–60
functional diagnosis of, 121
fixed, provisional cementation of, 216–220, *219*
disadvantages of, 216
in preventive therapy, 30–32
removable, maintenance of, teaching of, 134
space for, evaluation of, in assessment of occlusion, 58
transitional, 227–231, *230*
Protrusion, tooth and condylar guidance in, 116, *117*
Protrusive guidance, observation of, 58
Public assistance programs, treatment planning under, problems associated with, 25
Pulp, assessment of, prior to treatment planning, 220
conditions threatening vitality of, as criteria for clinical urgency, 125–126
health of, maintenance of, deep excavations of carious lesions in, 148–149
involvement of, as cause of tooth mobility, 54
Pulp testing, indications for, 54
methods of, 54–55
Pulp tester(s), 54–55, *55*
Pulpal disease, and periodontal disease, relationship of, 100–101, *100*
asymptomatic, 99, 100
definitive treatment of, 99
diagnosis of, evaluation of pulpal status in, 99
irreversible, 100–101
reversible, 99–100
Pulpectomy, in pulpal disease, 99
Pulpitis, irreversible, methods of treatment of, based on overall treatment plan, 124–125
serous, and purulent, medical model in, differential diagnosis of, 93
Pulpotomy, in pulpal disease, 99
"Pumice prophy," 134
"Pyorrhea," as example of well-known dental term, 20

Questionnaire, patient, occlusal/temporomandibular joint, *79–80*
Questions, in patient interview, 18–19

Radiograph(s), comprehensive, 36–46, *40–43*
dental, in dental records, 71
release of, 87
diagnostic quality of, 46
emergency, 36
nondiagnostic, *45*
Radiographic diagnosis, problems in, 44
Radiographic survey, guidelines for, 44–46
in adult examination, 36–46, *40–43*
scans following, 44
Radiography, in evaluation of temporomandibular joint, 119
Radioimmunoassay, 60
Reassessment of patients, intervals for, 44–46
Reassurance, verbal, in control of fear, 22
Recall system, in reinforcement, 28
Reception, in communication, 8–9
Record(s), centric-relation, interocclusal, with arbitrary hinge location and transfer, 64, *64*
with actual hinge-axis location and pantographic or analog records, 64–67
with actual hinge-axis location and transfer, 64, *65*
dental, 67–91
accuracy in, 70
example of importance of, 86
as legal document, 70
completeness and comprehensiveness of, 70–71, *71*, *72*
criteria for, 70–71
factors included in, 70
forms of, 70
importance of keeping, 86
in dental diagnosis, 108, *109*
legal aspects of, 86–87
legibility of, 70
own, evaluation of, 86
release of, guidelines for, 87
retention of, 87
and control of, 86–87
review of, advantages of, 70
signature of patient on, 87
written, 70
oral health progress. See *Oral health progress record (OHPR).*
patient interview, 78, *78*
special examination, 78, *79–82*
treatment, in dental records, 71
depth of detail for, 71, *72*
Record system(s), additional tools for, 78–83, *78*, *79–82*, 83t, *84–85*
commercial, criteria for selection of, 72
custom, approaches to design of, 72–78
clinical examination record and chart of, *73*
registration form of, *76*
treatment planning form and note space of, *74–75*
essential components of, 71–72
Referral, in control of fear, 22
Registration form, *76*
Reinforcement, motivation and, in prevention, 27–28
recall system in, 28
Resin, composite, acid-etch bonded, in misshapen teeth, 108

as compromise treatment, 227–231, *230*
Resorption, causes of, *98*, 99
Restoration(s), age of, as factor in failure of marginal seal, 106
anterior, patient preference for, 132, 136
anticipatory, 132–133
cast crown, in nonseparation fracture, 105
charting of, in adult examination, 52
defective, age of restoration as factor in, 106
charting of, in adult examination, 52
cost/benefit consideration, in, 106
dysfunction in, 105, *105*
hyperoccluding, 106–107
improper morphology in, 106
lack of or failure of marginal seal in, 105
clinical judgment in diagnosis of, 105–106
diagnostic factors in, 106
nonoccluding, 107
types of, 52–53
definitive, in goal-oriented treatment, 130–132
failure of, in uncontrolled dental disease, responsibility in, 205
goal of dentist in, 133, 205
interim, in major fractures, 104
maintenance of, 134
mechanical failure of, patient awareness of potential for, 204–205
nonesthetic, evaluation of, 108
prediction of useful life of, 204, 205
sedative intermediate (IRM), following deep excavation of caries, for restoration, *149*
sequence of, assessment of relative risk and, 130–132
efficiency in, 132
patient's felt needs and, 132
simultaneous anterior/posterior, indications for, 132
surface smoothness of, defects in, 106
technical failure of, as responsibility of dentist, 204
Restorative dentistry, preventive therapy in, 30–32
Restorative problem(s), diagnostic wax-ups in, 67, *68–69*
Restraint, diplomacy and, as important for dentist, 24
Restraining of patient, for maintenance of healthy oral environment, 134
Retruded contact position (RCP). See *Centric relation (CR).*
Review/reinforcement sessions, following establishment of healthy oral environment, 133–134
RIA testing, 60
Root(s), abnormal morphology of, 101
morphology, assessment of, in identification of key teeth, 162–165
Root-end pathology, assessment of, in adult examination, 44

Scans, following radiographic survey, 44
Sealants, 30
Sedative intermediate restoration (IRM), following deep excavation of caries, for restoration, *149*
Self-examination, in dental examination, 21
Setting, communication, changing of, 12
establishing of, 11–12
modification of, 12
Signature of patient, on dental records, 87
Shorthand, dental, 20
Silver amalgam, restoration with, as compromise treatment, *230*
Simple case(s), and complex case, in same situation with same teeth involved, compared, 160–162, *162*
examples of, 160, *161*
Smears, surface, as dental aid, 60
Snyder test, modified, 61
Socio-economic status, assessment of, in adult examination, 35
Soft tissue(s), condition of, in relation to oral appliance, 60
examination, in adult examination, 46–53, *48*, *51*
lesions, emergency/investigative treatment of, 135
Soft-tissue diagnosis(es), examples of, 94–95
findings in, 94
in multifactorial diagnosis, 94
management in, 95
Speech, observation of, in adult examination, 59
Speech patterns, abnormal, evaluation of, 121
Splint, occlusal-coverage, flexibility in use of, 136
tripod, 216, *216*
Splinting, cross-arch, 216, *217*
for stability of key teeth, 165
long-term, 209–216, *212–215*, *216*, *217*, *218*
of abutments, 216, *218*
provisional, of questionable teeth, 209, *210–211*
Stain(s), accumulated, in congenital pitting, *108*
disclosing, 61
etiologic factors in, 107–108
sources of, 49
tetracycline, *108*
Stress, mechanical, as factor in prognosis, 208
Study models. See *Cast(s), diagnostic.*
Sucrose, dental caries and, 49
Surgical procedures, for healthy oral environment, 128–129
Swallowing, difficulties in, 121
normal, 121
pattern of, assessment of, 59
Systemic disease. See *Disease(s), systemic.*
Systemic factors, as influence on prognosis, 208
Systemic treatment, steps in, 135

Telescope technique, with provisional cementations, *219*, 220
Temporomandibular joint (TMJ), abnormalities in, potentially pathologic, 119–120
and myofascial pain/dysfunction syndrome, 120
arthrography of, 119
dysfunction, changes in condylar guidance in, case illustrating, 117–118
evaluation of, 58–59
radiography in, 119
function of, and dynamic occlusion, 58
guidance of, in dynamic occlusion, 116
in maxillomandibular relationship, 114
normal, 119
problems, patient symptoms in, 59
treatment of, 59
sounds, 120
symptoms in, in occlusal pathology, 119
Terminology, dental, misleading substitutes for, 20
for interview, 19–20
Tetracycline staining, *108*
Thermal testing, for pulpal status, 55
Third party payment plan(s), 23–24, 25
phasing of treatment in, 155–159
alternate treatment approach and, 158
annual benefit limitations and, 155–158
dentist/patient/third-party stability for, 158
in determination of benefit by provider, 159
waiting periods and, 158
Thoughts, accurate expression of, 8
Tissues, soft. See *Soft tissue(s).*
Tongue, abnormal, 121
examination of, in adult examination, 47, *48*
habits, assessment of, 59
normal, 121
Tools, concealing of, during communication, 12
diagnostic, quality of, 53, *53*
Tooth(Teeth), alignment of. See *Alignment.*
array of. See *Array.*
cost-effectiveness of, as consideration for extraction, 183–184
extraction of. See *Extraction(s).*
guidance patterns, 115–116
inventory, in approaching complex cases, 166
examples of use of, *167–181*
key, as factor in prognosis, 208
creation of, 165–166

Tooth (Teeth) *continued*
favorable arch position of, 165
repositioning for, 165–166
identification of, 162–165
tooth inventory in, 166, *170*, *179*
stability of, assessment of, 162–165
increasing of, 165
misshapen, treatment of, 108
missing, nonreplacement of, in simplification of treatment, 185–189, *186–188*
movement of, in lateral excursion, 118
in simplification of treatment, 189, *190–196*
noncontributory, extraction of, 183
nonvital, not requiring treatment, 99
requiring treatment, 99–100
stained, etiologic factors in, 107–108
Tooth mobility, charting of, 54
Toothbrushing, as cause of abrasion, 103, *103*
Transplantation, autogenous, 165–166
Treatment, agreement, with consent statement, 90, *90*
compromise, in failure of treatment plan, 227–231, *228*, *229*, *230*
corrective, examples of, 136
dental, as elective, 6
preventive aspects of, 28–32
emergency/investigative, steps in, 135
goal-oriented, efficiency in, 127–134
establishment of healthy oral environment in, 128–130, *130–131*
following urgency-based treatment, 127
maintenance of oral environment and restorations in, 133–134
restoration of form, function, and esthetics in, 130–133
sequential steps in, 127–128
insufficient, discovery of, assessment of clinical urgency in, 126–127
investigative, in urgent dental or oral threats, 126
level of execution of, as factor in prognosis, 209
maintenance, commencement of, 136
examples of, 136
phasing of. See *Phasing of treatment.*
prediction of life span of. See *Prognosis.*
preparatory, examples of, 135
quality of, as factor in prognosis, 208–209
reducing steps in, example of, 127
redundancy in, avoidance of, 127
simplification of, establishment of anterior guidance in, 189, *197–198*
management of lost vertical dimension in, 189–203, *199*, *200–202*
nonreplacement of missing teeth in, 185–189, *186–188*
strategic extraction in, 166–185, *182*
tooth movement in, 189, *190–196*
situation, complex. See *Complex case(s).*
specific steps in sequence of, 134–138
flexibility in, 136
systemic, steps in, 135
temporary holding action, in failure of treatment plan, 227
time lapse between, to evaluate results, 148
urgency-based, 124–127
goal-oriented treatment following, 127
Treatment model, optimal, 143–145
phased plan, 143
as pleasing to dentist, 144
as pleasing to patient, 144
optimal approach for, 144
over indefinite period of time, 145
over 3-year period, 144–145
potential problems with, 144
time variable, 143, *143*
traditional, 143, *143*
Treatment plan(s), concerns of patient regarding, 21
failure of, alternative approach(es) in, compromise treatment as, 227–231, *228*, *229*, *230*
design flexibility in prosthetic appliances for, 221–223, *222*, *223*
endodontic recovery for, 220–221
long-term splinting for, 209–216, *212–215*, *216*, *217*, *218*
provisional cementation of fixed prostheses for, 216–220, *219*
provisional splinting of questionable teeth for, 209, *210–211*
role of dental laboratory in, 223–227
form for, *74–75*
in dental records, 71
options in, as function of time and money, 136–138
overall, type of immediate treatment based on, 124
presentation of, 21–25
procedures in, and fees for, forms listing, *137*, *138*
selection of, as influence on prognosis, 208–209
sequence of procedures in, 124–134
synthesis of, 124–139
with notation of patient acceptance, *88*, 90
written, for phased treatment under third-party coverage, 159
written review of, to be signed by patient, *89*, 90
Treatment planning, applied to patient's problems, 7
as independent process, 3
as orderly and systematic, 3
complex, principles of, 141–231
cost of treatment presented to patient in, 7
data base for, 4
decision of patient on, 7
diagnosis in, 4
effective plan in, 4
format for, *137*, 138–139, *138*
forms for, *137*, *138*
goal setting in, 1, 6–7, *6*
information for patient in, 7
integration of specialized steps in, 3
patient involvement in, methods of, 7
patient-oriented, 1–32
preventive approach to, 26–32
process of, 3–4
steps in, 124
systematic approach to, 33–139
Treatment record, in dental records, 71
depth of detail for, 71, *72*
Tripodization, 216, *216*

Urgency, clinical, criteria for, asymptomatic potential oral threats as, 126
dental or oral threats as, 125–126
systemic threats as, 125
treatment based on, 124–127
Urinalysis, 60

Verbalizing of findings, 19–21
Vertical dimension, lost, 189, *199*
restoration of, in simplification of treatment, 189–203, *200–202*
Veterans Administration programs, phasing of treatment in, 157
Vitamin C deficiencies, lingual ascorbic acid test and, 61

Wasserman test, 60
Water, fluoridated, 29
Wax-ups, diagnostic, 67, *68–69*
Wear, as factor in bruxism, 118
occlusal. See *Occlusal wear.*
Wear patterns, and excursive positions, 118
Welfare programs, phasing of treatment in, 155
treatment planning under, problems associated with, 25
Words, choice of, for description of dental conditions, 20
for good communication, 8
Working conditions, as factor in prognosis, 209
Working-side guidance, observation of, 58
Written materials, 12–14, *12*, *13*, *14*
Written plan, for phased treatment under third-party coverage, 159
Written summary of findings, in dental diagnosis, 108–110